MOBILE ROBOTICS IN HEALTHCARE

Assistive Technology Research Series

Volume 7

Previously published in this series

Vol. 1. I. Placencia Porrero and R. Puig de la Bellacasa (Eds.), The European Context for Assistive Technology
Vol. 2. K. Cullen and S. Robinson, Telecommunications for Older People and Disabled People in Europe
Vol. 3. G. Anogianakis, C. Bühler and M. Soede (Eds.), Advancement of Assistive Technology
Vol. 4. I. Placencia Porrero and E. Ballabio (Eds.), Improving the Quality of Life for the European Citizen
Vol. 5. L.H.V. van der Woude, M.T.E. Hopman and C.H. van Kemenade (Eds.), Biomedical Aspects of Manual Wheelchair Propulsion
Vol. 6. C. Bühler and H. Knops (Eds.), Assistive Technology on the Threshold of the New Millennium

ISSN: 1383-813X

Mobile Robotics in Healthcare

Edited by

Nikos Katevas
ZENON SA, Glyka Nera, Attikis, Athens, Greece

IOS
Press
Ohmsha

Amsterdam • Berlin • Oxford • Tokyo • Washington, DC

ISBN 1 58603 079 5 (IOS Press)
ISBN 4 274 90413 X C3047 (Ohmsha)
Library of Congress Catalog Card Number: 00-110850

Publisher
IOS Press
Nieuwe Hemweg 6B
1013 BG Amsterdam
The Netherlands
fax: +31 20 620 3419
e-mail: order@iospress.nl

Distributor in the UK and Ireland
IOS Press/Lavis Marketing
73 Lime Walk
Headington
Oxford OX3 7AD
England
fax: +44 1865 75 0079

Distributor in the USA and Canada
IOS Press, Inc.
5795-G Burke Centre Parkway
Burke, VA 22015
USA
fax: +1 703 323 3668
e-mail: iosbooks@iospress.com

Distributor in Germany, Austria and Switzerland
IOS Press/LSL.de
Gerichtsweg 28
D-04103 Leipzig
Germany
fax: +49 341 995 4255

Distributor in Japan
Ohmsha, Ltd.
3-1 Kanda Nishiki-cho
Chiyoda-ku, Tokyo 101
Japan
fax: +81 3 3233 2426

PRINTED IN THE NETHERLANDS

Preface

This book presents the conclusions of four years of a joint work of the *MobiNet* Training and Mobility of Researchers Network on mobile robotics technology for healthcare services. The book aims at: a) presenting the complementarity of the human factors and the demands for real-life applications based on the latest achievements of the robotics technology, and b) addressing the principles, the concepts, as well as the details for the design of robots that present autonomy/intelligence, and manipulability and/or maneuverability in the amounts required for effective collaboration with the human in healthcare environments.

The book is organised in fifteen chapters analysing topics covering all the related fields and including but not limited to: user and application requirements, human machine interfacing, mobile robots and manipulators, control architectures, navigation and sensing strategies, robot to smart building interconnection etc., giving technical details and hints to the reader on how to address real-life problems with the state-of-the art technology.

This book has been written because we see that the technology is there, mature enough to serve people in every day life problems. We see that that there is a weak link between what the technology may offer and how this could be efficient and useful in the hands of ordinary people. We would like to enhance this link between the engineering and the medical world, trying to bring together researchers and scientists from the very many disciplines involved, trying to learn from each other, to work together breaking the borders, bridging the gaps.

The work on this book has been inspired by mature professionals in our network, like Prof. Spyros Tzafestas and Prof. Pierre Rabischong, the first originating from the technology field and the second from the medical field, both being our passionate co-workers in the mobile robotics for the healthcare field. It has also been inspired by the fresh minds of the research fellows working in our network, offering their pure ideas and their innovative nature, motivated by the challenge of the new field.

This work was driven by our vision of technology in harmony with the human of the robotics of the next millennium. The scientific results of our efforts of the last four years may be found in the pages to follow. However, it is not clearly written in those pages that we are now *a team*; a team of young and mature researchers, from nine countries of Europe, from twelve laboratories devoted to various disciplines, we are Cedric, Simone, Cecilia, Magnus, Pierre, Fergal, Helmut, Andiana, Stanislao, driven by the same vision, knowing how to work together for the common goal. This is what we report as our major achievement.

Nikos Katevas
MobiNet Coordinator

Acknowledgements

The authors would like to acknowledge the support of the Training and Mobility of Researchers (TMR) Programme of the EC for the financial support provided under the contract ERB-FMRX-CT96-0070 (MobiNet) and the active contribution of the project officers, Christian Bernard and Panayiotis Moschopoulos.

MOBINET - TMR Project CT0070

***Mobi**le Robotics Technology for Health Care Services Research **Net**work*

The main objective of this research network is to concentrate the forces of European scientists in the prototype design of an autonomous mobile robot for health care services, using and developing innovative, on the state of the art techniques, as a result of the joint research activities. The aim of the proposed research network is to organise and establish an active workgroup of researchers for the mobile robotics technology and health care services, in a formal co-operative status. The outcome of the project will be the detailed design of the prototype of an autonomous mobile robot with high manoeuvrability and manipulability features. This prototype design will be the final deliverable, integrating the accumulated research results of four years.

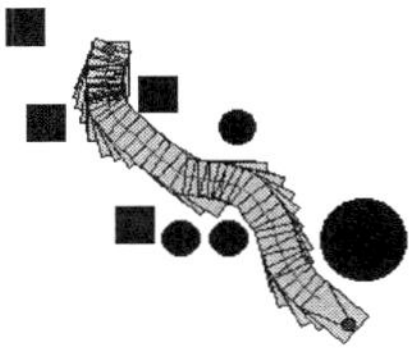

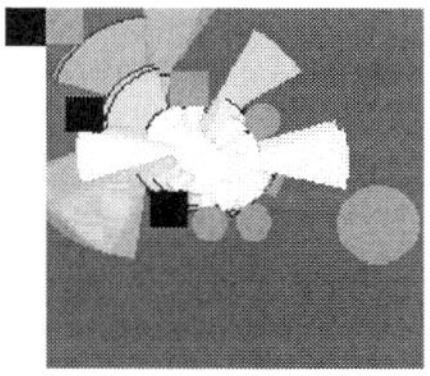

Operational features of the proposed mobile robot will include execution of complicated manipulation and transport tasks. Prototype will have fully autonomous operation. Environment perception will be realised with the onboard installed sensors like vision, ultrasound, infrared etc. The behaviour of the robot will be optimised for in-door health care tasks, interacting with the user by high level commands. All levels of autonomy will be addressed.

For further information please contact:

Dr. Nikos KATEVAS,
ZENON SA
Kanari 5, Glyka Nera, Attikis,
GR-15354 Athens, Greece.
tel: +30 1 6041582, fax: +30 1 6041051,
e-mail:nkatevas@zenon.gr

The Consortium

Zenon SA Industrial Automation
Athens, Greece

Fern Universitat
Hagen, Germany

National Technical University of Athens
Athens, Greece

Universidad Politechnica de Madrid
Madrid, Spain

FTB
WeetterRuh, Germany

University of Dublin
Dublin, Ireland

BIBA
Bremen, Germany

University of Reading
Reading, UK

Lund University
Lund, Sweden

University of Montpellier
Montpellier, France

Scuola Superiore Santa Anna
Pisa, Italy

TNO - TPD
Delft, The Netherlands

Contents

Preface, *N.I. Katevas* v

Chapter 1.
Mobile Robotics in Healthcare: the past, the present and the future, *N.I. Katevas* 1

Chapter 2.
User Requirements for Robotics in Health Care and Rehabilitation, *H. Heck, A. Prentza, E. Peruchon, N.I. Katevas and G. Lacey* 17

Chapter 3
Human-Machine-Interfacing for Control in Healthcare Robotics, *H. Heck, G. Lacey, A. Prentza, E. Peruchon and P. Rabischong* 45

Chapter 4
Mobile Robotics and Automation in Healthcare and Rehabilitation, *N.I. Katevas, W. Harwin, H. Heck, M.J. Aldon, U. Borgolte, G. Lacey, E. Peruchon, A. Prentza and J. Kontoulis* 73

Chapter 5
Control Architectures of Intelligent Mobile Robots, *S.G. Tzafestas and N.I. Katevas* 101

Chapter 6
Tackling Control Systems Complexity, *R. Sanz, M. Segarra, F. Matía and A. de Antonio* 137

Chapter 7
Mobile Robot Kinematics and Control, *U. Borgolte and N.I. Katevas* 161

Chapter 8
Global and Local Strategies for Mobile Robot Navigation, *N. I. Katevas, S.G. Tzafestas and F. Matía* 187

Chapter 9
Communicating Robots in a Healthcare Environment, *F.J. O'Hart, R.J. Greenane, G. Lacey and D. Wenn* 211

Chapter 10
State of the Art on Manipulators, *F. Weber, B. Driessen, G. Bolmsjö, S. Lauria and W. Harwin* 227

Chapter 11
Manipulator Control Architectures, *B. Driessen, W. Harwin, G. Bolmsjö and F. Weber* 253

Chapter 12
Case Studies on Mobile Manipulators, *B. Driessen, G. Bolmsjö and P. Dario* 269

Chapter 13
Sensing Strategies for Mobile Robots, *F. Matía, N.I. Katevas, F. Wawak and G. Lacey* 295

Chapter 14
Mobile Robots Localisation, *F. Wawak, F. Matía, N.I. Katevas, G. Lacey, W. Harwin and S. Lauria* 315

Chapter 15
Workspace Mapping for Mobile Robots, *F. Matía, N.I. Katevas and C. Peignot* 349

The Authors 369

Author Index 380

Chapter 1

Mobile Robotics in Healthcare: the past, the present and the future

by Nikos I. KATEVAS

Chapter 1

Mobile Robotics in Healthcare: the past, the present and the future

Nikos I. KATEVAS

1. Introduction

Robotics viewed from different perspectives, present images and reflections that are interpreted in various manners concluding to a fuzzy interpretation of the term. Although not a very clear term, robotics was always a popular term used by experts and non-experts in very many instances and occasions.

This chapter aims to contribute to the clarification of the term and to present the author's view-point of robotics and their future. The chapter begins with a presentation of robotics from the non-technical viewpoint. The departing point is the brief review of the robotics and its journey through out the times of the human-kind up to date, from the non-engineering perspective. The chapter continues with the author's view on the future of robotics. Major part of the chapter consists a guide for the reader on how to read this book and where he/she may find information of interest. The chapter concludes with proposals on how to boost the technology in (mobile) robotics and an open invitation to everybody that is interested to contribute to this future.

2. The Past

Robotics claim to be one of the most newly created sciences. However, one may find reports for robots in the ancient or even in the pre-historical times. *Myths of Egypt* describe statues that become alive when the gods transform material to live flesh. Similarly, in the *Greek mythology* there are several reports on robots, e.g. the story of romance of the artist Pigmalion who fell in love with his own creation, the statue of Galatea, to which the Godess of Love, Afrodite (Venus) gives life. In Iliada, Homer describes the "golden slaves" of Hephestus which help him to walk (Hephestus was one of the twelve ancient Greek gods lining on the holy mountain of *Olympus* – Hephestus was a disabled person and he needed support to walk.) Hephestus is also reported to be the one who developed the *human-like creature that embedded intelligence*, called *Talos*. Mmany other myths describe superhuman, human-like, of non-human nature creatures that acted (moved) according to the wishes of humans. Beyond the myths there are historical references on machines that present specific mechanical features and they embed a grade of intelligence. Some of those are results of the great ancient philosophers and engineers like *Archimedes* and *Heron*.

3. The Present[1]

The term *robot* originates from the Czech word *robota* which means the forced work performed by slaves. The first reference to robots by the term robots is not found in the engineering textbooks but in the play "*Rossum's Universal Robots*" written in 1921 by the Czechoslovakian writer Karel Capek (1890-1938). According to that play robots where human-like machines that where produced by the humans to have them operating in heavy and duly tasks. In the play the robots evolute against their creators and try to destroy human-kind. Although the play is highlighting the fight between the humans and the robots the play concludes positively. The robots and end are influenced by human feelings like friendship, taking and giving, and finally become a kind of human creatures. However, from the beginning of the century starting with the "Rossum's Universal Robots" (1921), later on in the famous film "Metropolis" (1926) till the end of the century, like in the popular TV series of "Star Trek" (70s-90s), as well as in very many other broadcasts, books etc. that heavily influence the public opinion, robots have always been *intelligent mobile (human like) machines* in the most cases acting as *a potential threat for human-kind.* There is one very sound exception. In 1942 in "*I, the robot*" Issac Asimov (1920-1992) presents robots as *assistants and partners of the human.* Asimov presented the *Three Laws of Robotics* that revised the ugly image of robots. It is the first reference of the term robotics. Asimov's laws bring back the ancient notion of human helpers that assist and by definition do not threat the human.

However even today robots are presented in arts as counter human machines. In technology the term robot is introduced in 1954. It is the year when George Devol Jr. applies for a patent of a machine that transports casts out of a casting machine. He refers to his patent with the term *industrial robot*. The first robot was built after a few years in 1958 by George Devol and Josef Engelberger. In 1961, Engelberger founds Unimation Inc, that is devoted to production and commercialisation of robots. In the next decades robots found application in several production and application fields. Later on the technologists managed to apply robots in several fields not exclusively industrial.

[1] Present is considered the 20th century

4. The future

Since the 70's robotics fights to get its position in science and industry. In science, robotics is recognised as the melting pot of several fields. In industry, robotics associated their name with the major advantage of flexibility in production. This flexibility made the robots the dominators in several applications where their counter part in hard automation suffered. However, the price for the flexibility was in the most cases the speed. Along with the time, robotics trended to new designs that presented features addressing particular applications. In 70's and 80's we saw the SCARA robots for parts assembly, cylindrical robots for torch welding, AGVs in warehouses etc. The blooming in robotics started in mid 80's when computer science and engineering offered the capacity required by the "soft" elements of robots to reach the maximum of their efficiency supporting the electromechanical system.

Even today robots keep their general-purpose nature. But what has happened all these years is that *robotics has motivated and inspired the research in the near by fields* due to the emerging demands and the need to increase the application range that robots should address. The inertia created produced results and today the traditional robots are equipped with products belonging in others sciences fields. Today AGVs (automated guided vehicles) has been transformed to LGVs (laser guided vehicles) because of the laser position estimator that replaced their original virtual cable rails buried in the ground. In addition the improvement in the robotics supportive fields (optics, electronics, computing etc.) have been enhanced by the embedded intelligence that is nested in each of the system that equips modern robots to provide the desired functionality.

It is by coincidence that the change over to the next *millennium* coincides with the closing of *the first circle of the robot history* and initiates the *start of the next generation.* Robotics begins the new loop of its contribution to the human-kind wealth of being. This happens by breaking into pieces the achievements of the last *40 years* and spreading them around various fields. At the time these lines are written *robots have already started their transformation from heavy, noisy, ugly machines to human assistive devices, helpers and companions of everyday activities*. Even in the very beginning of the 3rd millennium this new generation has already emerged and may be found as exceptional but existing products like toys (the SONY dog, LEGO robots) or high-tech developments (the HONDA humanoid). In the next years, if not already we will discover robotic elements well hidden in Hoover cleaners[2], wheelchairs, cars, and *everyday life appliances*.

If we would like to predict the life cycle of this new robotic generation we could safely quote a minimum time frame of *20 years*. These will be times were the *robots will be integral parts or our homes, businesses, education or entertainment environment*. There are signs and scientific reports on this future of robotics where the robots and their elements *will smoothly interact with humans, between themselves, with home appliances in order to help, support, serve, and perform according to the human wishes, fully adapted to the human needs in daily life activities.* Also, what we could be sure of is that *robots will go mobile* as much as

[2] (there are more that 20 years that several scientists or traders claim that have the solution to that, but only this year there is evidence of the existence of such a product announced by Electrolux)

possible and *they will be loosing their general-purpose nature in favour of the application they will be acting for*. And these will happen until the next generation arrives.

Mobility in services provided to citizens is the key issue for this new generation of robots; *modularity* is the second; and *interoperability* is the third. But beyond and above all is the issue of *ease and natural interaction with the human*. In the light of this robotic future this book addresses the issues that are related to *mobile robotics* in *healthcare applications*.

This book presents the conclusions of four years joint work of 12 European laboratories on mobile robotics technology for healthcare services. The book bridges the human factors and the demands of real-life applications to the achievements of the robotics technology. It is organised in 15 chapters analysing topics covering all the related fields and including but not limited to: user - application requirements, human machine interfacing, mobile robots' and mobile manipulators' control architectures, navigation and sensing strategies, robot - smart building interconnection etc. giving technical details and hints to the reader on how to address real-life problems. The book also performs a historical review and includes an overview of the current developments worldwide.

5. How to read this book

5.1 Introduction

The following sections briefly present the contents of the chapters and may guide the reader to the parts of this book that are more interesting for him/her. However, the overall book is structured in a manner that a reader interested in the overall field may follow from the beginning to the end in order to get information for all the related issues.

Each of the chapters concludes with discussions, suggestions and where appropriate guidelines for the reader (student, scientist, researcher or developer) interested in designing a mobile robotic system in healthcare sector. In order to help the reader the following sections include at the end of each one *a comment / suggestion on the chapter's content written in italics*. The reader may read this first to get the flavour of the corresponding chapter.

5.2 Chapter 2 - User Requirements for Robotics in Health Care and Rehabilitation

This chapter presents and analyses the requirements of the potential users of mobile robots in healthcare and rehabilitation. The presentation considers that robotics in *healthcare* aims to *the provision of a grade of autonomy* or a *service to people* that have permanently or temporally lost part of their physical and/or mental abilities. Also, the chapter considers robotics in *healthcare* as an assistant to the caregiving staff. More specifically, robotics in *rehabilitation* aims at providing people with a tool that (partially) compensates their disabilities. Under this perspective, it is the tool that helps the increment or the restoration of the user's abilities. The influence of robotics to the social rehabilitation as well as its influence to personal independence and subsequently to the quality of life are not neglected; in contrary are considered as the main objectives of rehabilitation robotics.

The chapter describes which the (potential) users are, the tasks and conditions to which they could successfully apply mobile robots and mobile manipulators. The chapter performs a detailed analysis on the potential tasks, categorises and prioritise them according to studies performed. The medical implications, ergonomic requirements, cost/benefit factors include some of the issues that are discussed. The chapter concludes with suggestions and important points for the researcher/developer interested in designing a mobile robotic system in the healthcare sector.

The chapter presents an analysis of the user requirements in applications in the healthcare domain. The chapter outlines and documents the importance of the requirements addressed. The reader may use this analysis in order to start working on a new development and try to fit his/her own application field to the tables given in the chapter. It is suggested that the user refers to this chapter as the starting point of a new application.

5.3 Chapter 3 - Human-Machine-Interfacing for Control in Healthcare Robotics

The chapter starts with the medical perspective analysing the physiological inputs and outputs that the humans use to interact with their environment. These physiological means are presented in relation to their influence to the control of devices. Unlike industrial robots that operate in well-defined, structured environments the *robotics in healthcare, and* especially in *rehabilitation,* are quite different. The *workspace* is the semi-structured or completely unstructured environment of hospitals, private homes or public areas like streets with traffic, shops or public buildings. The world is neither predictable nor static. In *rehabilitation robotics*, the user is quite often an integral part of the control loop.

The chapter performs a review of the devices for input and output for human-machine interaction. The review includes joysticks, trackballs, puff switches, keyboards and switches, touch screens, pads and pedals, data gloves, voice and speech recognition and synthesis etc. Also, the chapter presents behavioural models for human-machine interaction and the way they are applied to healthcare robotics. The chapter concludes to guidelines to select human-machine interfacing components for specific user categories.

The chapter provides medical documentation of the means, which the human use to communicate with the auxiliary world. Therefore the chapter may act as a reference for studies needed to bridge the human to a machine. Also, the chapter includes an overview of the devices available to human-machine interfacing. This may help the reader that needs a complete but not exhaustive reference of the devices in use in a health care application.

5.4 Chapter 4 - Mobile Robotics and Automation in Healthcare and Rehabilitation

The chapter performs an outline of the developments of robotic assistance devices for hospital fetch and carry services, in surgical procedures, and in physiotherapy etc. The focus is given on the overview of mobility and manipulation assistance for patients and people with motor impairments. The chapter presents examples of such prototypes/ products that have reached a mature stage of development.

It is argued that the provision of technology into these situations is difficult, not because the technology is not beneficial or cost effective, but because the purchasers are conservative, the demands complex and the benefits can only be measured by considering long term savings, something that healthcare provision does not cater for particularly well. Thus for example, mechanisms to transport people and goods safely around a hospital will have long term cost savings when considered as a means to increase efficiency of goods delivery, but will require a concerted effort by healthcare leaders to be realised. In addition to portering and transport applications we consider applications in the delivery of direct healthcare services such as the growing use of robots to assist in surgical procedures, and the emergence of possible robot assistance in the delivery of physiotherapy services. We also consider the use of mobile robot technology for assisting people with motor disabilities, as well as the provision of telemanipulation and telerobotic assistance for people with manipulation difficulties. Although the application areas for automation in healthcare is broad, there are often social and technical similarities. The purchaser of the technology is often not the final user. The technology may have multiple users each needing to access the services at different levels. There is a strong need for fast maintenance, good technical support, and comprehensive training.

The chapter presents an overview of systems/prototypes/products in the field of mobile robotics in automation of healthcare services and rehabilitation. The list of references in the chapter is neither complete nor exhaustive, but the reader may treat it as a collection of examples that compose the full image of the developments so far. In that sense the chapter is a good starting point for the reader that needs to see what other people have developed, what they achieved, how they plan to go on and get ideas and triggers for his/her own designs.

5.5 Chapter 5 - Control Architectures of Intelligent Mobile Robots

The aim of this chapter is to provide an introduction to the control architectures of *intelligent mobile robots* (IMRs) accompanied by a few implementation examples. IMRs constitute a subclass of *intelligent autonomous systems* (IAS) which have attracted over the years a great attention throughout the world with many industrial and every-day human applications. Currently the majority of working systems in practice have partial autonomy and a lot of effort is still devoted by research and development groups to further increase the level of autonomy. Compared with other types of robots, IMRs surely have a higher potential to replace the human in industrial and service applications (medical, domestic, etc.) due to their mobility, intelligence, manipulability and dexterity.

IMRs possess decision - making capabilities and use multi - sensory information about their internal state and workspace environment to generate and execute plans for performing difficult and complex tasks. System autonomy implies the ability of the robot to support the humans in their work as a human assistant does. To achieve this, the IMR needs an information processing system capable of detailing general task descriptions into sequences of primitive robot movements and handling unexpected uncertainties and / or faults, in addition to the required human-like sensoric and manipulating abilities. To construct a working-in-practice autonomous IMR, starting from the toy / research level, a modular approach should be followed independently of the particular control architecture that is adopted. Naturally, the basic steps of such a modular approach may be the following: a) complex task definition, b) complex task decomposition in simple (generic) tasks, c) task solving components' development and implementation, d) components' development and implementation, e) system integration.

The chapter presents the four classes of generic control IMR architectures, namely: hierarchical, nested, distributed, and behaviour-based architectures. Also, gives a short outline of three working IMR research prototypes which have been designed following the hierarchical and/or distributed/behaviour-based architectures, namely the KAMRO/KAMARA, ROMAN, and SENARIO. Finally, it provides concluding remarks on future prospects and directions for research.

The chapter presents a complete analysis of control architectures that may be used in intelligent mobile robots. The reader may find descriptions of hierarchical, nested, distributed, behaviour based control architecture as well as examples and applications of those. The chapter may be treated as a reference of mobile robots control architecture theory and may be used to identify the most appropriate control scheme for new designs.

5.6 Chapter 6 - Tackling Control Systems Complexity

Mobile robotics are in the common case complex systems composed by a variety of components needed to be integrated and controlled. Control systems complexity is increasing due to the need of performing tasks of higher difficulty. Complex controllers incorporate advanced sensors and actuators but most of the functionality is built using software technologies. In the case of intelligent control systems, as those used in advanced mobile robotics or strategic process control, the need of complex information processing leads to the use of heterogeneous software technologies to provide the needed functionality: digital signal processing, neural networks, fuzzy systems, communications, expert systems, artificial vision, etc. Development life cycles for these systems are not linear at all, with a high amount of prototyping and exploratory programming. New methods are needed to cope with the inherent difficulties in handling this type of system construction. Some ideas from advanced software engineering can be used to tackle this control systems complexity. Modular designs have been the key to these issues in other areas of engineering. In our business this means the identification of control-oriented information processing modular functions; the implementation of reusable modules; the design of product architectures; the construction of integration middleware; the reusability of designs; etc. Some insights, ideas and developments are presented in this chapter and we hope they can contribute to enhance the design and construction of complex intelligent controllers.

The chapter deals with systems complexity and how to identify, track and control it in both the design and development phase of a new mobile robotic system. The focus of the chapter is on the software complexity and the reader may find it helpful to refer to it when a complicated system is his/her aim. The development methodology presented, the examples and the design principles highlighted may be guide the reader in both understanding and designing of mobile robots for healthcare services.

5.7 Chapter 7 - Mobile Robot Kinematics and Control

This chapter introduces the basic concepts of mobile robotics. By way of introduction, a survey on the current state of the art is given, followed by application areas of mobile robots, and different implementation approaches for specific problems. Furthermore, sections both on wheeled mobile systems as well as on so-called walking machines are included.

Within the section on wheeled robots, different wheel configurations are discussed with regard to their advantages and disadvantages. Furthermore, co-ordinate systems, transformation matrices, and velocity calculations/Jacobians are addressed. The section on walking machines handles different models of walking, leg configurations, as well as possible fields of application of these systems. Different types of gait and static/dynamic stability are also discussed. Again, the section on control of mobile robots deals with wheel driven systems. Without going further into the concepts of control technology (this can be looked up in corresponding text books and is beyond the scope of this book), different control architectures are discussed, in particular for the lower level of control (motor control). The effects of mutual influencing in over-determined systems as well as resulting measures for the reduction of these effects are handled in a section on system coupling.

The chapter does a turn from the technical details to the application areas of mobile robots. In the first instance, different application scenarios are described, and current application fields are outlined. With respect to the specific situation in health care applications, suggestions for safety treatment are given. The chapter closes with a suggestion for the practical selection of a mobile robot, which may serve in the healthcare sector.

The chapter gives a complete overview of the kinematics concepts used in mobile robotics, but focuses on wheeled configurations. The reader who needs references on theory and details on kinematics constrains and equations governing robot's motion may use this chapter to address all variations of wheeled configurations. The chapter concludes to a set of guidelines for the reader who wants to design or study the kinematics of wheeled mobile robots.

5.8 Chapter 8 - Global and Local Strategies for Mobile Robot Navigation

Path planning or trajectory planning has been extensively studied by the scientific community and methods tackling the problem from various perspectives have been proposed. Initially the efforts were focused on the development of reliable off-line programming tools that would utilise exact geometric features of the environment, assumed to be available. However, navigating mobile robots introduces the need to heavily incorporate perception into the control loop and dropped the assumption of accurate and reliable environment representation. The first demand was to implement obstacle avoidance behaviour. Over the years, several control strategies for collision avoidance targeting mobile robots have been developed. These were based on information provided by environment perception devices such as ultrasonic sensors, infrared or visible light sensor, laser range sensors, cameras, tactile sensors etc. A great amount of effort has been given to develop systems that employ perception based on machine vision but the later was rapidly replaced by the use of simpler sensing principles targeting specific applications. Only in the last years it seems that all the related technologies are reaching the maturity required to realize navigation strategies based on machine vision meeting the efficiency demanded by real-time, real-life applications.

The chapter presents representative families of global and local strategies for mobile robot navigation. The overview of the families is neither exhaustive, nor complete. The chapter concludes, presenting case studies of the navigation control methods used in mobile robots for healthcare services. The aim is to present the methods and trigger the reader to select/combine one or more of those for the mobile robot he/she is designing. The reader is recommended to refer also to Chapters 13, 14 and 15 while reading this chapter.

5.9 Chapter 9 - Communicating Robots in a Healthcare Environment

Many new network technologies are now concerned with dynamically connecting devices to networks that may ultimately allow access to the Internet. The wide availability of the Internet has led most businesses going online into the dynamic world of e-Commerce. Manufacturing systems have large dedicated control networks to allow machinery to be controlled and audited by many different systems. In some cases these two technologies have merged to create a single virtual network populated by physical machines, people and agents that interact to perform complex tasks.

Under these principles the *intelligent building* infrustructure is used to integrate and service the communications. The particular demands of the robot architecture is discussed along with the issue of interlinking the robot navigation and the intelligent buildings. CORBA architectures are proposed as a solution to the software infrastructure issue. The chapter addresses also the topics of distributed multi-robot communication and control in conjuction with the use of the intelligent building infrastructure.

The chapter presents one of the most promising and impressive topics related to the future of (mobile) robotics: the integration of robotics with the intelligent building environment. By that mobile robots enhance their potential towards the goal of everyday home appliances. The reader is suggested to read the chapter and refer to the latest of the references in order to get the flavour of the latest achievements in the field.

5.10 Chapter 10 - State of the Art on Manipulators

This chapter outlines the state-of-the-art of manipulators and grippers. The main components and characteristics of manipulators are described and evaluated with respect to their applicability and relevance for mobile health care robots. Links, revolute and prismatic joints have been introduced as the building blocks of manipulators. Different types of drives and sensors are presented. The programming of robots and manipulators is explained with the characteristics of on-line and off-line programming. Robot oriented and task oriented languages and their basic features are presented.

The theory of grippers is based on the description of the grasping process and the explanation of grasping constraints. The form and force closure grip are introduced and principles of parallel jaw and multifingered grippers are analysed. The major issues in gripper control and different types of sensors used are outlined. The specific requirements of grippers in health care are compared with those in industrial applications. Various examples of existing grippers are presented.

The state-of-the-art on existing manipulators is presented by distinguishing three different concepts: workstations, wheelchair mounted manipulators, and mobile manipulators. For each category the specific characteristics are discussed. Different examples from each category are presented.

The reader is invited to read this chapter if he/she is looking for the state-of-the-art in manipulators and grippers. The chapter presents the gripping process and gripper configurations giving examples. It is a good starting point for the reader interested in (mobile) manipulators.

5.11 Chapter 11 - Manipulator Control Architectures

Since rehabilitation robots have to operate in the direct neighbourhood of humans, high demands are put on the control performance of the manipulator. The controller must move the manipulator to a destination (not too slow, and not too fast), guaranteeing safe behaviour. The manipulator must be able to operate autonomously carrying out pre-defined tasks. Think for example at fetching books from a known location, or opening a tap. For fetching objects in a structured environment, this autonomous behaviour is sufficient. However, service robots often work in unstructured, or at most partially structured environments. This means either an end-user, or an intelligent high-level controller (which uses sensors for gaining information about the unstructured environment), will directly control the robot.

The chapter gives an overview on widely used controllers in manipulators. The main emphasis is put on low-level controllers and on impedance controllers. The chapter provide a good theory reference on (mobile) manipulators control architectures.

5.12 Chapter 12 - Case Studies on Mobile Manipulators

The chapter presents three mobile manipulators: MANUS, ASIMOV, and MOVAID. Manus is a wheelchair mounted manipulator which is commercially available. At the time of writing of this book, Manus is in use by approximately 150 end-users. Also, the chapter describes the basic aspects of MANUS. ASIMOV targets the same application area, but is not commercially available yet. The chapter provides details about ASIMOV and its design process. The last manipulator described in this chapter is MOVAID. MOVAID aims to supply a mobile manipulator, which can assist end-users semi-autonomously. Technical details about MOVAID are presented and results from user trials performed are reported.

The chapter presents three of the most well known mobile manipulators in mobile robotics for healthcare services. The reader may find details about them, their advantages and disadvantages, their status and aims. The goal of the chapter is to stimulate the reader with new ideas, in particular towards modular designs.

5.13 Chapter 13 - Sensing Strategies for Mobile Robots

The chapter begins by introducing navigation sensors for mobile robots, including odometry sensors (strongly related with locomotion systems) and other navigation sensors such as proximity sensors, lasers and vision systems. The sensor calibration problem is also addressed. Following, a set of proposals for the integration of heterogeneous perception methodologies, sensor fusion and sensor redundancy techniques are presented. They will be useful for localisation and mapping tasks, which are discussed in the following chapters. The concept of virtual sensing is also introduced as an appropriate way to supply sensor information to the navigation module in a standard format. Finally, the selection, configuration and placement of sensors is discussed. This analysis concludes with the development of generic methodology that would be a proposed guideline for researchers on how to select, configure and place sensors on a mobile robot.

The chapter targets the reader interested in sensing techniques. The chapter describes the most well known sensing techniques and presents their use in mobile robotics. Therefore, it may be used as a reference for mobile robot environment sensing strategy design. The reader aiming at a new design may find guidelines on how to select, configure and place sensors on a mobile robot in order to achieve the desired functionality under particular constrains.

5.14 Chapter 14 - Mobile Robots Localisation

Vehicle localisation is a key requirement in mobile robotics. The expansion of sensor technology enables the manipulation of extensive environmental information. Without position estimation, only an instantaneous perception and a basic reactive control is possible, banning the possibility of path planning. Note that in the literature, the problems of perception and localisation are often disconnected. In this chapter it should be kept in mind that the localisation issue is working integrated with perception. In the design process of a localisation system, it is necessary to decide the kind of sensors to be used, the localisation method to be implemented, as well as the accuracy that is required for position estimation. Sometimes, the method just needs to provide identification of the room where the platform is, but more often, an accurate estimation of the position in the room is needed.

The chapter starts with descriptions of devices and techniques that provide position estimations of mobile robots. This may be helpful for the reader who needs references on the available techniques on robot localisation. Furthermore, the chapter gives application examples of those techniques, and presents guidelines on new designs that may operate in healthcare environments.

5.15 Chapter 15 - Workspace Mapping for Mobile Robots

The chapter starts by presenting a framework of methods of sensor fusion, for localisation and mapping purposes. Regarding the latter, the four components of the framework are related to: *environment models*, *local mapping*, *global mapping* and *geometric information updating*. The *environment model* is a 2D map that contains information about the world in which the robot is operating. Along the chapter the three mapping techniques are discussed: *occupancy grids*, *quad-trees* and *geometric maps*. Firstly, the chapter presents how geometric maps are generated by active vision sensors and the techniques used to add new objects to the environment. The main difficulties when identifying segments and objects are commented. Secondly, occupancy grids generated from both ultrasound sensors and active vision sensor are introduced as an appropriate technique for workspace modelling in unstructured environments. Spatial and temporal map fusion techniques are commented, as well as the main problems when identifying static objects. Thirdly, advantages of quad-trees are described. Also, experimental results with a real mobile robot elaborating maps dynamically are commented. The chapter ends with conclusions comparing the mapping techniques, and explanation on how to make use of their advantages in path planning by unifying the mapping models.

The chapter integrates the discussions and findings of the previous two chapters and the reader is invited to read them first unless he/she interested in particular to workspace mapping and holds knowledge on sensing and robot localisation techniques. The reader may refer to this chapter for getting information on workspace mapping techniques, including environment modelling. Although the chapter ends the book, it is of central importance for the reader interested in the integration of mobile robots. The reader is recommended to refer also to Chapters 8, 13 and 14 while reading this chapter.

6. Ideas and an Open Invitation

This book and the work for it is an example of collaborative work of people from different disciplines and several nations. The major scientific achievements are reported. However, it was of major importance that people from different backgrounds managed to cooperate and be productive and this is an achievement that might be not very much highlighted in the rest of the book, but it is difficult to reach, therefore we report that here. We considered that this is as a major achievement.

It is the authors' view that in order to improve the results the ordinary users of technology would like to have, we have to collaborate. If one considers that there is saturation in the results the technology delivers today, we see as a potential reason for that the limited collaborations between science disciplines that happen today. The proper approach to tackle a problem and deliver a proper solution is hidden when looking from one is e.g. the consumer's, the engineering, the medical, perspective. We consider that scientists, researchers, technologists, professionals, citizens (in random order) interested in providing solutions to real life problems or improving the achievements on a topic, should be ready to cooperate with other citizens, professionals, technologists, researchers, scientists, from other backgrounds, originating from other areas. We have to learn to work together, to learn from each other, to extract from each discipline the portion of knowledge and know how that is helpful in reaching the goal.

Therefore no barriers should be placed, no predefined conditions but one: we have to know that all contributors in such an effort have equal roles, share the same responsibility. It is not the engineering that is more important than the medical field or vice versa when the goal is a rehabilitation robot; it the goal that is dominating. The interest is not to register the results to one or the other field, but the results themselves, and further on, the new field that may emerge. It is only of short term interest that e.g. rehabilitation robotics have stronger relation to the engineering rather than to medical field. In the long term scientists in rehabilitation robotics will have their own field that would demand knowledge and efforts in both disciplines. This is only an example and soon enough we will be experiencing evidence of such merging. In the sections above, robotics has been described as the melting pot of various technologies, the point were several sciences contribute to give new results. Robotics should be also seen as the casting point of new fields, the point of birth of novel applications and sciences.

In an earlier section the future of robotics has been described *mobile*. The robots of the next generation has been described as being *partners and collaborators to the human*. The robots or the development emerging from the robotics of the future have been presented as being embedded in devices or *appliances for everyday use by ordinary people*. The vision is to reach the day where *all the bridges between the human and the robots will be built*, the day where *robots will be in harmony with the human*.

This is an open invitation to the reader that is interested in and/or being motivated from this future of robotics and the results that may occur. It is an open invitation to all scientists, researchers, citizens, regardless the discipline and background.. The reader is welcome to share with us views, ideas, visions, contacting us at nkatevas@noemon.net or nkatevas@zenon.gr. The aim would be to exchange experiences and/or ideas, or to potentially collaborate & contribute to the future of robotics or to the new emerging fields.

This concluding section offers an open invitation, but also share with the reader, thoughts on how the future of (mobile) robotics, might be promoted and triggered towards new scientific and application fields.

The *Robotics Olympics* is one of those thoughts. Robotics Olympics is perceived as an open worldwide competition organised at four years intervals - coinciding with Olympics - which brings together teams to compete with their robots in the classic athletic games. Robotics Olympics would be a great opportunity for scientists to deal with complicated problems demanding collaborations. However, the event has to respect the classic principles of the Olympics and by no means trend to a fair of fancy machines. Therefore, the task of setting up the rules themselves is a challenging as well as delicate task. The rules have to be designed to be both socially and scientifically correct. Organisation of such an event as the Robotics Olympics is a challenge for scientists visioning the mobile robots of the next generation.

Another thought towards the very same goal, is the set-up of a network of citizens interested in the (mobile) *robotics future*. The *Robots and the Future* network would include citizens wishing to influence as well as contribute to the future of mobile robots. *The Future and the Robots* should equally give floor to scientists and researcher from all the involved disciplines of technical or social sciences. *The Future and the Robots* should include all the range of citizens interested in the future of robots either being consumers or manufacturers of robots. In order to accumulate the view and opinions of eventually all network participants without exclusions, the network could be organised in a set forums. Scientific forums, social forums, ethics forums, consumers forums are some of the forums being considered as helpful in the network. All those forums may be met in a major network event to be performed yearly. In order to produce exploitable results, each forum will have to conclude to a consensus and report that deals with specific topics. Also, each forum will have to address and report its view on the finding of the other forums. The focus of the *Future and the Robots* would educate scientists and citizens in synergistic actions, to train them to walk in a common way. The aim of the *Future and the Robots* would be to produce the critical mass of scientists, researchers, and citizens coming from various origins that will envision and describe the future robotics and the ways to achieve it.

7. Acknowledgments

The author would like to acknowledge the support of the EC, under the TMR Project FMRX-XT96-0070 without which this book would not be in the readers' hands. Also, the author would like to thank all and each one of the participants of the network for their active contribution to the project aims and their devotion to the common goal.

Chapter 2

User Requirements for Robotics in Health Care and Rehabilitation

by Helmut HECK, Andriana PRENTZA, Edouard PERUCHON, Nikos KATEVAS, Gerard LACEY

Mobile Robotics in Healthcare
N. Katevas (Ed.)
IOS Press, 2001

Chapter 2

User Requirements for Robotics in Health Care and Rehabilitation

Helmut HECK, Andriana PRENTZA, Edouard PERUCHON,
Nikos KATEVAS, Gerard LACEY

1. Introduction

Robotics in *healthcare* aims the provision of a grade of autonomy or a service to people that permanently or temporally lost part of their physical or mental abilities. It might be the case that these people need to interact with the robot in order to get the service required.

From another point of view, robotics in *healthcare* aims at assisting or releasing the care giving staff in/from certain tasks in a hospital environment or in institutional care. Such a robot may be operated or commanded by a nurse to do some standard tasks or by a patient who seeks assistance usually provided by a nurse or care giving person. – The robot in healthcare is used as a *service robot* and economic reasons may be the driving factor for its application.

More specifically, robotics in *rehabilitation* aims at providing people with a tool that (partially) compensates their disabilities. In this application, the robot is not a *service provider* but a tool that increases or restores the user's abilities to perform certain tasks and, by this, (re-)activates the disabled person. Social rehabilitation, as well as increment of personal independence and quality of life are the main objectives of rehabilitation robotics.

According to these differing objectives, the application areas "health care" and "rehabilitation" are treated separately in the following – although a significant number of the requirements are identical for both application areas – and are described from the "users' perspective". This chapter describes who the (potential) users are, the tasks and conditions to which they could successfully apply mobile robots and mobile manipulators.

2. User Needs for Mobile Service Robots in Healthcare

There are no well-known, well-defined user requirements for autonomous mobile service robots in hospital/rehabilitation environment that are based on long term experiences because of the rarity of such systems. Some hospitals use guided mobile systems for transportation of meals or cloths, e.g. HelpMate™ by 'HelpMate Robotics Inc.' [5,6,7]. However, these are not equipped with a robot arm.

Therefore the process of user needs analysis has to be quite interactive and incremental, starting with presenting the researchers' ideas of autonomous mobile service robots to potential users and showing some potential capabilities of such systems. From this point, users can start to think about tasks to be performed by a service robot.

One thing should be clear: Hospitals etc. are organised in such a way that human care givers or service personnel are able to perform all typical tasks. Therefore service robots cannot be expected to be "a must" for such establishments in the sense that they can perform tasks that human beings are not able to do. Potential benefits of service robots can mainly be expected to be economic and practical on one hand, and to contribute to quality of life for disabled users, on the other hand.

2.1 Application Sites

Potential application sites of mobile service robots are establishments for ill, disabled or elderly people, like:

- hospitals
- rehabilitation clinics
- residential homes and independent living centres for elderly & physically disabled people
- sheltered workshops for physically disabled people

One should be aware of the fact that most of the hospitals and many of the rehabilitation facilities work under conditions characterised by work-overload, stress, time-critical tasks, changing personnel etc.

Furthermore, these facilities can be regarded only as partly structured (from the technical point of view) where at any time and at any place situations that have not been foreseen by the developers of the system may occur.

2.2 Stakeholders

Four groups of stakeholders have been identified, summarised in the following table.

Table 1. Stakeholder groups

Stakeholder group	Role
Potential users: • Care giving personnel • Service personnel • Patients: ill, elderly or disabled people	This is the target group of a mobile service robot, people who shall get assistance by the system.
Decision makers: • Administrative manager • Medical manager • Technical manager • Works council	These people decide about the purchase / application of a mobile service robot.
Other potentially involved persons in the establishment (application site): • Technical service personnel • New patients, visitors etc. not familiar with the mobile service robot	These people do service work for a mobile service robot or just meet the system when visiting the establishment.
Potentially involved persons from external companies/institutions • Manufacturer • Dealer • Maintenance service provider • Researcher	These people have economical, technical or scientific interest in the mobile service robot.

2.3 Requirements for Mobile Service Robots

In principle, a mobile service robot should be viewed more as an assistant to the personnel in hospitals or rehabilitation facilities, rather than a replacement of service or care giving personnel.

Potential functional tasks – How a robot can help the care-givers and the patients

The following list of potential (assistive) functional tasks of a mobile service robot, summarised in the three following tables, was elaborated from the results of discussions with representatives of :

- care giving personnel in a rehabilitation hospital
- managing and care giving personnel in sheltered workshop for physically disabled people
- severely physically disabled persons
- hospital patients

The description of the tasks does not take into account whether the mobile robot is technically able to accomplish the task. The description presents the potential demands of the users.

The tables that follow indicate the type of task to be performed by the robot, the initiating persons and persons being involved as well as the priority of the task in the hospital, residential home etc. for disabled people.

3: high prioprity
2: medium priority
1: low priority
0: no demand

P: patient (ill person, disabled or elderly person)
C: carer (nurse, occupational therapist, medical doctor etc.)

Table 2. Tasks with patient involvement

Tasks with patient involvement	Initiated by	Persons involved	Priority in hospital	Priority in workshop	Priority in dormitory
Care giving tasks					
• personal hygiene assistance controlled by the patient	P	P	0	1	1
• feeding assistance controlled by the patient	P	P	1	2	2
• measuring of blood pressure	C,P	P	1	2	1
Transportation tasks					
• drinks to patient	P,C	P,C	3	3	3
• meals to patient	C	P,C	2	1	2
• dishes from patient	P,C	P	3	1	3
• medicine/fever thermometer to/from patient	C	P,C	0	0	0
• pushing patients in wheelchairs/bed to medical application rooms	C	P	3	1	3
Manipulation tasks					
• picking up objects from the floor	P	P	1	3	3
• fetching objects from a shelf etc.	P	P	1	3	3
• preparation of meals	P	P	0	1	3
• assembling, e.g. of dishes in a cupboard or of boxes in a shelf	P	P	0	3	3
• simple manual office work	P	P	0	3	3
• holding objects in a fixed position	P	P	2	3	3
• holding a video camera to a place where the user cannot look at	P	P	0	3	3
• giving water to home plants	P	P	0	2	3
• open a door	P	P	0	3	3
Service tasks					
• guidance of (new/ disoriented) patients or visitors in large buildings	C	P	3	1	1

Remarks on Table 2

The tasks listed as "Manipulation tasks" shall be performed only with direct control of the user in manipulator mode.

Tasks with direct contact of the robot to the body of the patient have relatively low priority. The reason for this is that there is a general reluctance to have the robot arm very close to the body (major safety concern). The priorities will change as soon as service robot systems have proven their reliability and safety. It is very important for these tasks that the robot is directly controlled by the user (as a manipulator).

Table 3. Tasks close to the patient

Tasks close to the patient	Initiated by	Persons involved	Priority in hospital	Priority in workshop	Priority in dormitory
Monitoring / surveillance tasks					
• directed monitoring of the patient	C	C	3	2	2
• directed search for a person in a building	C	C	0	3	1
Transportation tasks					
• transport of materials, goods, medicine in the station	C	C	3	2	3
• directed transport and handling of materials, goods, tools at the workplace and between workplaces	P	P	0	3	3
Service tasks					
• cleaning a patient's room/ workplace	C,(P)	(P)	2	2	2
• cleaning bathrooms, toilets, living rooms, floors, etc.	C,S	(S)	2	2	2
• collection of garbage, dishes etc.	S,P	S,P	1	3	3

Remarks on Table 3

Especially in a workshop for disabled people, it is important that the service robot can be controlled directly by the user, not operating in autonomous mode. The aim in this context is to give the disabled user more independence and enable him/her to perform more tasks as well as increase their complexity. This will result in a reduction of care giving needs during work and in a higher productivity of the staff.

Table 4. Tasks far from the patient

Tasks far from the patient	Initiated by	Persons involved	Priority in hospital	Priority in workshop	Priority in dormitory
Transportation tasks					
• meals/dishes between central kitchen and stations	C,S	C,S	3	2	2
• clothes between laundry and stations	C,S	C,S	3	1	3
• material, goods, medicine between storage rooms and stations	C,S	C,S	3	2	3
• patient documentation between station and application rooms	C	C	3	3	3
• beds, furniture between station and disinfection room	C,S	C,S	3	2	2
Service tasks					
• cleaning and disinfection of used furniture (beds, chairs, sideboards etc.)	S	S	3	3	3
• disinfection of medical instruments	S	S	3	0	1
• handling of chemicals (e.g. for chemotherapy)	C	C	3	0	0
• work in faeces room (cleaning of urinals, putting devices into cleaning machine etc.)	C	C	3	3	3
• preparation of drinks and special meals - kitchen tasks	C	C	1	1	2
• simple manual office work	C	C	3	0	0

<u>*Remarks on Table 4*</u>

Robot tasks far from the patient aim to reduce the staff's workload in tedious, unhealthy, and time-consuming simple manual work, allowing care-giving personnel to spend more time providing personal care for the patients.

Economic requirements

At least one of the following items might be the reason for applying a mobile service robot (each might be applicable at a specific case):

- more economic operation in comparison to man power (in long term periods)
- reliable, accurate, flexible and faster than a person (in special tasks)
- able to work under unpleasant or unhealthy conditions (infectious environments, chemicals, work at night)
- enables the disabled persons to effectively perform some tasks

The above are arguments derived from a strictly technico-economic point of view of robotics in healthcare. The aim of robotics in healthcare is definitely not to replace the human care giver but to reduce his/her workload and enhancing his/her role towards a social partner.

General requirements

The following requirements are of a more general nature; they also take into account that the mobile service robot will operate very close to humans and will mainly be operated by non-technically qualified persons:

- increase individuality of the patient / disabled user
- not decrease personal contacts and communication
- safe operation with respect to patients/persons and objects
- easy to operate
- easy to learn operation
- easy to adapt to environments
- only few changes of environment necessary
- reliable
- manual operation in case of power supply failure
- consistent in operation
- low maintenance needs
- low hygiene maintenance needs (cleans itself)
- pleasant (noise, design, voice/display)

3. User Requirements for Personal Manipulation and Mobility Robotic Aids in Rehabilitation

Thanks to the progress in the domain of intensive care and the increase of early admissions in rehabilitation centres more and more very severely injured persons survive – however, often with severe impairments. As a consequence, therapists are facing daily an increasing number of multi-handicapped persons with a high level of dependence.

The problem is to meet the daily needs of individuals presenting severe upper limb deficiencies, allowing them for extremely restricted mobility and manipulation capabilities, while trunk and lower limbs may be fully functional (a combined disability of upper and lower limbs is sometimes the case).

Current development of mobile robotics capitalised on the huge progress during the last decade of industrial robotics technology, open promising prospects of application in the medical field. Nevertheless, designing robotic systems to assist people with special needs e.g. the motor disabled individuals, requires a good knowledge of the context within which they will have to operate. In the medical field, applied robotics is still "in the starting block" because, although such an advanced technology seems to be very attractive for the severely handicapped, the potential applications are as yet poorly defined. Good knowledge of the application domain is essential to efficiently guide the technological effort.

3.1 Medical Indications for Robotic Aids in Rehabilitation

Potential users can be classified according to their capability to interact with the robotic mobility aid-system. The ICIDH (International Classification of Impairments, Disabilities and Handicaps) considers three interrelated concepts as consequence of disease: *impairment*, *disability* and *handicap*. Impairment is characterised by any loss or abnormality of psychological, physiological or anatomical structure or function. Disability is a temporary or permanent consequence of impairment. Handicap is a disadvantage resulting from impairment or disability that limits or prevents the social, professional or cultural role of an individual. Whatever be the cause, a motor disorder may lead to dependence, and searching for technical solutions to overcome any motor deficit requires deep awareness of the physiological, psychological and medico-social framework.

Based on the definition of impairment, users can be classified according to the type of functional loss. Each category corresponds to particular functional needs and demands for robotic assistance.

Loss of lower limb control

Patient types:

The group is mainly represented by paraplegic patients. Aetiology is either spinal cord injury, tumour, or degenerative disease.

Expected functionality:

Although these patients, generally with full upper-limb functional ability, are able to move using simple devices (classical manually propelled wheelchair, walking apparatuses, etc.), the functional electrical stimulation (FES) of paralysed muscles can be used as a means of producing motor activities including standing and walking.

Loss of upper limb control, associated to locomotor disorders

Patient types:

The group is essentially composed of cervical spinal cord injury patients (tetraplegic). It also includes other pathologies leading to a motor deficit of the four limbs (quadriplegia), associated or not to abnormal movements or tremors:

- cerebral palsy, multiple sclerosis, Parkinson disease, neuromuscular disorders (myopathies, muscular dystrophy) and
- severe diseases effecting locomotive capabilities such as polyarthritis, poliomyelitis, etc.

Loss of upper limb control can be initially partial, allowing the patient to perform some manipulation tasks or to control a wheelchair using an appropriate command.

Other patients can be secondarily and/or provisionally unable to perform any effort towards autonomy as a result of:

- occurrence of intercurrent complications (cardiac),
- ageing,
- specific deficiency precluding use of some existing command modes which is

sometimes the case of:
–arthropathy (joint pathology) of the cervical spine, precluding well known chin
–or occipital command,
–aggravation of spasticity increasing stiffness of the upper limb muscles,
–aggravation of the visual disorders, in multiple sclerosis for instance,
–fatigue, characterising neuromuscular pathologies (myopathy, poliomyelitis, etc.).

Expected functionality:

Patients of this group should benefit by the use of semi-autonomous mobility aids (given an appropriate human machine interface). Particular attention should be paid in the customisation of the system. In medical institutions (e.g. rehabilitation centres) as well as in non-medical institution (e.g. retirement houses), the collective use of a semi-autonomous powered wheelchair will enable the patients to move easily from one place to another (given easy individualisation of the human machine interface).

Moreover, for bed-ridden or severely disabled patients there is a need for multipurpose systems with high level of autonomy, associating mobile robotics and telemanipulation.

Clinical case:

Mr. X, 35 years old, has complete and bilateral tetraplegia (C5 level). He uses a chin control device to control a powered wheelchair. Severe arthropathy of the cervical spine generates cervical pain resistant to most analgesics and local infiltration. He is frequently bed-ridden because of pressure sores. Celibate and living at home with his mother, he never leaves his home except for hospital admission. Recreational activity is limited to TV and radio and he has very few friends.

Two problems have to be considered. First, the arthroplasty of the cervical spine and secondly the need for frequent confinement to bed.

This example shows a patient potentially able to be independent by using a powered wheelchair and some technical aids and who has reached a higher degree of disability because of recurrent complications. This patient could benefit from a powered wheelchair with semi-autonomous control and an appropriate command interface allowing the cervical spine to keep at rest. Moreover, when confined at bed, he could appreciate using remotely controlled manipulation aid-systems to perform a set of pre-programmed tasks.

Loss of spatio-temporal orientation

Patient types:

This category includes patients suffering from:

- mental and neuropsychological impairments,
- vigilance disorders related to traumatic brain injuries (coma and post-coma patients),
- stroke,
- psychiatric disorders,
- ageing, or
- visual deficiencies.

Expected functionality:

These patients are unable to perform any effort towards autonomy and require "intelligent" mobility aids with high degree of automation. Semi-autonomous navigation could be applicable, provided that the system includes the possibility of automatic switching to the autonomous mode in the case of an inconsistent command or a complete loss of orientation. Such a system could be used within an institutional environment for collective application. It could be considered as a "taxi-wheelchair" designed to transport patients directly from one department to another within for instance a rehabilitation centre .

3.2 Technical Solutions: Robotic Aids

Allowing motor disabled persons to reach a desired target or to perform a particular task can be achieved through different techniques, depending on the real domain of application (home, institution) and the clinical profile of the user.

Robotic systems used for healthcare can be classified in two main categories: the mobile technical aids for patient or manipulator transportation, and the active orthosis and prosthesis, which provide patients controlled bipedal locomotion.

Mobile Technical Aids

i) Powered wheelchairs:

Generally electrically driven, these wheelchairs are devoted to the transportation of disabled persons. The features of the command interface depend on the patient's ability to transmit command orders to the system (joystick, button box, voice, etc.).

Some systems incorporate intelligence into the navigation system from transducers analysing on-line the environmental features, in order to perform risk and obstacle avoidance [12] and provide permanently the control system with position data.

A representative example is the SENARIO project of the Telematics/TIDE programme [19]. The project developed a user-oriented approach of a robotic wheelchair (*see also* Chapter 4), able to operate in two different modes [9]:

- the *semi-autonomous* mode, from which the user can freely choose the pathway, the system observes the wheelchair perimeter, informs the user about the presence of obstacles, the risk level, and takes decision in case of necessity,
- the *autonomous mode*, in which the system moves on pre-defined pathways, or cruises autonomously reaching a selected target.

A manipulator (robot arm) is sometimes mounted on the wheelchair (MANUS [11,2]) (*see also* Chapters 4, 10 and 11) providing the patient with manipulation functionality.

ii) Remotely controlled mobile unit with on board manipulator:

Designed for severely disabled & bed-ridden persons, the system associates a mobile robot and a manipulator capable of performing a set of defined domestic tasks [3], remotely controlled by the patient from bedside workstation.

A representative example is the MOVAID system [18] (*see also* Chapters 4, 10 and 11). The robot was implemented in the frame of a Telematics/TIDE programme, and has undergone clinical evaluation. It is an example of a modular and multipurpose aid system, which could provide the severely disabled with daily time segments of complete autonomy.

The system includes a navigation control system, docking capabilities on workstations (bed-side, kitchen board, etc.) and an 8 DOF manipulator.

iii) Robot mobility aids for the frail visually impaired:

Designed for persons with both visual and mobility impairment, the system provides the user with the ability to safely navigate in domestic familiar environment. The user is physically and navigationally supported by the system.

A representative example is the PAMAID system. The majority of the PAMAID system [14] (*see also* Chapter 4) development was undertaken in the Telematics programme of EU. Current research is assessing the clinical merit of the system and on increasing the system functionality. The system includes a user pushed version and an autonomous robot version. The user interface and obstacle avoidance system are key to the systems' usability.

Active Orthosis and Prosthesis

Systems of this type can be divided into two main categories: *walking machines* with motorised joints running as an active exoskeleton – and *neuroprostheses*, external or implanted, based on the functional electrical stimulation of the paralysed muscles.

i) Walking machines:

They are generally motorised lower limb orthoses worn by the patient, enabling him to move on short distances within instrumented environments. A prototype was implemented in 1990 in the frame of EUREKA/CALIES project at INSERM U103 Laboratory [17,4]. It consisted of 6 electrical motors located at the hip, knee and ankle joint level, providing the lower-limb impaired patient with standing-sitting and bipedal walking functions. The user must be able to maintain balance by using crutches. Gait generation signals are provided by an on-board computer and computed and controlled by joint goniometric transducers and foot switches. Due to energy consumption problem, these devices do not provide satisfactory solution to wide range walking assistance, but constitute efficient tools for gait retraining and rehabilitation.

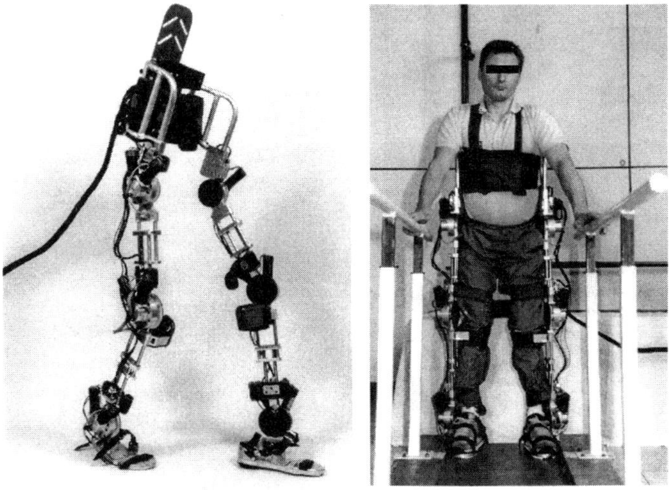

Figure 1. Walking machine for paraplegic patients (INSERM-U103)

ii) Neuroprosthesis:

Neuroprostheses are external or implanted devices [16] applying functional electrical stimulation to the paralysed muscles.

The PARASTEP® [10] performs sequential stimulation of locomotor muscles and enables people with spinal cord injuries to stand and ambulate short distances independently. The patient maintains upright posture thanks to a walker. Stimulation is applied to the quadriceps for knee extension and to the peroneal nerve for global flexion of the leg, through external surface electrodes. The patient controls the stimulation sequence by acting manually on switches placed on the walker. Additional stimulation of the gluteus muscle is envisaged to produce trunk straightening as well as in order to improve the quality of the motion.

An improvement to the above-described device is the EXOSTIM system (currently under development). EXOSIM will lead to smoother movements. In this system, controlled modulation of the stimulation signals will minimise the electrical energy applied to the muscles and noticeably improve the quality of the gait.

Similarly, the SUAW (BIOMED 2) research project [1] aims in restoring the gait function of at spinal cord injured patients, by the use of implanted stimulation devices. Stimulation is directly applied to the muscular nerves or muscles by the means of neural or epimysial electrodes. These electrodes require very low electrical energy. The implanted unit consists of a miniaturised multichannel stimulator controlled by radio signals transmitted through the skin. Present stage of the research is the control of pre-programmed gait sequences from joint goniometric sensors and plantar force transducers. A portable programmer, in which the intelligent part of the system is located, adapts the functionality of the neuroprothesis to each patient. Recently, surgical implantation of such open-loop neuroprosthesis was carried out on a paraplegic patient, and the system is currently being tested in clinical environment.

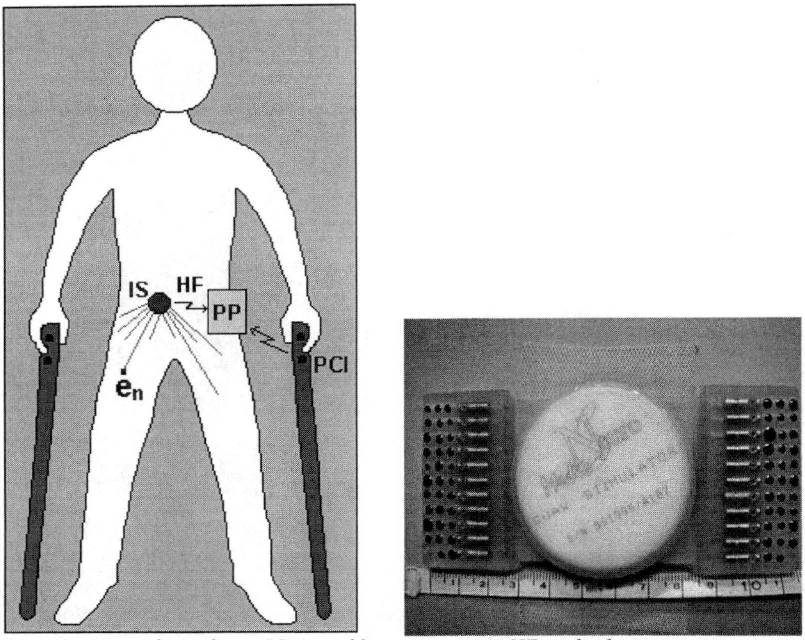

PCI: patient control interface – PP: portable programmer – HF: radio frequency transmission – IS: 14 channel implantable stimulator, Neuromedics S.A. (diameter: 5 cm) – e_n : electrode n.

Figure 2. The SUAW implantable stimulation system

3.3 Requirements for Applications – Case Studies

In the following, requirements for applications are summarised and further explained in case studies.

Major basic requirements

Despite the promising prospects of application of robotics to the rehabilitation domain, designers of robotic aids have first of all to take into consideration a basic set of recommendations imposed by the clinical context. They have also to keep in mind the main objective of the medical application of robotics: *to contribute to autonomy and quality of life, and assist disabled persons to live a more self determined life at home and/or in an institution.*

Any rehabilitation strategy aims at assisting the disabled individual to reach the maximum level of independence. The basic principle relies on the necessity to utilise at best the remaining capabilities of the user to command the system. This feature is a necessary condition for acceptance and for retraining the disabled subject. It constitutes for him/her a challenge for enhancing autonomy and consequently the quality of life.

Effectiveness:

Effectiveness is the extent to which the functionality of the device improves the disabled person's living situation, enhances his/her functional abilities and/or independence.

Reliability:

Reliability is the prime prerequisite of user's (patient, therapist, carer, doctor etc.) acceptance. Efforts towards independence constitute real challenge for the patient both on the physical and the psychological level. Lack of reliability can have an inhibiting effect against the patient's willingness to be further involved in any other activity.

Safety:

Special attention has to be paid to the safety and comfort. The probability that the user may issue a command that drives the system in a dangerous situation must also be considered. The system should be able to deal with erroneous commands. This is imperative, both, for patient's system acceptance and general security in a public institutional environment. The patient must feel safe in any dynamic situation, whatever the environmental conditions are [9].

Adaptation:

Medical application of mobile robotics poses the major problem of interfacing mobile systems to patients. The generally limited functional and/or mental capabilities of the user moves the efforts to the system designer side. The available functionality of the system must fit "on line" the ability of the user, which could vary according to therapy and/or training effect over the time.

Moreover, considering the extreme variability of the user's command capabilities, the command interface must be able to receive a wide range of command devices.

Generally, the limited functional capabilities of the user and the diversity and variability of the clinical cases and functional profiles necessitate high degree of flexibility of the aid-system. In addition, the robotic aid must be able to be installed and operated within various environments.

Aesthetic factors:

They are generally considered as criteria of less importance. In fact they have a surprisingly noticeable effect on the patient's psychology and on his/her relationship to the system. A noisy and bad-looking device will constitute a serious obstacle to acceptance.

Manoeuvrability, Manipulability:

Accessibility and easiness to operate are also essential factors appreciated both by the patient and the therapist, and will enhance the acceptability of the robotic assistance.

Ethical factors:

They are mainly related to unaccompanied patient transportation. This especially applies to patients with restricted ability to communicate, or oversensitive to physical or psychological risks. However, there are several other factors that are included in this area but are not discussed here.

Cost/efficiency ratio:

This has to be carefully estimated, to tackle the challenging issue of robotic assistance for all.

User requirements for a personal assistive robot

It is evident that there are demands for applications that increase the independence of the disabled. The following are applications that have been reported as desired to be delivered by robotic devices [21, 8, 20]:

- eating
- drinking from various sized glasses
- cleaning the mouth (during a meal)
- washing the face
- cleaning the teeth
- shaving
- applying make up
- playing (board) games
- painting & drawing
- turning pages of a book or magazine
- playing with toys, e.g. lego™
- picking and place small objects
- playing mouth-organ
- smoking cigarettes or the pipe

For these applications it is not really necessary that the robot substitutes a human care giver, although it would be desirable. The user already benefits from the robot when he can do something on his/her own without the help of another person. This increases his/her self-confidence and it is a good motivation for more independent activities. By using the robot for tasks that he/she could not previously perform without help, he/she becomes more active than a passive person who receives care. Real independence in tasks is gained only if the robot supports the complete sequence of actions without the need for any assistance from another person. *The user should be autonomous in performing certain tasks*. The situation where a caregiver has to assist the robot to assist the user should be avoided!

Many of the above mentioned tasks are performed in front of the user's face, some with contact to the user or even inside his/her mouth, like brushing teeth. For this, a totally *safe operation* of the robot is required, giving the user at any time the chance to interrupt the robot's action and to remove the end-effector away from his/her body.

When introducing an assistive robot to a disabled person, it is necessary to give him/her the time to get *confidence* in the robot - especially for the safety critical tasks. Therefore it is advisable to start with simpler applications e.g. tasks far from the user's face.

Aesthetics is an important aspect in daily use of the robot because the robot becomes a part of the furniture at home. It should not look like clinical/medical equipment, but should have a home appliance like design. It has been proposed by disabled people to give especially children (or their family members) the chance to individually paint the robot's surface.

Although the reduced quality provided by the robot for certain tasks is accepted (e.g. eating with the robot, is not that efficient as being fed by a care giver) – for the sake of independence – there is a strong requirement that *personal hygiene tasks*, e.g. cleaning teeth, should not be of lower quality compared with a human care giver – for medical reasons. This is certainly a big challenge for robot developers.

The control of the manipulator should be as direct as possible by the user, i.e. preferably in a joystick mode – assuming that the task can be performed in a reasonable time. Therefore the human-machine-interface has to be as versatile and adaptable to the user's abilities as possible – including single/multiple switch, joystick and voice recognition as input options to make operation more efficient. Speech output or a graphical display should be present to guide the user/care giver through the adjustment procedure or option menus.

All (automatic) operations of the robot should be done with minimal movements; the movements should be smooth and as silent as possible; the trajectories must be predictable and understandable by the user. If the teaching of certain robot postures is necessary, then this teaching should be done easily by moving the robot by hand to the teach-in positions.

Usually the tasks mentioned above are performed at different places in a person's home: living room, dining room, kitchen, bathroom etc. This requires that the robot, (if it is to support the tasks), is mobile or at least moveable. Mobility could be achieved by moving the robot system with the user's (electrical) wheelchair, by an autonomous mobile platform, or just by a moveable platform.

For many of the tasks the robot arm has to reach over the user's legs or body, face, especially when the disabled person sits back in his/her wheelchair.

For some of the tasks, like washing or shaving, it is acceptable that the robot is positioned in front of the user. However, when the disabled person uses the robot in a communicative situation, e.g. at meal-time when talking with other people or when playing a board game with a partner or when watching TV, then it would be much better to position the robot beside the user. This would be much more natural from the user's point of view, because from the side position the robot would substitute the function of the user's arm – instead of substituting an arm of a care giver in the front position.

User requirements for a robotic mobility aid (e.g. intelligent wheelchair)

Robotic mobility aids have to provide the people suffering from disabilities (physical and mental) with an easy and safe transportation means. More specifically, when focusing on potential user's point of view, a robotic mobility aid has to contribute to:

- facilitating the mobility of persons with serious motor disability (tetraplegic, elderly, etc.),
- allowing displacement for physically disabled persons with additional mental handicap by providing a supervising mode.

Generally speaking, potential users may present several kinds of disability, for example, locomotion disabled persons or mentally retarded children with associated physical disabilities, muscular diseases (myopathy, muscular dystrophy), tetraplegia or multiple sclerosis. Different characteristics of the users have to be considered, as the following:

- different types of workspace: home, office, hospitals, shops, etc.,
- different kinds of users: disabled persons with all the possible variety of disability, and care givers belonging to medical and socio-professional staff,
- different kinds of disability evolution: temporary (post-surgical), stationary, increasing (elderly people).

User classification:

The user requirements for a robotic mobility aid (user interface, operating mode), and more specifically for a robotic wheelchair depend on the user's ability to drive his/her vehicle. Different user groups can be defined as follows (Figure 3):

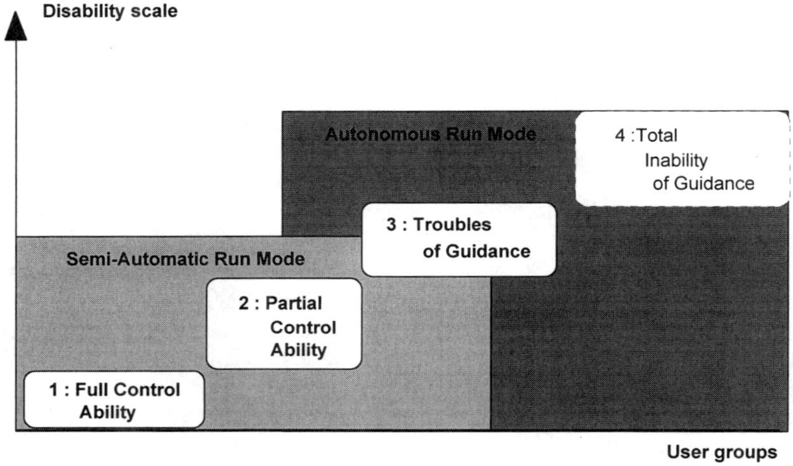

Figure 3. Different operational modes for the various user groups

Full Control Ability:

- Users: Individuals with at least one upper limb ability and no mental impairment. Examples: elderly people, weak people, etc.
- Operating mode: manual or (eventually) semi-autonomous.
- User interface: manual control (joystick).
- Description: The user drives the wheelchair himself without any special difficulty.

The system may act as risk observer, task which can be decomposed in the two following activities:

- risk detection and warning of the user (from a warning beep for example),
- risk avoidance (if the user did not react to the warning signal).

Partial Control Ability:

- Users: Individuals without limb mobility, but with remaining control sites (eg: head mobility), safe intellectual ability and sufficient perception capabilities (sight, hearing, tactile). Example: tetraplegic people.
- Operating mode: semi-autonomous or autonomous
- User interface: adapted manual control (chin or tongue-based control, vocal control...)
- Description: In addition to the previously mentioned activity, the system has to inform the user about inconsistent orders (involuntary tremors for example) and ignore them.

Guidance Problems:

- Users: Individuals with troubles in environment perception, e.g. temporary visual impairment, disorientation or memory loss. But users must still have capability to make decisions, especially when much manoeuvring is required, e.g. in a bathroom.
- Operating mode: essentially automatic operating mode on pre-defined paths.
- User interface: Sophisticated Control Panel (sip-and-puff or speech recognition).
- Description: If the user experiences problems during long and difficult navigation, while maintaining his/her perception of the local environment, he should be able to switch from autonomous to semi-autonomous mode, for obstacle avoidance for example. If the wheelchair follows a pre-defined path under the user control, it may be interesting to envisage a warning system if the trajectory leaves the planned path.

Application environments:

Robotic mobility aids may be used in different environments. From the user‘s point of view, types of environment can be the following:

- home,
- working environment (office),
- hospitals and specialised institutions,
- outdoor (streets, shops, etc.).

Potential user tasks:

The distinction between people that need a robotic mobility aid and people that do not need it, may be performed observing their ability to perform the following tasks:

1. *On / off:* It is the simplest action to be performed on the wheelchair, including emergency stop.

2. *Guidance control:* Obtained by the directional control of the robot through a joystick (forward/backward and left /right).

3. *Cruise control:* Speed control is obtained by the same command as the guidance control. Speed control is a function of the joystick position. Speed command laws are often non-linear, in order to permit a best precision for the lower speeds. A "dead zone" is associated to such a law allowing ignoring unintentional actions (shock, tremor). Speed is also limited by the power control.

4. *Risk detection and avoidance:* When the user pilots his/her wheelchair, he watches over the surroundings. He/she must detect obstacles, estimate risks (approaching stairs, for example) and must also anticipate events (a dog or child darting across the trajectory). The system must ensure the safe movement of the user (the highest priority) but that movement should also be comfortable. The Risk Avoidance system (path planner) has to plan smooth curves from the starting point to the target.

5. *Obstacle avoidance:* After the detection and localisation of an obstacle, the user reaction can be:

- stop and wait the opening of the passage, eventually call for help,
- avoid the obstacle by a walk around, or
- keep the way free by pushing the obstacle.

6. *Orientation, locating:* When considering long trajectories (e.g. longer than five meters), it will be necessary for the user to know his/her position in the environment. He needs two elements: a general knowledge of his/her environment and several cues to detect and identify it. The more the environment is unknown, the more difficult the task will be to perform and a learning stage will be necessary. Some people can find this bearing less easily than others. It concerns:

- children or elderly persons,
- persons suffering from memory loss,
- persons suffering from perception troubles (hearing, seeing, etc.),
- persons suffering from orientation troubles.

7. *Path planning:* A successful trajectory joining a point to another is the combination of several actions and of knowledge to choose the way. It will be necessary to know the general environment and to estimate many choice criteria such as distance, time, fatigue or risk. The trajectory is built step by step. The resulting trajectory is composed of several shorter sections marked with beacons. Each extremity of segments is characterised by a specific action that implies a decision. Some people have specific problems when such a kind of decision occurs: memory loss or incapacity to decide.

8. *Navigation:* When the path is chosen, the person must follow it. Then he/she must be able to find his/her bearing from the environment and from the way that was chosen first. He/she must estimate the realised distance. He/she must also remember performed steps and anticipate next cues showing the right way. He/she will necessarily have to face to unpredictable events such as:

- lack of cues
- existence of obstacles leading to loss of the initial path (modification in order to reach goal is necessary)
- the way loss, which can be resumed by the loss of all known beacons

Ergonomic requirements:

The most important consideration in the development of any robotic mobility aid and especially of a robotic wheelchair is that the wheelchair should "fit" the user. If he/she feels uncomfortable with the chair and avoids using it, then the wheelchair will fail its intended purpose, regardless of the technological sophistication incorporated in its design [13,15].

The persons that need to use a wheelchair may suffer from numerous disorders, such as Paraplegia, Hemiplegia, Spinal cord injuries, Parkinson's disease, Cerebral Palsy, Muscular Dystrophy, Brain Damage, Stroke, etc. The wheelchair provides the mobility that has been lost because of disorders such as the ones mentioned above. However, wheelchair-bound persons who spend a large part of the day on a chair need to feel comfortable while using it, otherwise they might reject its use and prefer to stay in bed, with all the negative results that this implies. For the wheelchair user to feel comfortable while using the chair for a considerable amount of time, (something especially important for the users of most powered wheelchairs), the wheelchair design has to follow a number of ergonomic principles and incorporate the largest possible number of customised features for the benefit of each user.

The main reason that wheelchair users feel sometimes uncomfortable in their chairs is the absence of correct ergonomic design, which can compensate the disorder, and the problems caused by it. These are mainly posture problems, which are created either by the disorder itself or by incorrect wheelchair design. There are a number of disorders that cause posture problems, such as Brain trauma, which may result in defects of power, muscle tone, co-ordination and sensation. Other possible problems are contractures and deformities, decubitous ulcers (pressure sores), reduced ability and performance, infection, tiredness and discomfort.

"Good posture" is a consideration that has to be taken into account. Generally, we talk about a "good posture" when the body segments are balanced in a position of least strain and maximum support. Posture is maintained by righting reflexes originating in the mid-brain area, namely the labyrinthine reflexes, body righting reflexes on body, neck righting reflexes, body righting reflexes on head, and optical righting reflexes.

Since a "good" posture means that there is efficient energy expenditure, we can state that:

- static and erect postures should be avoided,
- when seating, proper supports should be available to replace the function of the muscle groups which are relaxed,
- the centre of gravity of each body segment should ideally be vertical above the area of the supporting base and near its centre.

For the persons who cannot maintain upright position and require the use of a wheelchair there are the following needs:

- The wheelchair should "fit" the user.

- It is important to fix the pelvis orientation while seated.
- It is also important to maintain the lumbar curve for stress relief.

Generally, two groups of postural instability can be recognised, the first is a forward curvature of the upper trunk and the second is backward curvature of the upper trunk. The seating problems that most of wheelchair users face to can be summarised as follows:

- The body slumps or arches.
- The trunk may fall to one side.
- There is lateral trunk flexion along with the mentioned trunk movements.
- The head may flop forward, backward or sideways.
- The body generally is falling and it is trying to find its own level of support.

In the case of seated postures, factors such as the position of the body mass relative to the support, muscle forces, possible bracing of the body, and the inertia of the body dead weight have to be considered. To ease posture problems while seated, it is important:

- to have frequent changes of position,
- to employ a rest for the elbows and the forearms,
- to assure that the minimum possible pressures are applied to the body flesh,
- to have support for the lumbar region so that the lumbar erector spinal muscle can be relaxed, and
- to make sure that there is little pressure on the anterior aspect of the thigh by varying the height of the seat in relation to the length of the lower legs.

Summarised, the following recommendations have to be followed in order to maintain postural stability:

- The person sitting on the wheelchair has to be supported in a position that reduces the tendency of the body to slide, and balance the trunk.
- Stress on spine has to be reduced.
- The body /seat interface has to be firm and of adequate area.
- The centre of gravity of the person has to remain within the base area.
- It is essential to have equal weight bearing through both ischial tuberosities.
- There should be provision for support of the lumbar spine.
- The height of the armrests is important because they also serve the stabilisation of the trunk.
- The use of a tray can take weight off the shoulder girdle and provide stability.

To satisfy these conditions, a forward position of the trunk over the base should be evaluated. In the most of demanding cases, like Cerebral Palsy, the trunk can be supported along the anterior surface with a breastplate. Also, the flexion of the trunk should occur only about the hip joint, and not about the lumbar spine.

In order to get an assessment for a seating support system, several factors have to be taken into account. The main factors as these have been identified in the SENARIO intelligent wheelchair [19] are:

- body size and shape
- posture
- balance
- perceptual problems
- continence
- muscle weakness
- ability to get out of the wheelchair
- oedema
- confusion

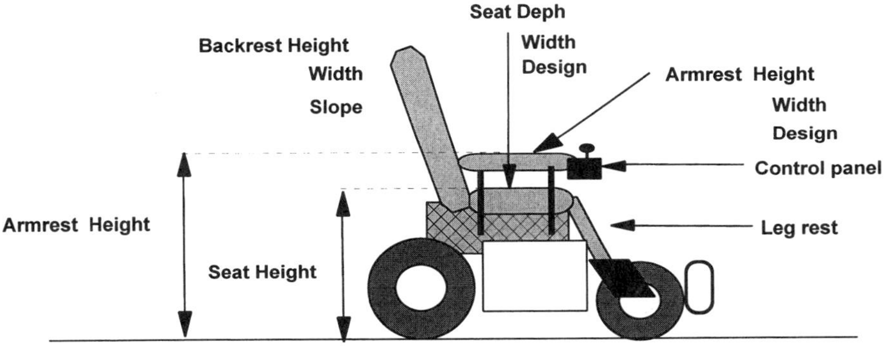

Figure 4. Ergonomic elements description

The following criteria can be used for selecting and specifying the appropriate wheelchair (Figure 4)

- *Seat Height.* The feet should be flat on the floor when the knees are at a 90-degree angle.
- *Seat Depth.* The sacrum should be in contact with the backrest gap.
- *Seat Width.* The seat should be wider than the person sitting, so that seating position can be changed easily.
- *Backrest Height.* It should be high enough to support the shoulders and the head of the patient.
- *Backrest Width.* It should be broader than the shoulder width.
- *Backrest Slope.* It should provide sufficient support in lumbar region and allow neck movement.
- *Backrest Shape.* It should support the base of the scull and not the back of the head.
- *Armrest Height.* It should be low enough to make the wheelchair easy to push (if that is possible). If the person seated uses the armrests, the force on the knees can be reduced when he/she rises.

- *Armrest Width.* It should not be too narrow so that activity is restricted, but it should not be too wide either so that it is hard to get out of the chair.
- *Armrest Design.* Armrests should have a flat top and rounded edges and sufficient width.
- *Wheelchair Leg support.* It should be possible to position the feet under the front of the chair. The support should be well padded (to avoid slipping).

The wheelchair ideally should be light enough to be lifted into a car. This is not possible with powered wheelchairs, and consequently a special car, which can accept powered wheelchairs, must be used.

In addition to the general criteria listed above, there are special conditions that require special design considerations. The selection of the type of persons that can use the wheelchair will dictate which of those design elements will be incorporated into the chair design.

4. Conclusions

Designing robotic systems to assist motor disabled individuals requires first of all rather good knowledge of the real framework within which they have to operate. Interfacing mobility and /or manipulation aids has to be performed taking into consideration the user's clinical profile and functional ability. Possible applications are light/heavy loads transportation, manipulation and surveillance, according to specific classes of impairments and disabilities. Some practical examples of application in real clinical environments were suggested, emphasising the physical, physiological and ethical constraints of applying such techniques in a domestic or institutional environment.

It is obvious that (with existing technology) *a robot in healthcare able to perform all the mentioned potential tasks would be too expensive and too complicated to use* – if at all possible. Therefore researchers and developers should focus on one or two of the task categories taking into consideration whether the above mentioned "General Requirements" can be achieved. Only if they can be fulfilled for certain tasks in principle, then a more detailed functional requirements analysis combined with an economic cost/benefit analysis should be made.

At the present state of development of robotic aid systems, assessment and validation procedures have to be initiated. Especially, collecting users‘ impressions about the capacity of the system to contribute to autonomy and self-determined life is of prime importance.

Evaluation has to be performed with systems that meet the basic criteria of technical reliability and safety, which is not the case for laboratory prototypes. This poses the industrial problem of manufacturing of small series of devices.

Evaluation must also be carried out in terms of efficiency and cost/benefit ratio in comparison with the employment of a human caregiver. In most cases human aid is definitely a necessity since it seems difficult to imagine a patient living alone with a mobile robot, even fully responding to all needs. A realistic prospect should be a solution providing the motor disabled person with few hours per day of complete autonomy.

5. References

[1] BIOMED 2, SUAW Project: Stand Up and Walk, Demonstration project (1996-1999).

[2] Bühler Ch., Heck H., Nedza J., Schulte D., "MANUS Wheelchair-Mountable Manipulator – Further Developments and Tests", *Manus Usergroup Magazine*, January 1994, Vol. 2, No. 1, pp. 9-22.

[3] Dario P., Guglielmelli E., Alotta B., "Mobile robotics aids". *Proc. of the Workshop on Robots for the Disabled and Elderly people*, Nagoya, Japan 1995, pp.16-24.

[4] EUREKA, CALIES Project: Computer Aided Locomotion by Implanted Electrical Stimulation 1989-1995.

[5] Evans J. et al., HelpMate™: "A Robotic Materials Transport System", *Robotics and Autonomous Systems,* 1989, Vol. 5, pp. 251–256.

[6] Evans J.M., "HelpMate: An Autonomous Mobile Robot Courier for Hospitals". *Int. Conf. on Intelligent Robots and Systems IROS* '94, 1994.

[7] Evans M. "HelpMate: A Service Robot Success Story", *Service Robot,* Vol. 1, No. 1 (1995).

[8] Heck H., Bühler Ch., Bolmsjö G., "Development of New Applications for a Personal Robotic Aid to Assist Physically Disabled People", *Proceedings of the 2nd MobiNet Symposium on Mobile Robotics Technology for Health Care Services*, Edinburgh, Scotland, 23 July 1998, pp. 61–73.

[9] Katevas N., Tzafestas S., Bishop J.M., Preuss R.., Rabischong P., Koutsouris D., Ikonomopoulos A., Papakonstantinou G., Tsanakas P., Uzunoglou N., "SENARIO The Autonomous Mobile Technology for the Locomotion Handicap: Operational and Technical Issues", Placencia Porreo I. ,Puig de la Bellacasa (eds.), *The European context for Assistive Technology.* IOS Press, Amsterdam, Oxford, Tokyo, Washington DC (1995), pp. 371-374.

[10] Klose K. John et al., "Evaluation of a Training Program for Persons With SCI Paraplegia Using the Parastep®1 Ambulation System: Part 1. Ambulation Performance and Anthropometric Measures", *Arch. Phys. Med. Rehab.,* 1997, Vol. 789-93.

[11] Kwee H., "Integrating Control of Manus and Wheelchair", *Intern. Conf. on Rehabilitation Robotics,* ICORR'97, Bath, 14-15 April 1997, pp.91-94.

[12] Longhi S., Leo T., Zulli R., "On-line collision avoidance for a robotic assistance system", *Proc. of the IFAC Workshop on the Human-Oriented design of Advanced Robotic systems*, DARS'95, Wien 1995, Vol. 1, pp. 89-95.

[13] Mulcany C. M. et al., "Adaptive Seating for Motor Handicap", Rehabilitation Engineering Unit, Chailey Heritage hospital, North Chailey, Lewes, East Sussex.

[14] O'Neill A-M., Petrie H., Lacey G., Katevas N., Karlsson M-A., Engelbrektsson P., Gallagher B., Hunter H., Zoldan D., "Establishing Initial User Requirements for PAM-AID: a Mobility and Support Device to Assist Frail and Elderly visually Impaired Persons", I. Porrero Placencia ,Billabio E. (eds.), *Proceedings of the Third TIDE Congress. Improving Quality of Life for the European Citizen: Technology for inclusive design and equality*. IOS Press, 1998.

[15] Pope P. M., "A study of Instability in relation to Posture in the Wheelchair – Proposals for the Improvement of the Unstable Postural condition and some cautionary notes", Royal Hospital and Home for the Incurables, Putney.

[16] Rabischong P. "Les Neuroprothèses". *Pour la Science,* 1995, Vol. 217, pp. 98-100.

[17] Rabischong P., Rabischong E., Péruchon E., Micallef J.P., "Computer Aided Locomotion by Implanted Electrical Stimulation", The CALIES project, Popovic D.B. (ed.), *Proc. Advances in External Control of Human Extremities*, Belgrade 1990, pp. 491-494.

[18] TIDE, MOVAID Project n° 1270: "Mobility and Activity Assistance systems for the disabled", 1994-1997.

[19] TIDE, SENARIO Project n°1045: *Sensor Aided Intelligent Wheelchair Navigation*, 1994-1997.

[20] Topping M., "A Brief Overview of the Development of Handy 1 a Robotic Aid to Independence for the Severely Disabled", *Proceedings of the 1st Forum for European Rehabilitation Robotics (FERR)*, Wetter/Ruhr, Germany 1995.

[21] Topping M., Heck H., Bolmsjö G., "An overview of the BIOMED 2 RAIL (Robotic Aid to Independent Living) project", *Proceedings of the Intern. Conference on Rehabilitation Robotics*, ICORR '97. Bath, England, 1997, pp. 23-26.

Chapter 3

Human-Machine-Interfacing for Control in Healthcare Robotics

by Helmut HECK, Gerard LACEY, Andriana PRENTZA, Edouard PERUCHON, Pierre RABISCHONG

Mobile Robotics in Healthcare
N. Katevas (Ed.)
IOS Press, 2001

Chapter 3

Human-Machine-Interfacing for Control in Healthcare Robotics

Helmut HECK, Gerard LACEY, Andriana PRENTZA,
Edouard PERUCHON, Pierre RABISCHONG

1. Introduction

While *industrial robots* usually work in well-defined, structured industrial environments, the sequence of their movements and actions following a prepared program, partially including real-time sensor information, but without the necessity of further human interaction, with the exclusion of human beings from the robot's workspace for safety reasons – the situation for *robotics in healthcare, and* especially in *rehabilitation*, is quite different:

The *workspace* is the semi-structured or completely unstructured environment of hospitals, private homes or public areas like streets with traffic, shops or public buildings. The world is neither predictable nor static. It may change during the application of the robot in an unforeseeable way: other people, animals or e.g. cars may suddenly become obstacles on the intended way of task execution. Re-planning of action or even re-defining of goals may become necessary.

This requires in the common case *interaction* with the user. In the intelligent wheelchair example, the user has to be active in steering the robot to a high level of "online action planning", and furthermore the active participation of the user is required with respect to his/her "perception system". Especially the visual capabilities of seeing and interpreting the environment and the actual actions/movements of the robot in real-time. In *rehabilitation robotics*, the user is quite often an integral part of the control loop.

Furthermore the disabled user (in case of rehabilitation robotics), or the patient (in case of health care robotics) is often present inside the *workspace* of the robot, e.g. in eating and drinking assistance by the robot, or the human being is the target of the robot's action, e.g. in body washing and personal hygiene tasks. This requires an extremely high standard of safety.

In contrast to these stringent requirements, from an ergonomic point of view, there are the *abilities and skills of the users*. There are no well-trained technicians or robotics engineers in a healthcare setting as would be in typical industrial robotics applications. But they are nurses, patients and disabled persons; none of whom will have had a fundamental training in robotics, and in case of the "disabled" users they additionally have a great variety of individual disabilities.

This obvious "gap" between the requirements and the users' abilities makes the human-machine interface the most crucial and important part of the robotic system (from the users' point of view). The present chapter tries to give an overview on the physiological means and devices to control a robot as well as some guidelines to select human-machine interface components for specific users.

2. Physiological Means for Control of Devices

2.1 Normal Physiological Means

Control of a device requires *physiological output* by the user, which has to be consciously expressed in order to act on a command interface.

Starting from this assumption, any physiological activity can be used to generate a command signal. However, control of the device's functioning cannot be performed without feedback from any *sensory input*, consciously perceived and analysed.

Physiological outputs

Physiological outputs have to be managed according to the number of degrees of freedom required to activate the command system, from simple push button to six degrees of freedom systems. Various outputs can be considered:

Segmental motor actions:

Action means either force application on the command interface or movement, which requires contact perception and/or movement identification in terms of direction, amplitude and velocity. It is important to point out that *the skin* [13] covering all the segments of the body and fixed in places, plays the crucial role of position transducer, leading without visual control to conscious identification of position and movement of all body segments. That is mainly related to the Ruffini corpuscles located within the dermal part of the skin. They consist of a central fibrous system surrounded by a capsule more or less fixed to the connective tissue of the derma and to which myelinated nervous fibres convey the specific skin stretching information. Activation of any joint creates some tension strength in the periarticular skin generating a signal related to joint position or movement. In addition, a high-level control loop is located between area 4 of the precentral gyrus, i.e. the frontal cortex of the brain and areas 1, 2, 3 and 5 of the postcentral gyrus of the parietal lobe (Figure 1). The first area represents the "motor keyboard" in which all the 600 muscles of the body are topographically represented with a major importance for the face and upper limbs. Post-central gyrus areas represent the "sensitive keyboard" with all parts of the skin topographically integrated. This high-level control loop belongs to the statokinesthesia (statokinetic sense), which is the conscious perception of the position and movements of all body segments. It allows a person to be consciously integrated in the 3D space.

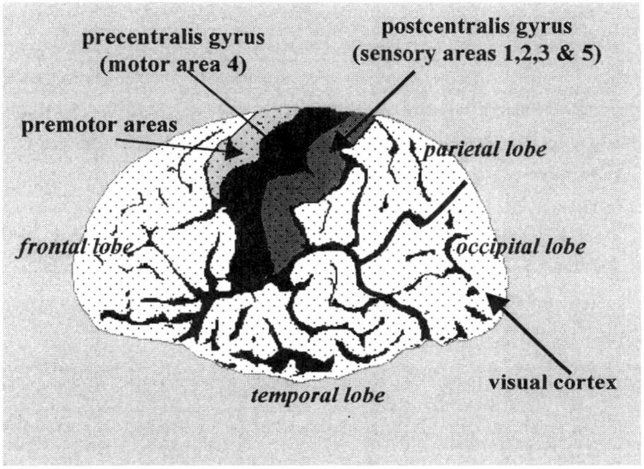

Figure 1. The brain. Sensory and motor areas for control of movement

Learned motor programmes for complex co-ordinated (bilateral) movements of eye, head and hand are stored within the premotor areas in the frontal lobe.

The use of the *vision* is perfectly complementary and provides more precise information for the control of the visible body segments. Therefore, any body segment can be used to command and control a device. But, in fact, some of them are more precisely controlled by the central nervous system, which is the case of the hands. The central projection of the group of muscles controlling the hand in the motor keyboard and the cutaneous representation are largely more important than for the lower limbs. The hand is indeed the most precise and flexible command interface. Different segmental motor actions can be used to command assistive devices.

Hand output:

The hand can be used to touch a button, to push or pull a device, to grasp a joystick or to activate a series of keypads without limitation of number. Adding all the degrees of freedom of the upper limb can allow for wide and complex movements, to activate a lever in space or to manipulate a stick. Any kind of movement in all directions (including controlled rotation) can be done by the upper limbs and the hand. The command signal can be generated from on-off or proportional force contact, without movement, or from controlled segmental displacement. Moreover each finger, with its four degrees of freedom can also be used separately as a command organ.

It has to be noted that in some specific situations where fingers are unusable, shoulder or wrist movements may constitute valid command means.

Lower limb output:

The control in position and movement of the foot can be also very precise with more power but with less possibilities than for the hand, due to poor grasping capability and the smaller number of available degrees of freedom. But the foot or the knee can be used properly and efficiently to act on specifically designed control devices.

Head output:

Head movements are normally linked to eye movements for the visual exploration, and require mainly two degrees of freedom: for vertical and horizontal rotation. Micrometric activation systems are located at the head/cervical spine junction, forming a real cardan joint. In addition, different groups of muscles of the cervical spine can move the head laterally which constitutes another available degree of freedom [39].

The vestibule contributes to the static and dynamic positioning control of the head, as well as the skin of the neck. Finally, head movements are very precisely and consciously identified by the brain and can serve as a control of a device.

In addition, displacements of the mandible and chin from head or jaw movements can be used to accurately move adapted control devices.

Eye movements:

Humans have two eyes to see one image. This is related to the *stereoscopic vision*, which requires perfect co-ordination and adjustment of the two eye movements and positions. Some basic technical principles have to be identified in order to understand the exact conditions of use of eye movement as control output [30]. The two eyeballs are included within a fibrous sac called the Tenon capsule, which is laterally fixed inside the orbit by fibrous anchoring. The movement itself is generated by four recti muscles oriented along two different axis, vertical and horizontal, pulling backwards the eyeball during horizontal scanning movements. The retropulsion component of the recti muscle action is compensated by some antepulsion action of the superior oblique muscle. This explains the complex dynamic equilibrium process of the eye positioning and movement, resulting from the simultaneous action of six muscles. The muscle co-ordination on both sides is performed by the different nervous nuclei and nervous pathways of the brain stem, which is the junction between the brain and the spinal cord and the location of the main automatisms of the head. Nevertheless, accurate adjustment of both eyes cannot be achieved with the muscular co-ordination only. A high resolution reference visual point (135000 cones/mm^{-2}), the macula, located in the retina on the optical axis, allows the brain to exactly adjust the angle co-ordinates of both eyes in order to perform the fusion of the two images for stereoscopic vision. In other words, the image is guiding the whole visual servomechanism, including the eye-head co-ordination. The last allows head and eyes to move together in such a way that the stereoscopic vision, which is lost over 40% of eye movement amplitude, can be conserved. In addition, the fixation of the gaze on a particular mobile or immobile object, is performed by a centre located in the frontal lobe of the brain. Various pointing techniques using accurate positioning of the gaze have been designed and successfully tested to controlling assistive device interfaces [6].

Tongue movement:

The tongue is equipped with 17 muscles, allowing this organ to move in many directions and to push on the teeth or on any kind of device located inside the mouth or at few centimetres outside of it. The mucosa covering the tongue is very richly innervated and contains numerous mechanoreceptors, thermal and taste receptors. The normal activity of the tongue is devoted to the mastication of sounds to create phonemes and also to the swallowing functions. The ability of the tongue to precisely identify the shape and consistency of an object [21] justifies its possible use as command interface.

Voice control:

Phonation is a basic function of the human species, which occupies a very large area of the brain. Two major functions are concerned.

First, *the comprehension of oral and written language,* requiring a large memory cerebral zone, in which all the visual symbols (numbers, letters, words and sentences) are stored, as well as sounds and phonemes corresponding to all the listened sentences, possibly in different languages. This corresponds to the Wernicke's area of the brain (Figure 2) within the parietotemporal lobe. This area is largely connected with the primary visual cortex in the occipital lobe and with the primary auditory cortex in the temporal lobe.

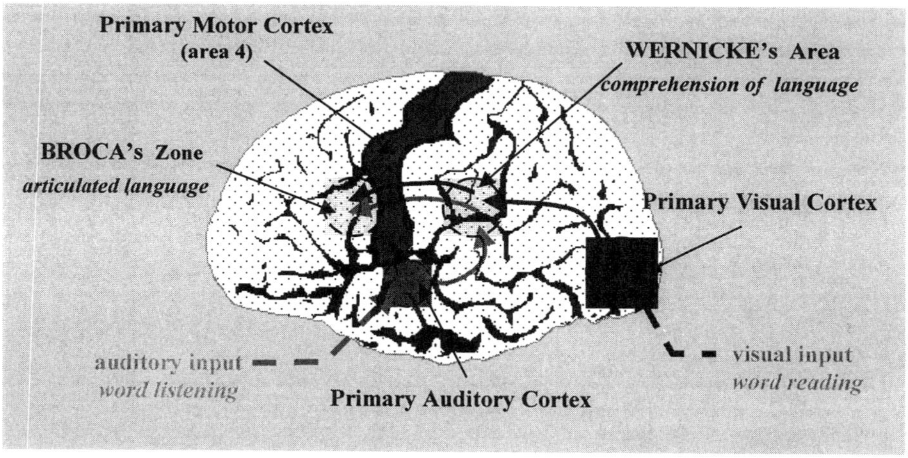

Figure 2. Language comprehension and articulation – the Wernicke-Geschwind model

Second, *the articulation of language*, which requires the action of 35 different muscles, results from the modulation of the sounds coming from the larynx, acting as a "voice processor", and going either to the nose or to the mouth for a specific construction of phonemes, words and sentences. Related brain area is located in the base of the gyrus precentralis i.e. within a frontal zone of the brain: the Broca's zone. Comprehension and articulation of language are perfectly complementary functions. The full reception-emission process can be activated without speaking, which represents the "internal language". Not only the voice corresponding to a particular command language can be used as control output [33] but also sounds, cries or whistles.

Capture of physiological signals:

Many organs are generating micro-currents during their activation and the modern physiological measurement techniques allow us to use these functional signals as command outputs. That is the case of all the striated muscles which generates myoelectrical signals during their active contraction [12]. Such signals can be directly collected from surface or implanted electrodes (Electromyography) [38]. Moreover, brain electrical activity (Electro-encephalography) or peripheral nerve activity (Electroneuroraphy) could be used as command signals. Electro-oculography which consists in capturing changes in the standing potential between cornea and retina related to eye movement, has been successfully experimented to command an external device [16].

Physiological inputs

The most efficient way to control a device is to operate in the close-loop mode, allowing real time regulation by means of retroaction or sensory feedback.

Three main sensory inputs are concerned. First, the *visual inputs* which are very precise and can be selected in terms of shape, colour or movements. Second, the *tactile inputs* can be proportional to the level of force feedback, or can be of on-off type in relation with a contact feedback. Third, the *auditory inputs* can be modulated in terms of sound intensity or frequency. Auditory feed-back could also be supplied via synthetic voice.

2.2 Dysfunction of the PMCD

For any alteration of physiological outputs or inputs, the command interface must adapt using the remaining capabilities of the impaired functions. Depending on the nature of the device to be controlled, it will be useful to determine the minimum number of degrees of freedom necessary to achieve the control procedure as well as the required amplitude of the command output. Few major pathological entities can be identified.

The paralysis:

Paralysis is the loss of the voluntary muscle command, which can affect either half of the body (hemiplegia) or the lower limbs (paraplegia), or the four limbs (tetraplegia), or even the articulated language (aphasia). The pathological deficit can be of vascular, (thrombosis, haemorrhage), traumatic, tumoral, or infectious origin. A loss of skin sensitivity can be associated, generating asomatognosia which is the loss of the sense of body segment spatial position, due to the disconnection into the brain or spinal cord of the goniometric cutaneous pathways. Another complication is the spasticity [5], which is the increasing of stiffness of the joints during movement or passive mobilisation of joints. This is due to the lack of central control of the fusorial servomechanism, where the muscular sensors called "muscular spindles" act as tensiometres. Some associated perturbation of the equilibrium in standing up or sitting posture, with or without vertigo, can oblige to adapt the command interface. The solution has to be found in the remaining able part of the body. In case of high tetraplegia in which limb movements are impossible, voice, eye or head movements can be used as control output.

The abnormal movements

Some neurological diseases like Parkinson or multiple sclerosis can generate a tremor [14] in limb extremities. Filtering of these abnormal oscillations can be performed in order to get a usable command signal. The choreiform or athetosic [29] movements which are oscillations of the body of greater amplitude are more complicated to be modified or filtered and in many cases, other physiological means like sound control have to be tested.

Sensorial deficits

In case of blindness, the tactile sense can be overdeveloped and easily used for device control. Deafness doesn't allow for including auditory feedback in the closed loop system, but the ability of deaf persons to lip-reading can be exploited to analyse some even complex visual feedback. The most complex situation is the polysensorial deficit which has been seen during wars, combining complete blindness and deafness. In this case, only the skin contact can be used as an interface for the patient, not only to control a device, but also to understand the explanations needed for the control procedure.

Mental deficits

There is a great diversity of pathological syndromes and etiological factors, which can be clinically observed. But, two important aspects have to be taken into consideration. Firstly, the ability of the person to understand how to use a substitution or an assistive device. This can be linked to intelligence weakness or deep memory dysfunction, like in Alzheimer disease or in post-coma patients. Secondly, the proper use of the command interface can be altered substantially by some behavioural perturbations or some real incapacity to precisely control a movement selected for monitoring a device. In case of unpredictable behaviour of a psychiatric patient, the crucial problem of safety has to be analysed with great attention in order to avoid physical damage during the inappropriate and possibly dangerous use of a device.

3. Devices for Input and Output for Human-Machine Interaction

This section gives an overview of input and output devices currently used to control mobile robots. With input/output devices the user is able to transfer commands and information to connected devices, the user's physical manipulations are being tracked and physical feedback is being provided representing the results of those manipulations. Generally speaking, input devices constitute the robot's interface to external sources of information, such as active user operation, his/her monitoring system, the environment of the user, or the network. On the other hand, output devices aim at providing the necessary interface for data to be transmitted out of the system, and for prompts generated by the system.

Input and output devices designed to provide interface to users are of particular interest as in many cases robots are used to provide assistance to disabled people. Current technology provides a wide range of input/output devices to cover needs of disabled people, in addition to the devices used for interaction with non-handicapped users.

New technologies can significantly increase the efficiency of user interfaces and thus result in better utilisation of robots used in critical applications such as surgery. In these cases, the optimisation of the user-machine interaction can play a prominent role in improving the quality of the result produced by the use of the robot.

In addition to input/output devices used for interaction between robots and people with no disabilities, this section is also concerned with devices used for enabling disabled people to make efficient use of robots which, in most cases, play an important role in the quality of everyday life.

Diversity in the needs of disabled people call for the design and integration within the robot systems of a variety of input/output devices to better suit the needs of their users.

This section is first giving an overview of input devices paying special attention to devices used by disabled people, whereas the second part discusses output devices including output devices for people with disabilities.

3.1 Input devices

Until now man-machine interfaces have been dominated by input devices such as mouse and keyboard. In recent years, however, great efforts have been made to improve man-machine interaction substantially. For many applications, the additional use of video- and speech-based input could result in significant gain in naturalness, simplicity and effectiveness. New ways of controlling machines including speech, face and gesture recognition are being developed.

The most common ones are: keyboard, mouse, joystick, switch input, head pointing and eye gaze, voice and gesture, touch and myo-electric control.

Joysticks

Joysticks (Figure 3) allow control of several analogue (proportional movement joysticks) and switch (switch type joysticks) functions with one hand e.g. speed, guidance control of the robot etc. A joystick uses mechanical linkages to adjust two variable resistors, one for forward/backward motion and one for side-to-side motion. The change in resistance in each axis is interpreted and translated to x- and y-coordinates. There are also 3-dimensional joysticks that are used for example as a standard input device for driving an omnidirectional wheelchair. However, not all persons are able to operate this kind of joystick. There are people that are able to operate only switches instead of a joystick.

Another type of joystick is the force-reflecting joystick with different degrees of freedom which is used for example by surgeons providing force and tactile feedback.

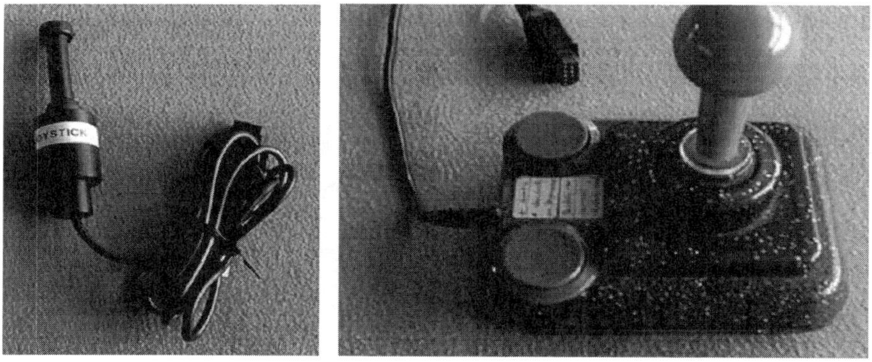

Figure 3. Different types of joysticks

Mice, trackballs and head pointing devices

Besides the conventional hand-operated computer mice, which can be used as input device, there are also available head- and voice-operated devices that can substitute mice in controlling the movement of a pointer on a screen.

Trackballs (Figure 4) can replace the mouse in computer systems where rapid, accurate pointing functions are desired and in environments where a mouse cannot be used due to space limitations, harsh environments, or other factors.

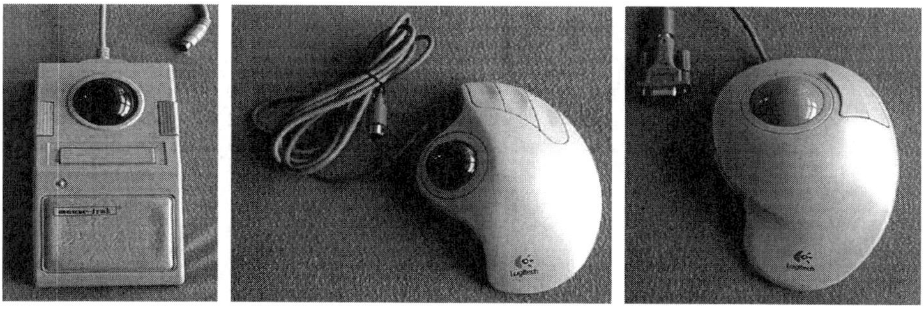

Figure 4. Different types of trackballs

In the head-operated devices the user's head movements are translated into mouse pointer movements. These devices require the user to wear only a small, reflective pad that is stuck to the user's forehead or glasses. This reflects infrared light that is emitted from a device mounted close to the user's computer monitor. The light reflected from the head-mounted pad is used to determine head orientation, from which appropriate signals are generated to emulate a standard serial mouse. Figure 5 shows a type of head-operated device.

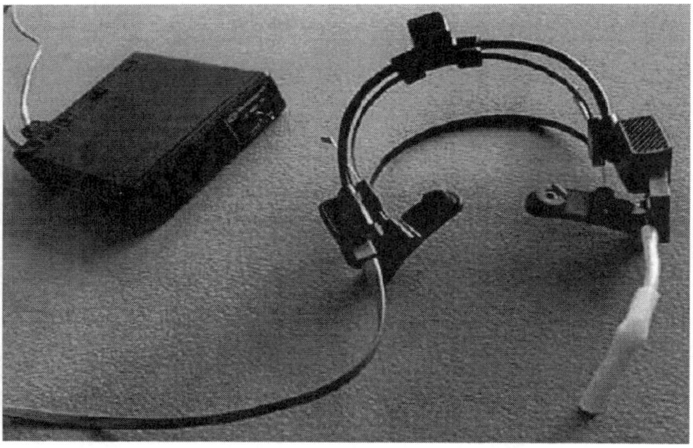

Figure 5. A head-pointing device with a puff switch

Switches and buttons

A wide variety of switches are available. In most cases, a switch is available or can be designed for an area of the body or muscle group where the individual can produce an internal movement or action. Examples of how switches may be activated include pushing small buttons or large plates, sipping and puffing on a tube, wrinkling the eyebrows, blinking an eye or making contact with a metal plate. There are many types of switches available which make it possible for a person with limited or uncontrolled movement to operate a mobility/aid system.

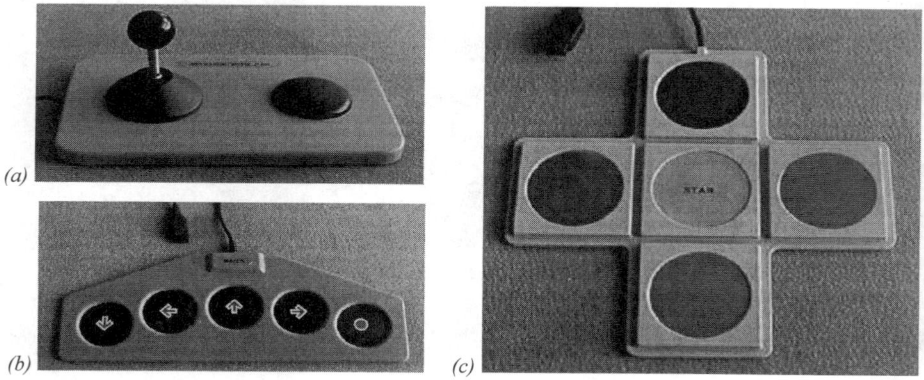

Figure 6 (a-c). Different types of switches: multiple switches

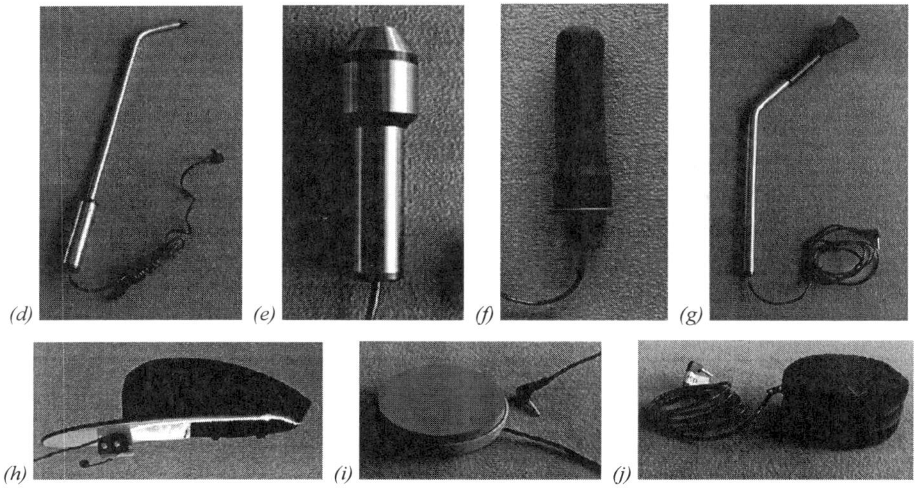

Figure 6 (d-j). Different types of switches: single-/double switch systems

In Figure 6a, one can see a convenient switch for people who can manoeuvre a *joystick*, but need a large one. The joystick has four positions, and pressing the raised pad activates the fifth switch. It is a very rugged switch.

Figures 6b and 6c show *five-buttons systems* with coloured stickers. These large buttons can be operated also by feet.

Figure 6d shows a *sip and puff switch*, which is activated by any small change in air pressure (caused by pursing the lips, moving the tongue, etc.). The user sips or puffs on the mouthpiece, and the change in air pressure is transferred along the tube to a switching unit. This unit activates one switch for sipping, one for puffing.

An extremely sensitive switch, which requires only *skin touch* for activation - no force necessary is shown in Figure 6e. One switch is activated by touching the barrel, and the other by touching the cone at the top.

Figure 6f shows a *grip switch*; the switch in Figure 6g can be operated by *coarse movements*. The switch in Figure 6h is to be operated by an *eyebrow*.

Pressing on the top foam surface activates the switch in Figure 6i. The smooth and soft surface makes this a nice switch for *head or cheek activation*. A light touch on the bellows sends air pressure to the switching unit where the change in pressure activates a switch. For example, the user selects the desired drive code for a wheelchair by activating a light touch switch concealed in the headrest. Tapping makes selection gently with the back of the head.

The *pillow switch* in Figure 6j can be used by persons able to perform only coarse movements.

There are also *capacitive touchplate* systems, which have individual capacitive touch plate channels. The touch plate is operated from the body's capacitance and requires only contact - no pressure. There are many versions available with a variety of positions and sizes to adapt for limited range of motion or force output.

A *mercury switch* is activated depending on different positions of the user's head. Operators are enabled to move a wheelchair merely by tilting the head in space in the desired direction of travel. The degree of head tilt directly controls the speed of the wheelchair similar to a standard hand operated joystick control.

There are also switches available that are being activated by any *muscle movement*, for example by raising the forehead muscles. When any surface in contact with the switch moves, the wafer sends a signal to the switch unit. There are also eye switch devices, which can detect *eye movement* in two directions and generate one or two switch closures as output.

Tongue switches can be operated by tongue, nose, chin, cheek, finger or other movement.

Finger flex switches are switches built into a partial glove. Bending fingers certain degrees activates the switch.

Voice activated switches are switch units with a self-contained microphone. When the microphone detects a sound (such as speech), the switch is activated.

Keyboards

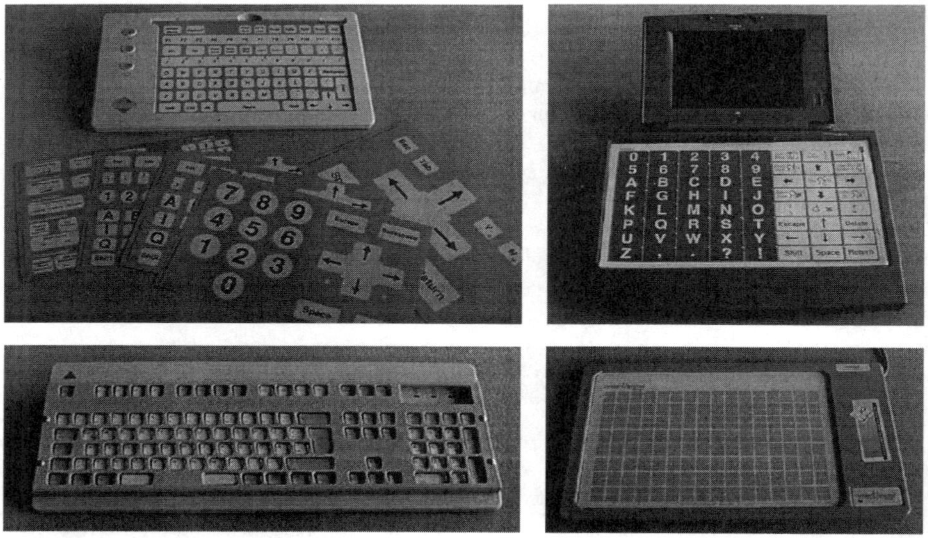

Figure 7. Different types of keyboards

A user can move a robot manually using the arrow keys on the keyboard (Figure 7). Keys can be programmable to store various commands. There are keyboards available with keys that require a very little touch to be activated. Some special keyboards have exchangeable overlays for different applications.

User actions on the keypad can be interpreted by a control unit, which permits sending the corresponding command to the robot as well as recording the action in a logfile. Input adaptations are also used by the visually impaired to improve accuracy and efficiency during data entry. The most frequently used device is the keyboard. Modifications include home key indicators (dimples/dots or felt appliqués) and key replacement (larger, more unique) for the often-used keys.

Touch screens and touch pads

The *touch screen* interface allows direct selection of the desired item displayed or it can be used as a single switch for scanning access. They rely on a pressure or capacity that is applied by pushing on a membrane that lay over the screen (Figure 8a).

In case of direct selection a touch screen is possible. Different scan systems can be used like row-column, linear etc. The scan time and speed can be personalised.

Touch pads (Figure 8b) give the capability to simply glide the finger over the touch pad's surface and gently tap on the pad or click on the buttons to perform all mouse functions.

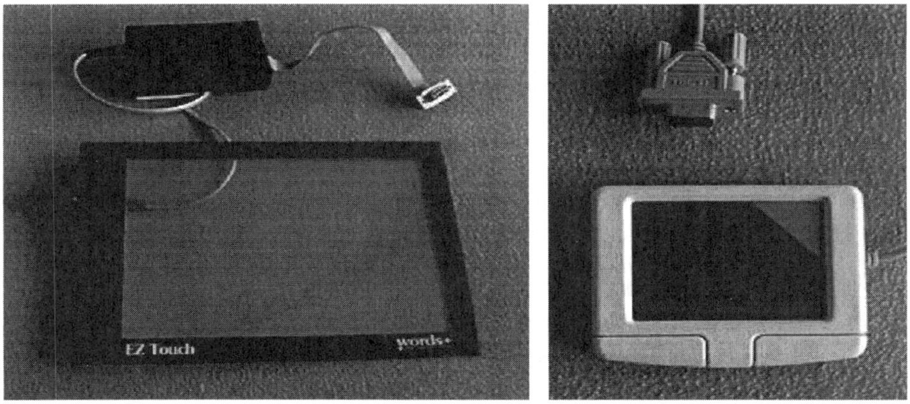

(a) *(b)*

Figure 8. Touch screens (a) and touch pads (b)

Pedals

Foot pedals (Figure 9) can be programmed to emulate keyboard keys (Shift, Control and Alt by default) or mouse-clicks. They eliminate the need for controlling mouse clicks by hand.

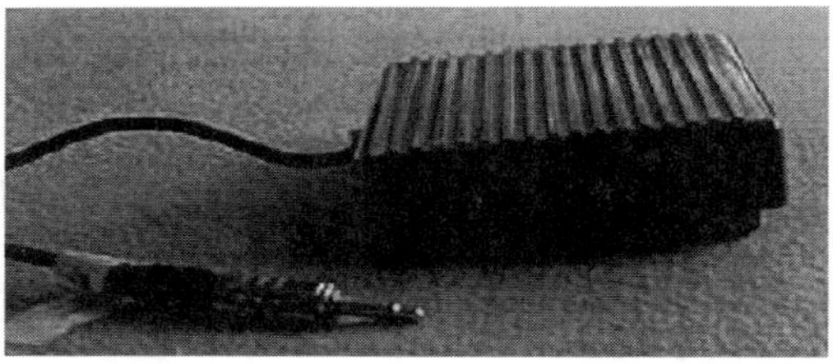

Figure 9. Foot pedal

Datagloves

A "*Dataglove*" is an input device that converts hand gestures and positions into computer-readable form. Sensors mounted on a lightweight lucre glove monitor flexion and extension of the fingers and the position and orientation of the hand. The microprocessor-based control unit acquires data from the Dataglove and transmits it to the host. Dataglove opens up new ways of interacting with computers in robotics and telemanipulation.

Voice and speech recognition input

Using *speech* as main command input enables even the inexperienced human to utilise the service robot. There exist *speech-recognition control systems* that can be used by quadriplegics to control their power wheelchair. A throat microphone picks up the vibrations of the vocal cords when the user speaks the commands. In some cases a headset microphone can also be used. There exist speech recognition devices that have the ability to recognise a number of commands. The main interface element of the device is an automatic speech recognition module. The module is capable of recording and interpreting user commands and provides the required control signals for the target device control systems. The system understands basic commands such as start, stop, etc. There is a panic override system (hand or blow/suck device operated) in case of any undesirable action resulting from incorrect command interpretation.

Speech-recognition system can be used by micro-surgeons in operating rooms, to control the movements of their surgical microscopes by giving voice commands.

Ultrasonic head control

The user operates by tilting his/her head forward or backward, left or right - movements analogous to the manipulation of a joystick. The electronic control signals generated from the calculated head position mimic are similar to those produced by a joystick. The signals can be used to operate a variety of devices including an electric wheelchair, a communication aid, or a robotic arm. This type of input is used by high level quadriplegics who can still move voluntarily only their head and neck muscles.

Two transducers generate inaudible high-frequency sound waves that propagate through the air toward the user's head. Energy reflected by the head is detected upon its return to the transducers. The distance from each transducer to the head is calculated from the elapsed time between transmission of the sound and the reception of the echo. Ranging measurements from both transducers allow the two-dimensional determination of the user's head position.

3.2 Output Devices

Speech output or a graphical display can be used as *output options* to guide the user through the different procedures or option menus. Tactile output is an alternative method of output, which utilises the tactual sense of the user.

LCD output devices

The Liquid Crystal Display (LCD) output devices provide visual display of text or graphics. Dynamic information from/about the system (like speed or battery power of the wheelchair) and diagnostic readouts are displayed on the screen.

There is also an option available of a scanning LCD device, so that patients who can only utilise certain devices (e.g blow/suck device) for control will be able to use the system. They are flat, consume low power, lightweight devices, therefore they are the first choice for portable applications.

Speech synthesisers

Voice output through the use of synthetic speech module using a speakerphone can provide feedback to the user and dynamic information from/about the system (like speed or battery power of the wheelchair). Different voices (e.g. male and female voices or different speakers) can be used in analogy to the use of highlighting or colour on visual displays to highlight similar features as these do. The speed of the speech and the character of the voice can be personally adapted.

Tactile devices

Tactile output is an alternative method of presentation that utilises the tactual sense of the user. Tactile displays may be divided in two classes: the so-called softcopy displays, and hard-copy displays. Soft copy means that the tactile stimulus is temporary, whereas in hardcopy the stimulus is made permanent, usually as a raised pattern on paper. Tactile displays are normally perceived with the fingertips, but other parts of the body, such as the skin of the back have been used.

4. Models of Human-Machine Interaction

In this section the background to the adaptive Human Machine Interfaces (HMI) is described in terms of Human Supervisory Control [36]. The focus of much Human Supervisory Control research has been to optimise the performance of aircraft and pilots [26]. However the principles used to analyse human machine interaction are also useful in developing assistive technology. Of most importance are the ways that tasks can be decomposed into sub-tasks and then shared between humans and machines.

4.1 Principle Ways of Interaction

Supervisory control

The definition of a supervisory controller as provided by Sheridan [36] is one in which "one or more human operators are intermittently programming and continually receiving information from a computer system which itself closes an autonomous control loop through artificial effectors and sensors to the controller process or task environment". This definition is very broad covering systems as different as chemical plants and robots on the surface of Mars. For the purpose of this discussion Sheridan's definition may be restricted to a human-machine system in which a single user and a single machine are involved in a closely coupled feedback loop. Interaction with the environment is achieved directly and/or via the Human-Machine Interface (HMI) as shown in Figure 10. The controller supports the user in completing their task and provides updates to the user on the state of the environment.

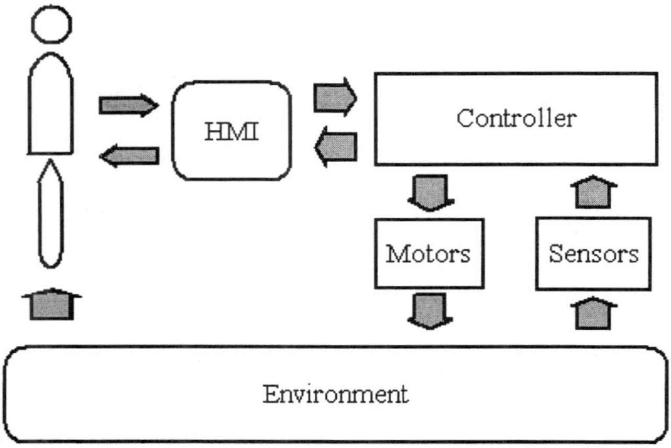

Figure 10. Schematic of the Role of the Human-Machine Interface (HMI)

A supervisory controller could be compared to the corporate structure [35]. The directors (*the operator)* determine the company goals and delegate these goals to their subordinates (*the controller)*. The nature of this delegation can be by way of general targets to subordinates who are quite autonomous as to how they achieve them, or the directors may provide detailed instructions and may also undertake some of the work themselves. In a supervisory controller multiple levels of control exist, resulting in multiple nested control loops [18]. Thus even within a single user system multiple interacting control loops are likely.

The role of a controller in a Human-Machine system is to extend human performance or to reduce the physical or cognitive load on the user. The controller may perform some function beyond the user's capability or may act as a backup in case the user makes a mistake. The way in which tasks or sub-tasks are delegated within the controller can be described using concepts of *Traded Control* and *Shared Control.* They can be used to distinguish between the situations where a system is under the direct control of the user, completely autonomous or controlled by a combination of automatic control and human input.

Let us say that the primary output of the system is the heading of a car. In *traded control* the heading is completely determined by driver input or, when cruise control is turned on, by the automatic controller. No combination of the two is ever used to determine the heading. In *shared control* the driver would set some of the control variables and would have influence over at least some of the remainder but would not have direct control over the heading.

Adaptive interfaces in human-machine systems

Human-Machine systems are expected to work in a wide variety of situations. Often the human is required to control the adaptation to new conditions by modifying control parameters or by changing the system goals. Much of the previous research into machine adaptation uses measures such as the operator performance [37] or environmental conditions [34] to drive the adaptation scheme. The aim of such systems is to optimise the overall performance of the human-machine system in some quantifiable way, often ignoring the effects of these changes on the operator.

Another approach to adaptation is to aim to maintain the cognitive load at the optimum level according to a psychological model of human performance under stress [17]. At the heart of such methods is the user model that attempts to measure the cognitive load quantitatively, in real time and measure the benefit of adaptation against a quantifiable performance measure.

Adaptation can be achieved by allocating tasks automatically between the user and the operator on the basis of overall system performance [27]. For example the NavBelt guidance system for the blind [37] had two control modes, a guidance mode and an image mode. The guidance mode gives the user acoustic signals to indicate the safe path in a cluttered environment. The image mode presents a stereo image of the distance to objects. Adaptation between the modes is achieved by measuring the information throughput of the human-machine system.

A shared controller can be modelled by an expert system [27, 4]. The study by Aretz *et. al.* [4] investigated the provision of automated support for fighter pilots performing defensive manoeuvres. The system provided fixed and adaptive levels of assistance. Interestingly, no quantifiable performance improvement was measurable between the two. Users while using the adaptive system reported lower cognitive loads. This was countered by a preference for fixed rather than adaptive assistance. The work by Morris *et. al.* [27] showed that overall performance was better with an automatic aid but subjects preferred the manual aid. Recent work by Horvitz *et. al.* [20] have demonstrated a working expert system to provide assistance to users of Excel. While the aim is to improve user performance currently no results are available verifying that this is the case.

Human-machine control architectures

In human supervisory control the overall architecture of the system is of critical importance. Adaptability can be achieved but at the cost of having a complex system. The way in which the various sub-systems inter-operate can have a significant bearing on the tractability of a problem. Early manual control theory developed models of human-machine interaction for the automotive and aerospace industries. With the advent of electronics these models were expanded to cover the entire human-machine system. Early models, such as McRuer's crossover model [26], were subsequently extended by Optimal Control Theory. Filters such as the Kalman Filter estimate the current state and thus the optimal decision can be made [22]. Human-Computer Interface (HCI) models are mainly used to evaluate the ergonomics of the keyboard and pointing devices [15, 9]. However, Rasmussen in [32] describes a more general three layer model (Figure 11), which is based on knowledge based activities, rule based activities and skill based activities.

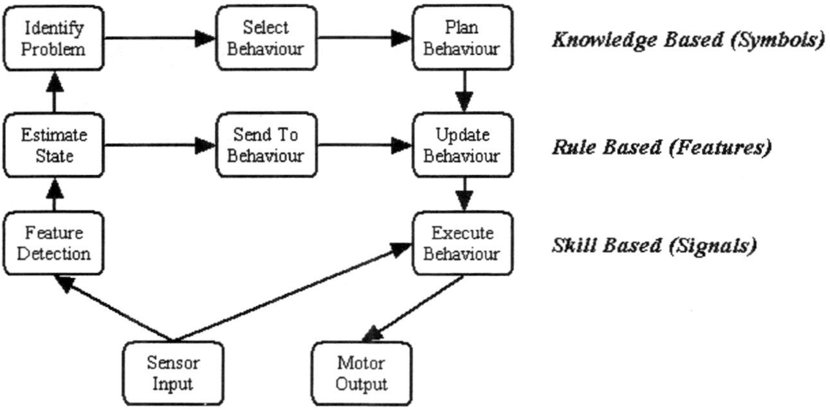

Figure 11. An abbreviated version of Rasmussen's Model (after Sheridan)

Albus [1] describes a more complex multi-layer architecture, NASREM, for robot control in which the operator interface is a central part. This has been applied in tele-operator interfaces [2]. Bonasso *et. al.* [7] propose a three tiered architecture, 3T, similar to Rasmussen, which incorporates variable autonomy. The level of autonomy is attached to the context of the current task being executed. The layers represent skills, the sequencing of skills and a deliberative layer that performs planning.

Layered approaches are common in robotics architectures. Brooks in [8] proposed a multi-layered system of task achieving behaviours. This celebrated paradigm has achieved some success in creating complex autonomous systems [10, 19, 25]. This paradigm avoids complex internal representations thus exhaustive trial and error is required to find the set of sensor features that can be directly coupled to actions. However if the environment is changed such that one of these features is altered, such as changing the colour of the carpet [19], then the behaviours fail.

Behaviour based systems have difficulty adapting to new situations because of the fixed priorities between behaviours. Several approaches have been suggested to provide flexibility: Kosecka and Bajcsy [23] used the supervisory control theory of Ramadge and Wonham [31] to control mobile robots, the desired behaviour is specified in Discrete Event Systems (DES) syntax, these are then synthesised with the system capabilities to form *controllable desired behaviours* which are then executed. Crowley [11] proposes a hybrid approach that provides flexible sensing by the use of the VAP architecture where vision algorithms are selected based on their performance on the current task.

4.2 Context Aware User Interfaces

The need to control a wide variety of devices in the user's environment is in tension with the desire to provide a simple and coherent interface. Associated problems arise when users make erroneous inputs causing devices, such as wheelchairs, to produce erratic behaviour. A possible solution to both of these problems can be found by making the computer system aware of the context of the interaction. This mechanism can be demonstrated with the following simple example: The user is driving a wheelchair fitted with a context aware user interface; it has a single switch that the user uses to turn lights on and off. As he drives into his/her kitchen the switch input is directed to the lights in kitchen, likewise in the bedroom the switch input is directed to the bedroom lights. The context in this instance is the user's position in the house and it is used to re-map the destination of the user input.

This simple example demonstrates how position can be used to re-map the destination of a switch input. The functionality described could be implemented using a simple line of sight communications medium such as infrared. However if we extend this example by having several different lights in the room we need to add more context information. For example the user's preference for bright lights in the kitchen during meal times but background lighting in the late evening. Now user preferences and the time of day have become part of the context used to re-map the user input.

When the context used to define a user input is sufficiently rich we can then begin to identify unusual or out of context inputs. For example during daylight hours the user very rarely uses the lights in the kitchen – if his/her light switch is activated during this time it can be highlighted as an unusual occurrence possibly indicating that he needs assistance. Again user preferences can be used to determine the nature of the response, if he is nervous about fainting the response could be to initiate a call for help, alternatively it could simply be ignored as an erroneous input.

Just as the tension exists between the need to provide a simple interface to many devices in a smart home through the use of context sensitivity there is also a need for consistency. Context aware applications have the ability to alter their functionality based on erroneous sensor data or for spurious reasons. Probabilistic or Fuzzy methods can be used to control the sensitivity of an interface to uncertain sensor data. However, context aware applications require flexibility in their design to allow users and carers to customise their functionality performance to user preferences and needs.

5. Guidelines and Selection Criteria for HMI

The design, selection or adaptation of a human-machine interface is a complex task. Especially in rehabilitation robotics where the robot is used as a "personal robot" it is individual:

- with respect to the user who has individual abilities, disabilities and needs,
- with respect to the robot which may have a programmable functionality,
- with respect to the task to be supported in the specific environment of the user.

5.1 The Process of Designing an Individual HMI

The task of designing an individual HMI consists of several problems:

- the assessment and training of user's abilities
- the selection and adaptation of HMI operation methods and strategies
- the selection and adaptation of HMI devices
- the selection and programming of the robot's functionality
- the restriction, preparation, and structuring of the task execution and the environment.

Within the HMI design process a common solution to these problems has to be found. Unfortunately there is no linear sequence to solve the problems one after the other. Each "solution" of one problem can influence the other four problems. Therefore an iterative approach, starting with the assessment of the user's capabilities, is necessary. It has been observed that the outcome of such a process is more successful when it has been undertaken by a multi-disciplinary team consisting of professionals with specialist expertise in particular aspects of medical rehabilitation and the related technology.

5.2 Guidelines for the Assessment of Users' Capabilities

The goal of assessment is to objectively estimate the physical, mental, and sensory abilities of a person in order to optimally use them as command or feed-back for control of the robot. The quality of assessment of the physiological potential is of prime importance to designing suitable human-machine interfaces.

The remaining motor activity

The remaining motor activity has to be evaluated in terms of amplitude and direction of movement, force intensity, and power. This leads to the identification of the different available degrees of freedom and to the determination of their usability. Appropriate measuring instruments are based on the use of force sensors, accelerometers or goniometers, giving directly quantitative evaluation of the relevant parameters.

Computerised optoelectronic systems for 3D movement analysis of moving body segments constitutes a powerful means for assessing human mobility. They can be used for assessing the various physiological means for control of devices previously presented:

- *head movements*
  flexion-extension, horizontal rotation, lateral flexion
- *eye movement*
  vertical and horizontal scanning
- *upper limb movements*
  shoulder movements (up and down, forwards-backwards)
  elbow-forearm movements (flexion and extension)
  wrist movements (wrist dorsal and ventral flexion, pronation and suppination, etc.)
  grasping ability (two finger pinch, lateral or palmar grasp)
  combined activation of upper limb joints (hand push-pull effect)
- *lower limb movements*
  knee abduction adduction (frontal plane)
  foot plantar and dorsal flexion (vertical plane)
  combined activation of hip, knee and ankle joints (foot push-pull effect)

The remaining sensory inputs

The remaining sensory inputs can be assessed by using specific sensors and testing procedures and equipment:

- *vision*
  visual acuity (keenness of sight)
  visual field
  chromatopsy
  stereoscopy
- *hearing*
  audiometry
  binaural hearing
- *touch*
  cutaneous spatial resolution
  perception threshold
  thermal sensitivity

Other remaining physiological functions

Specific measuring systems are available to quantitatively evaluate:

- *breathing*
  inspiration and expiration flow and pressure
- *voice*
  phoneme identification
  sound intensity
  voice resolution, frequency
- *muscle function*
  muscle electrical activity (EMG)
- *reaction*
  reaction time

The patient's mental status

The user's mental capacity can be evaluated from appropriated tests regarding:

- cognition
- learning
- memory

5.3 Matching of User Capabilities, System Functionality and Application Constraints

After or in parallel to the assessment of the user's abilities, a pre-selection of potential input/ output devices can be made. The remaining functional capabilities of a disabled user have to be classified according to their practical usefulness and their controllability. The technical requirements of a HMI have to be defined taking into consideration:

- the efficiency of the selected mode of activation in the various conditions of use,
- the comfort of the user in terms of physical and/or mental fatigue, to avoid the rejection of the control procedure,
- the patient safety, by evaluating the potential risk in using given control device.

There exist well elaborated procedures to do this in a systematic way, e.g. in [3, 28] for alternative computer access or more general in [24] for assistive devices. However, special procedures for HMI devices for rehabilitation robots do not exist so far.

It should be noted that neither the user's capabilities, nor the system's functionality, nor the constraints given by the environment and application are static factors:

- The user may increase his/her abilities by training and by practical experience, or the capabilities may decrease due to a progressive disease.
- The system's functionality may be definable. Some robot systems provide the possibility to modify, to enhance, or to restrict their functionality via programmable functions.
- The application environment may change at all. Or it may be modified (structured) by purpose in order to simplify the application task.
- The application task may be widened or modified.

This implies that there is no static optimal configuration of the HMI. The HMI of the robot should be updated from time to time

6. Conclusions

The large variety of disabilities and the diversity in the needs of disabled people call for the design and integration of a variety of input / output devices within the robot systems to better suit the needs of their users.

Different segmental motor actions can be used for commanding and controlling an assistive device, for example hand, lower limb, head, eye and tongue movements. There is also the possibility of voice and puff control, or of capturing physiological signals generated by different organs and using them as command signals.

Sensory feedback is also necessary for an efficient way of controlling a device, allowing real time regulation. Three main sensory inputs are concerned: visual, tactile and auditory inputs.

Different input devices (keyboard, mouse, joystick, switches, head pointing and eye gaze, voice and gesture, touch and myoelectric control) and output devices (graphical displays, tactile and speech output) exist which enable people to make efficient use of robots, depending on their abilities.

For any alteration of physiological outputs or inputs the command interface must adapt using the remaining capabilities of impaired functions.

The models of human-machine interaction are not yet systematic. Detailed guidelines and selection criteria for human-machine interfacing have to be developed. The quality of assessment of the physiological potential is of prime importance to design suitable human-machine interfaces. The remaining functional capabilities of a disabled person have to be classified according to their practical usefulness and their controllability and there has to be a matching of user capabilities, system functionality and application requirements/constraints.

7. References

[1] Albus J. S., "An Engineering Architecture for Intelligent Systems", *Proceedings of the AAAI Fall Symposium*, November 1996, AAAI Press, MIT.

[2] Albus J. S., McCain H. G., Lumia R., "NASA/NBS Standard Reference Model for Telerobot Control System Architecture (NASREM)", National Institute for Standards and Technology, NISTTN 1235, 1989, Gaithersburg, MD, USA.

[3] Anson D. K., "Alternative Computer Access – A Guide to Selection", F. A. Davis Company, Philadelphia, 1997.

[4] Aretz A. J., Hickox J. C., Kesler S. R., "Dynamic Function Allocation in Fighter Cockpits", *Proceedings of the Human Factors Society 31st Annual Meeting*, 1987, pp. 414-418.

[5] Ashby P., D. McCrea A., "Neurophysiology of spinal spasticity", R.A. Davidoff (ed.), Handbook of the spinal cord, Vol.4/5, New York 1987, Dekker Marcel, pp. 119-143.

[6] Bach-y-Rita P. et al., "Form perception with a 49-point electrotactile stimulus array on the tongue", *J. Rehab. Res. & Dev.*, Vol. 35, No. 4, October 1998, pp. 427-430.

[7] Bonasso R. Peter, Kortenkamp D., Whitney T., "Using a Robot Control Architecture to Automate Space Shuttle Operations", *9th Conference on Innovative Applications of AI (IAAI97)*, July 1997.

[8] Brooks R. A., "A Robust Layered Control System for a Mobile Robot", *IEEE transactions on Robotics and Automation*, Vol. 2, April 1986.

[9] Card, Newell, Moran, "The Psychology of Human Computer Interaction", Lawrence Erlbaum Associates, 1983.

[10] Connell J., "A Colony Architecture for an Artificial Creature", PhD Thesis, MIT, August 1989, also as MIT AI Lab Technical Report AITR-1151.

[11] Crowley J. L., "Integration and Control of Reactive Visual Processes", *Robotics and Autonomous Systems*, 1995, Vol. 16, pp.17-27.

[12] De Luca C. J., "The use of surface EMG in biomechanics", *Journal of Applied Biomechanics*, May 1997, Vol. 13, No. 2.

[13] Edin B. B., "Strain-sensitive mechanoreceptors in the human skin provide kinaesthetic information", O. Frannzen, R. S. Johansson, L. Terenius (eds.), Somesthesis and the Neurobiology of the Somatosensory Cortex, Birkhäuser Verlag AG, Basel, 1996, pp. 283-294.

[14] Findley L., Capildeo R., "Movement disorders: tremor", Oxford, Oxford University Press, 1984.

[15] Fitts P. M., "The information capacity of the human motor system in controlling the amplitude of movement", *Journal of Experimental Psychology*, 1954, Vol. 47, pp. 381-391.

[16] Gips J., Olivieri C. P., Tecce J. J., "Direct control of the computer through electrodes placed around the eyes", Smith M. J. and Salvendy G. (eds.), Human-Computer Interaction: Applications and Case Studies, *Fifth International Conference on Human Computer Interaction*, Orlando, FL, August 1993, Elsevier, 1993, pp. 630-635.

[17] Hancock P. A., Chignell M. H., "Mental Workload Dynamics in Adaptive Interface Design", *IEEE Transactions on Systems, Man and Cybernetics*, July 1988, Vol. 18, No. 4, pp. 647-658.

[18] Hess R., Nally Mc B.D., "Automation Effects in Multi-Loop Control System", *IEEE Transactions on Systems, Man and Cybernetics*, 1986, Vol. 16, No. 1, pp. 111-121.

[19] Horswill I., "Specialization of Perceptual Processes", Phd Thesis, MIT, 1994, also as MIT AI lab Tech Report AITR-1511.

[20] Horvitz E., J. Breese, Heckerman D., Hovel D., Rommelse K., "The Lumiere Project: Bayesian User Modelling for Inferring the Goals and needs of Software Users", *Proceedings of the 14th Conference on Uncertainty in AI*, July 1998, Morgan Kaufmann, Madison, WI, pp. 256-265.

[21] Jacob R. L. K., "What you look at is what you get", *Computer*, July 1993, pp.65-66.

[22] Kleinman D. L., Baron S., Levison W.H., "An optimal control model of human response", *Automatica*, 1970, Vol. 6, No. 3, pp. 357-369.

[23] Kousecka J., Bajscy R., "Discrete Event Systems for Autonomous Mobile Agents", *Robotic and Autonomous Systems*, 1994, Vol. 12, No. 3-4, pp. 187-189.

[24] Lee K. S., Thomas D. J., *Control of Computer-Based Technology for People with Physical Disabilities – An Assessment Manual,* University of Toronto Press, 1990.

[25] Mataric M. J., "Interaction and Intelligent Behavior", *PhD Thesis*, MIT, August 1994, also as MIT AI lab tech report AITR-1495.

[26] McRuer D. T., "Human dynamics in man machine systems", *Automatica*, May 1980, Vol. 16, No. 3, pp.237-253.

[27] Morris N. M., Rouse W. B., Ward Sh. L., "Studies of Dynamic Task Allocation in an Aerial Search Environment", *IEEE Transactions on Systems, Man and Cybernetics*, May 1988, Vol. 18, No. 3, pp. 376-389.

[28] Nordic ,*Guidelines for Computer Accessibility,* Nordic Cooperation on Disability, Vällingby, 1998.

[29] Penny J. B., Young A. B., "Huntington's Disease", Jankovic and Tolosa (eds.), *Parkinson's Disease and Movement Disorders,* Williams & Wilkins, 1993.

[30] Rabischong P., "Anatomical substrate of motion and vision", *6th Advanced course of the European Society of Neuroradiology, Functional Neuroanantomy of Motion and Vision,* Scotti G., Le Bihan D. (eds.), Milan September 18th 1996, pp. 9-23.

[31] Ramadage P. J., Wonham W. M., "The Control of Discrete Event Systems", *Proceedings of the IEEE,* January 1989, Vol. 1, No. 77, pp. 81-97.

[32] Rasmussen J., Pejtersen A. M., Goodstein L. P., *Cognitive Systems Engineering,* John Wiley & Sons, 1994.

[33] Ross D., "Personal freedom: a wearable interactive universal access device", *Proceedings of the 19th Annual RESNA Conference*; 1996, Salt Lake City, UT. Washington, DC: RESNA Press, 450-2.

[34] Rubin K. S., Jones P. M., Mitchell Ch. M., Mspert O.F., "Inference of Operator Intentions in Supervisory Control Using a Blackboard Architecture", *IEEE Transactions on Systems Man and Cybernetics*, July 1988, Vol. 18, No. 4, pp. 618-637.

[35] Sheridan T. B., "Task Allocation and Supervisory Control", *Handbook of Human Computer Interaction,* Helander M. (ed.), North-Holland, 1988, pp.159-173.

[36] Sheridan T. B. Telerobotics, *Automation and Human Supervisory Control,* The MIT Press, 1992.

[37] Shoval S., Borenstein J., Koren Y., "Mobile Robot Obstacle Avoidance in a Computerized Travel Aid for the Blind", *Proceedings IEEE Robotics and Automation Conference*, May 1994, San Diego, California.

[38] Slack M., Berbrayer D., "Myoelectrically Controlled Wrist-Hand Orthosis for Brachial Plexus, Injury: A Case Study", *J. Prosth. and Orth.*, 1991, Vol. 4, No. 3, pp. 171-174.

[39] Winters J. M., Peles J. D., Osterbauer P. J., Derickson K., Deboer K. F., Fuhr A. W., "Three-Dimensional Head Axis of Rotation During Tracking Movements: A Tool for Assessing Neck Neuromechanical Function", *Spine,* 1993, Vol. 18, pp. 1178-1185.

Chapter 4

Mobile Robotics and Automation in Healthcare and Rehabilitation

by Nikos KATEVAS, William HARWIN, Helmut HECK, Marie Jose ALDON, Ulrich BORGOLTE, Gerard LACEY, Edouard PERUCHON, Adriana PRENTZA, John KONTOULIS

Mobile Robotics in Healthcare
N. Katevas (Ed.)
IOS Press, 2001

Chapter 4

Mobile Robotics and Automation in Healthcare and Rehabilitation

Nikos KATEVAS, William HARWIN, Helmut HECK, Marie Jose ALDON, Ulrich BORGOLTE, Gerard LACEY, Edouard PERUCHON, Adriana PRENTZA, John KONTOULIS

1. Introduction

Levels of automation can vary from simple control systems such as patient hoists, to complex, multiaxis robots. In this chapter we outline social and technical issues that relate to automation in hospital and home healthcare services and highlight examples in a wide range of applications ranging from portering services in a hospital to manipulation assistance for people with motor impairments.

There is a strong potential for automation and technology assistance for people requiring healthcare assistance, either in a home or hospital environment. This chapter outlines some possible areas where work is ongoing in seeking out the best technological solutions to the specific problems that are encountered in this non-industrial environment. It is argued that the provision of technology into these situations is difficult, not because the technology is not beneficial or cost effective, but because the purchasers are conservative, the demands complex and the benefit can only be measured by considering long term savings, something that healthcare provision does not cater for particularly well. Thus for example, mechanisms to transport people and goods safely around a hospital will have long term cost savings when considered as a means to increase efficiency of goods delivery, but will require a concerted effort by healthcare leaders to be realised. For success it will be important that the provision of such a service is fully integrated into a functional hospital information technology system so that progress of goods can be monitored by the users, and help is given to the patients and staff. There is a considerable danger that such systems are either seen as a sop for providing high quality information electronically such as medical records, or that it is seen as unnecessary because in light of advanced IT provision, an impractical philosophy where food delivery is concerned. Consideration of full integration of IT within a hospital environment is discussed in the final section of this chapter on intelligent buildings.

In addition to portering and transport applications we consider applications in the delivery of direct healthcare services such as the growing use of robots to assist in surgical procedures, and the emergence of possible robot assistance in the delivery of physiotherapy services. We also consider the use of mobile robot technology for assisting people with motor disabilities, as well as the provision of telemanipulatior and telerobotic assistance for people with manipulation difficulties. Although the application areas for automation in healthcare is broad, there are often social and technical similarities. The purchaser of the technology is often not the final user. The technology may have multiple users each needing to access the services at different levels. There is a strong need for fast maintenance, good technical support, and comprehensive training.

2. Robotic Assistance for Hospital Fetch and Carry Services

There is a great potential to automate the process of hospital deliveries. As described in chapter 2, transportation tasks in hospitals concern a large variety of needs, from heavy loads of clean or dirty linen to light sets of drugs or sterilized instruments. Most "semi-automated" existing systems (not semi-autonomous systems), which operate today in indoor environments, are located by using a network of wires buried in the floor or another similar technique. Other possible solutions are to install dedicated delivery mechanisms such as vacuum tubes or tracks in an interstitial floor. These solutions limit the size of goods that can be carried and affect the flexibility of the delivery system, for example it is not possible to carry blood products in vacuum tubes because of the complexity of dealing with the biological hazard should the container break in transit.

Thus, over the last decade, an alternative approach based on the autonomous robots has been developed. Two mobile robots systems for fetch and carry tasks in hospitals are discussed as well as a tracked aerial delivery system. HelpMate designed and built by TRC (now Helpmate Robotics, Danburry, CT, USA), FIRST developed by a French consortium including ITMI/APTOR (Grenoble) and the LIRMM (Montpellier). Aerial is a concept that emerged from the ARIADNE project at the University of Reading.

2.1 HelpMate

Helpmate is an autonomous transport system designed for healthcare environments e.g. hospitals [8]. The robot is designed for hospital environment and is equipped with ultrasonic sensors, a vision system and an internal map of the environment for navigation.

The HelpMate robot addresses issues of flexibility and allows transportation of materials like X-rays, medical specimens, equipment, meals etc., however its limitations include the cost and the operating speed. On the other hand HelpMare can negotiate with elevators, and therefore change floors, needs no track to be installed in the facility, and operates through an easy to use user interface.

Much of the cost of the HelpMate is due to the high level of processing and sensing required by the robot to allow it to navigate in cluttered environments. The slow speed is necessary for reasons of safety and in addition the robot has to contend with occasions where an emergency medical team need to travel along the corridors at high speed, or when hospital visitors try to block a passing robot. Several solutions are provided to the above mentioned problems either technical or managerial (e.g. the robot is not allowed to operate in medical emergency routes). However, the cost factor still remains and leads the enterprises commercialising it to select a hiring policy to interested customers. This policy makes the overall operation of Helpmate cost-effective and therefore quite attractive. Developed in the USA by TRC Inc. was the first commercially available device in the sector. It has established a user base of about 80 hospitals worldwide. Helpmate was initially manufactured and commercialised by TRC Inc. in early 90s and later on by Helpmate Inc. in the USA. Some years later it was commercially available by OTIS, also in Europe, and lately has moved to Pyxis Corporation.

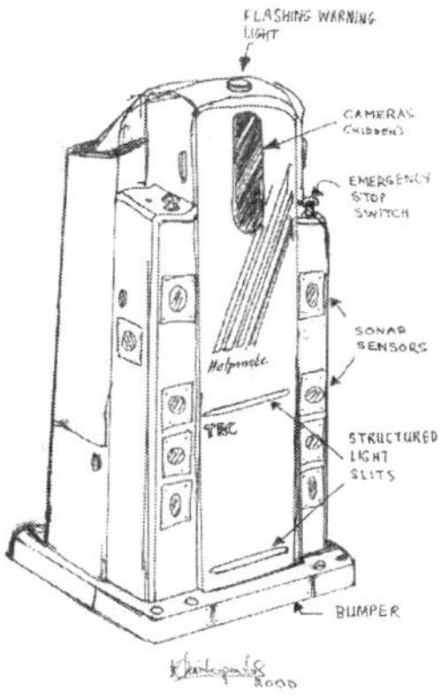

2.2 FIRST - Transport Robot in Hospital Environments

FIRST is a prototype of a self guided robot designed to transport and handle heavy trolleys containing meal trays, linen, drugs or waste weighing up to 300 kg [1]. It is able to navigate autonomously within a hospital environment, without external guide tracks. It has to load or unload trolleys, to carry them between different hospital departments, running along more or less narrow hallways, and using standard lifts. A learning system allows an off-line acquisition of a network of simple standard trajectories that connect a set of predefined stations. The robot stores the paths followed, and also undergoes a training phase. The path followed is instantaneously modified if an obstacle is present, as it possesses obstacle avoidance algorithms. The loading/unloading and the entry to the elevator are performed in a completely automated manner. The key to navigation is an efficient perception and localization system able to provide on-line the path-planner with data necessary to plan an accurate and collision free trajectory.

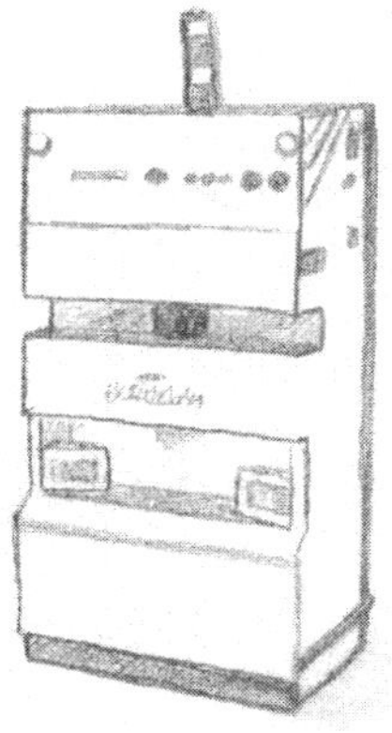

2.3 Aerial Delivery Pod Concept

A solution that reduces the complexity of the robot hardware, and the level of sensing requirements and increases the speed of delivery is to move the robots out of the human environment, for example a track based system that could be installed in interstitial floors or be suspended in unused corridor ceiling spaces. Although similar to the vacuum tube mechanism used in some hospitals, it differs in several important ways. Of particular importance is that unlike a vacuum system, the pod can control and monitor its acceleration and is sufficiently accessible to allow safe, rapid, and reliable delivery of fragile materials or materials that may be a biohazard. Also a vacuum tube system has limited intelligence as to the destination or priority of goods. A high speed delivery system can use autonomous and independent pods on an aerial track and is shown in figure 1. The algorithms for path navigation developed [13] so as to allow rapid and fault tolerant goods delivery with the ability to track progress through the delivery network are available.

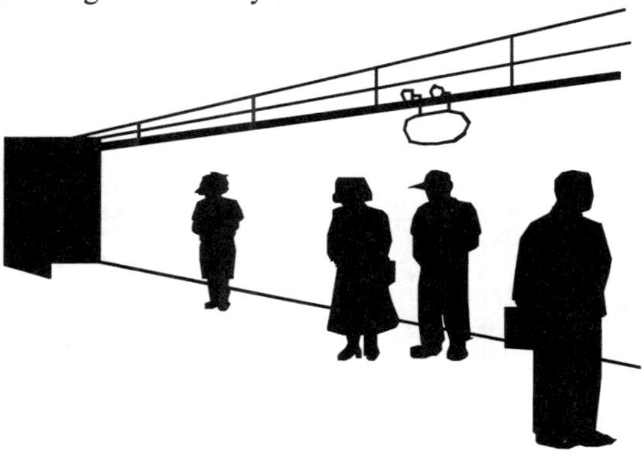

Figure 1. Concept of aerial delivery pod system

3. Robotic Assistance in Surgical Procedures

Although not central to the focus of this book, there is a growing interest in automation and robotics to assist surgical procedures. Studies for robotic surgery started slowly fifteen years ago, but today the new technologies offer powerful solutions for surgical procedures requiring careful planing and accurate execution. Some industrial systems are currently under clinical evaluation in hospitals.

Many medical or surgical interventions requiring minimal-access, precision or repeatability can take advantage of robotics and computer assistance [5]. For instance, the use of a robot and/or an appropriate guidance system make feasible:

- repetitive data acquisition tasks [20] or execution of a predefined operative strategy,
- complex surgery on difficult to reach organs or for which a human operator would have poor or no visibility,
- accurate positioning and fixing of surgical tools, such as probes (microsurgery).

Future possibilities in surgery include scaling large movements of the surgeon into small movements of the robot and the ability to increase the dexterity of the surgeon in minimal invasive surgery.

Computer Assisted Interventions include three phases:

- The *perception*, which uses standard medical imaging devices (radiology, echography, MRI, etc), as well as nonstandard sensors (Doppler effect, pressure or tactile sensors). Image processing and multidata matching are used to model data in a common reference frame.
- The *decision*, which aims to define an optimal operative strategy based on the interpretation of the available sensor data,
- The *action*, which consists in performing the intervention with a guiding system.

Robot devices for assisting surgeries can likewise be classified into three categories:

1. *passive systems*, providing the human operator with numerical and graphical data in order to make feasible an on-line comparison between the simulation of the task and its actual execution (e.g. visual feedback on the position of a tool on pre-operative images),
2. *semi-active systems*, constraining physically the action to follow a predefined strategy. The final control depends on the human operator (e.g. laser-guided alignment for spine surgery, stereotactic neurosurgery using a mechanical guide, passive arm with mechanical constraints with a fixed point developed for laparoscopy),
3. *active systems* make use of an autonomous robot supervised by the operator and controlled by redundant sensors (e.g. ROBODOC currently used in trials on humans for automated implant of hip prosthesis, HIPPOCRATE, a position and force controlled manipulator for 3D echography of arteries [1], and teleoperated robots used for microsurgery).

The use of robots in surgical applications has economical and safety [7] implications which must be taken into consideration during system design.

4. Robotic Assistance in Physiotherapy

An emerging area for healthcare robots is to assist in the process of providing physiotherapy. Thus for example, cerebral vascular accidents or stroke are a leading cause of disability with a prevalence of about 140 per 10,000 of the population. The associated incidence is approximately 20 per 10,000 per year with two thirds of incidence in people over 65 years of age. Early intervention and intensive therapy improves the outcome of people recovering from a stroke and if therapies can be machine delivered they can both improve the intensity of the therapy thereby effecting the outcome, or reduce the level of physiotherapist intervention thereby saving direct healthcare costs.

For people with upper limb hemiplegia it is possible to consider both unilateral and bilateral therapies where intelligent assistance from a robot is able to provide varying degrees of compensatory movements for the affected side. Examples of this work include the MIME system [14] where a dummy automobile steering wheel is driven by an electric motor and has force sensors to measure the force contribution the patient can apply with their affected hand and their normal hand. Thus soon after the rehabilitation process is begin the patient is able to move the steering wheel primarily using muscles in their normal hand, the affected hand is essentially passively moved. As the patient progresses through their physiotherapy treatment the program can be adjusted to require greater force from their normal hand thus encouraging the person to make use of their affected hand to `steer`. Hand eye coordination is encouraged as the movement of the steering wheel controls a `computer game` like simulation of driving along a road. Although no quantitative study has been done the assumption is that a physiotherapy program of this nature can be more effective in providing treatment yet require less intervention from the physiotherapy staff.

Unilateral physiotherapy rehabilitation can also be achieved and the MIT-MANUS provides a mechanism to allow a person recovering from a stroke to move their hand in reach and grasp like task with unusual force pattern overlaid so as to determine the nature of and recovery of the neuro-motor system [15]. The concepts for retraining reach and grasp activities in a way that encourages motor relearning are also explored in the EU GENTLE/S project [12] and is shown in figure 2.

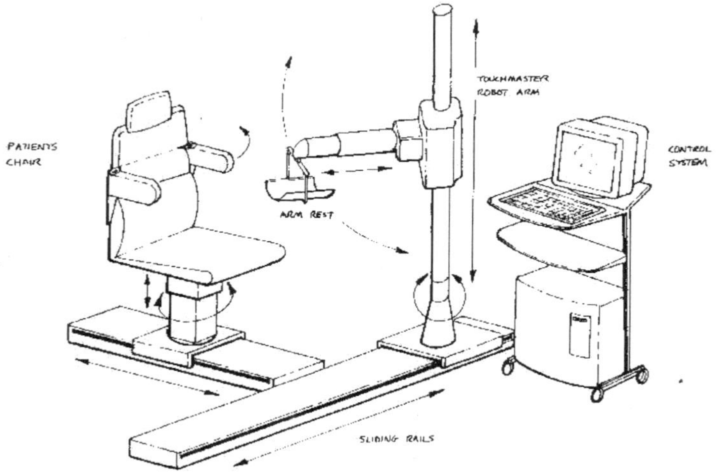

Figure 2. Gentle/s, machine mediated rehabilitation

5. Mobility Assistance for Patients and People with Motor Impairments

Autonomous and intelligent wheelchairs have often been considered as a possible application for mobile robotics technology in healthcare and rehabilitation. It is still a matter for research to determine the level of automation, and the needs for different client groups. Thus a young motor disabled person might require some basic shared control concepts to assist in the process of learning about how the world works, leading on to safe independent mobility. Alternatively where the person is profoundly disabled, more autonomous wheelchair navigation features would be attractive. Some early commercial technologies are available such as using line following to teach children to operate a wheelchair joystick without risk of collision. The evolution of technology has to meet the diverse needs of the targeted users. Safety is also a critical issue as the greater autonomy given to the wheelchair, the greater the cost of providing adequate levels of safety. The following sections present a collection of prototypes and commercial systems.

5.1 FRIEND - Functional Robot Arm with User Friendly Interface for Disabled People

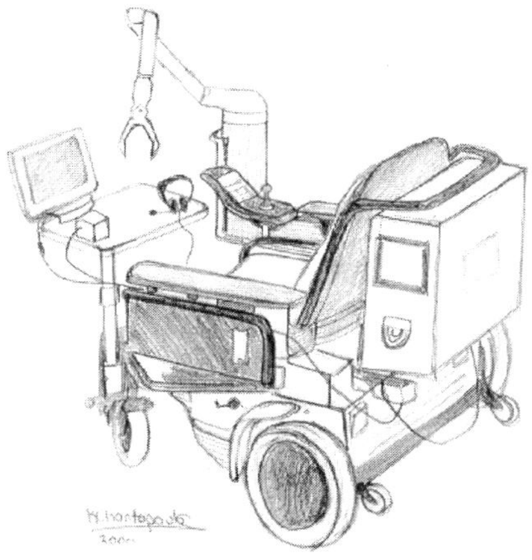

FRIEND is a laboratory prototype developed by the Institution of Automation of the University of Bremen, Germany. The aim of the system is to provide support to disabled persons both at home and at work. The system has been built on a commercial wheelchair (Sprint, MEYRA) and has been equipped with the MANUS manipulator. FRIEND is governed by a central processing unit (a personal computer) attached to the back of the wheelchair which hosts all the control modules, namely, robot·controller, command interpreter, administration module for the pre-programmed motions and man-machine interface. There are two operation modes: i) pre-programmed motions (the robot executes programs stored in the systems memory) and ii) user-controlled robot movements. There is no obstacle avoidance functionality implemented but there is position estimation, which enables path tracking (required for the point-to-point control of the mobile robot). The system uses a multimedia user interface, which accepts high-level commands. The work in FRIEND was focused more to the manipulation tasks (visual servoing of the manipulator and visual object recognition were included in plans of future work) rather on the mobile robot navigation. More information may be found at http://www.ipa.fhg.de/srdatabase/friend.html.

5.2 VAHM - Autonomous Vehicle for Disabled Persons

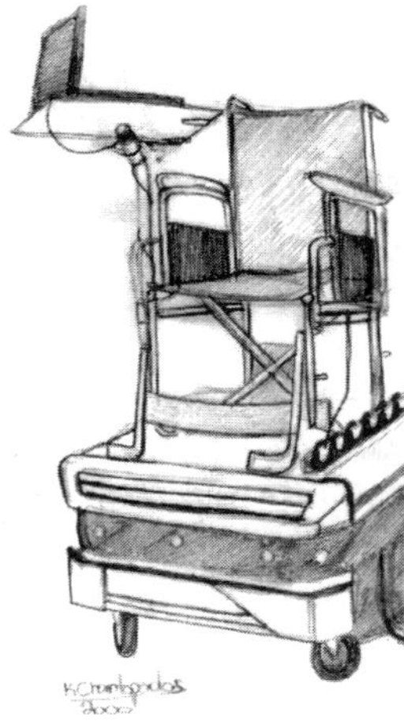

VAHM is the acronym of "autonomous vehicle for disabled persons" in French. The VAHM prototype was developed in University of Metz in France. The prototype met two major releases. VAHM-1 [4], was developed in 80s and was built on a mobile robot equipped with ultrasonic and odometry sensors, along with a conventional chair placed to the top of the robot (see the drawing beside). The prototype achieved three modes of operation: manual motion, assisted motion, and autonomous motion. In manual mode the user drives the robot as a conventional powered wheelchair, in assisted motion the control is shared between the user and the system (the sensors readings are contributing to the decision of the selected direction) and in autonomous motion the robot takes over the full control of the system implementing autonomous navigation with obstacle avoidance behaviour. The path planning method employed was based on the artificial (potential) fields principle (*see* Chapter 8).

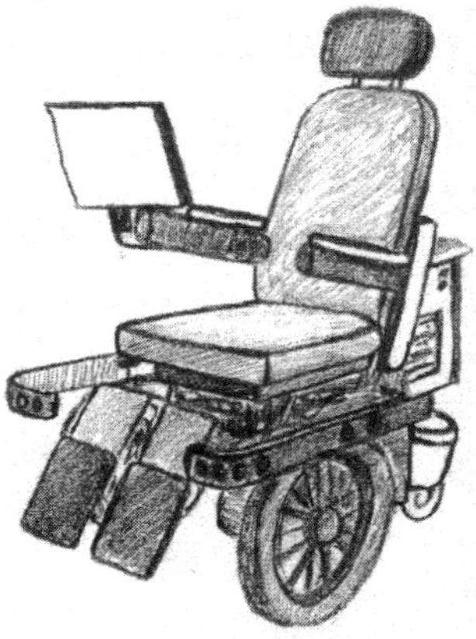

After achieving the results as above the research team proceeded to VAHM-2 [3]. In this project the system was built around a commercially available wheelchair (PowerPush, Swiss). The wheelchair was equipped with ultrasonic sensors, and a user interface was installed on-board (see drawing beside). All the required processing power was placed at the back of the wheelchair. As its ancestor VAHM-1, VAHM-2 had three modes of operation: manual controls (by passing the embedded intelligence and driving the system as a conventional wheelchair), assisted controls (where the system presents behaviours such as wall following, free space following, direction following, initial position return) and goal oriented control (where the system navigates autonomously towards the desired goal).

5.3 The Smart Wheelchair

The Smart Wheelchair [19] is a development of the Call Centre of the University of Edinburgh for children with severe and multiple disabilities who could not use ordinary mobility aids. The first prototype was built in 1987 and undergone several user tests in real-life environments. The Smart Wheelchair can be driven by single or multiple switches; a scanning direction selector; proportional joystick; and communication aid or laptop computer. The concept is highly modular and the Call Centre has developed a set of so-called tools that can be configured on the chair to provide a desired behaviour. The modularity principle addressed the mechanical, the electrical and the functional aspects of the wheelchair. For example, bumpers were installed to protect the user and the environment. On collision the wheelchair stops and takes an avoiding action (e.g. stop, back off, turn around obstacle etc.). The track follower enables the system to trace reflective lines on the floor or through tight situations like doorways etc. Call Centre supports the wheelchair with a full set of training material on how to operate the wheelchair.

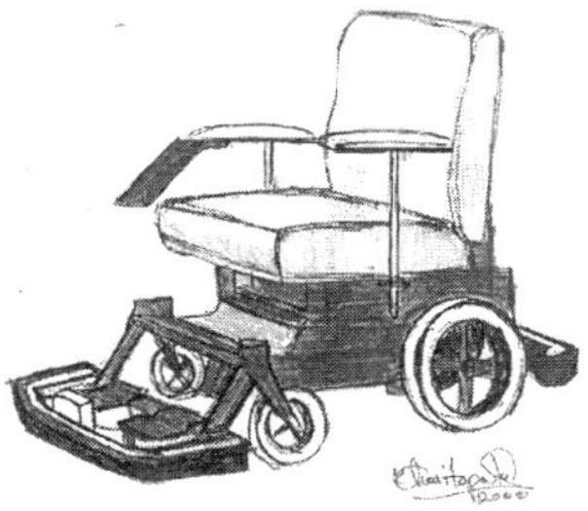

The Smart Wheelchair is commercially available by either Call Centre or Smile Rehab Ltd. which manufactures the wheelchairs. More details on Smart Wheelchairs may be found at http://callcentre.education.ed.ac.uk/Smart_WheelCh/smart_wheelch.html

5.4 NAVCHAIR

NavChair [18] is a laboratory prototype of the University of Michigan, USA of a 3 years project started in 1991. The project achieved obstacle avoidance and wall following functionality cruising in high speeds (0.8m/s). The system employs a set of ultrasonic sensors to collect information about the local environment. The system operates in semi-autonomous mode, where the machine shares controls with the user. The algorithm governing the motion is the well-known Vector Field Histogram (VFH) obstacle avoidance algorithm (*see* Chapter 8) [2]. More information maybe found at http://www-personal.engin. umich.edu/~johannb/navchair.hml.

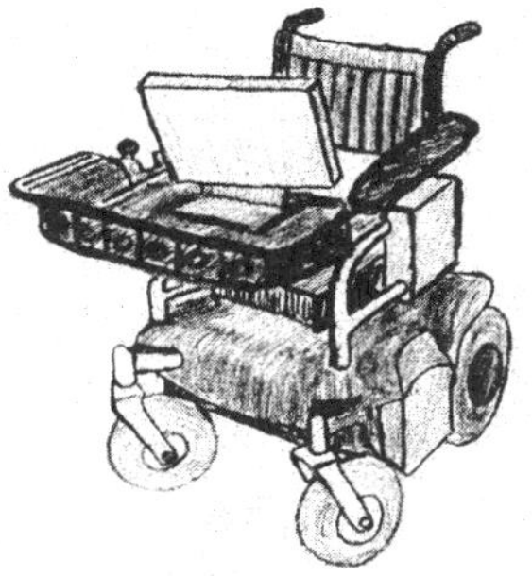

5.5 TINMAN

TinMan is a development of the KISS Institute for Practical Robotics. The institute along with other sponsors (MITRE Corporation, Apple Computer, and Vector Mobility) supported the development of a driver assistive system for powered wheelchairs. The system reached two major prototypes, TinMan I and TinMan II (see drawing beside). The system was controlling the inputs coming through the joystick and modified the instructions to the motion controller of the wheelchair in order to implement an obstacle avoidance behaviour. More infromation on Tin Man may be found at www.kipr.org/robots/tm.html

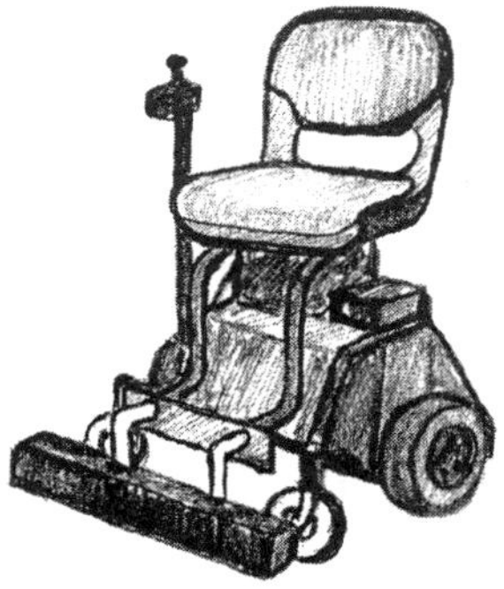

5.6 Wheelesley

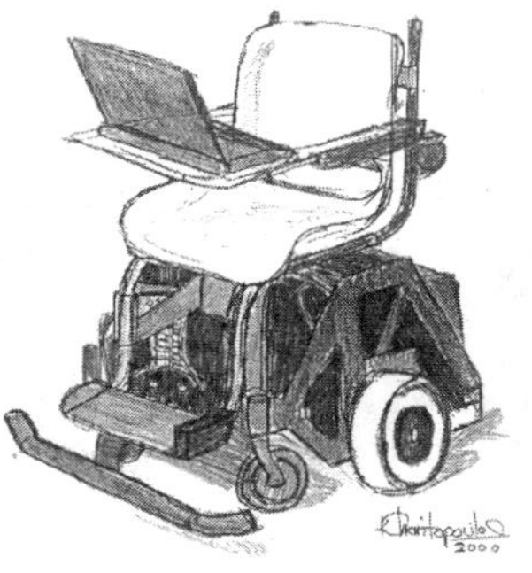

The Wheelesley project started at Wellesley College in January 1995 but later on the work continued at MIT. Some of the development on Wheelesly were based on experiences gained in TinMan robot. Wheelesley is a semi-autonomous robotic wheelchair system. The user issues general directional commands to the system through the on-board interface. The robot presents obstacles avoidance and wall following behaviour. Wheelesley supports three modes of operation: manual, joystick and user interface. In the manual mode, the wheelchair is controlled as a standard wheelchair. In joystick mode, the user issues general directional commands while the system performs collision avoidance. In the user interface mode, the user may interact solely through the user's interface. More information may be found at www.ai.mit.edu/people/holly/wheelesley or http://www.kipr.org/robots/tm.html.

5.7 VTT Wheelchair Drive Assistant

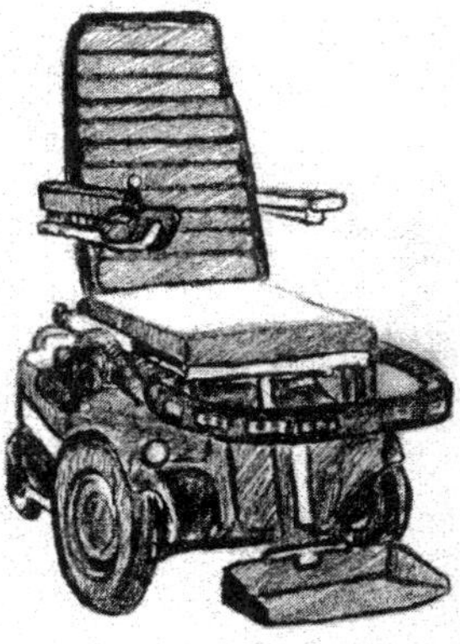

VTT Wheelchair Drive Assistant (obstacle avoidance module) is a development of the Adaptation Training Centre for Disabled and VTT Automation, Finland. The project's purpose was the development of an obstacle avoidance module. The implementation has been based on a behaviour-based concept and environment perception via ultrasonic sensors. System operates in two modes: guidance mode, and active mode. These two modes are different instances of the same algorithm, which calculates the potential field of the wheelchairs environment. Beyond the sensor typical ultrasonic sensors placement in a ring (as shown in the drawing besides) VTT developed a highly compact ultrasonic sensor unit that was combining four sensor heads (receivers and transmitters). The system has been tested on wheelchair of deferent manufacturers with similar results. More information may be found at http://www.vtt.fi/aut/kau/results/tracker/

5.8 INRO - Intelligent Wheelchair

INRO it is a development of FH Weingarten, Germany that performed with the support of the national research project INRO (INRO stands for *Intelligenter Rollstuhl* which means intelligent wheelchair in German) [21]. The system integrated on a commercial wheelchair (Genius, Meyra) the following subsystems:

a) a ring of five ultrasonics for obstacle avoidance, indoor navigation and convoy driving,

b) an active marking system to detect low and concave obstacles, c) a differential global positioning system for outdoor navigation.

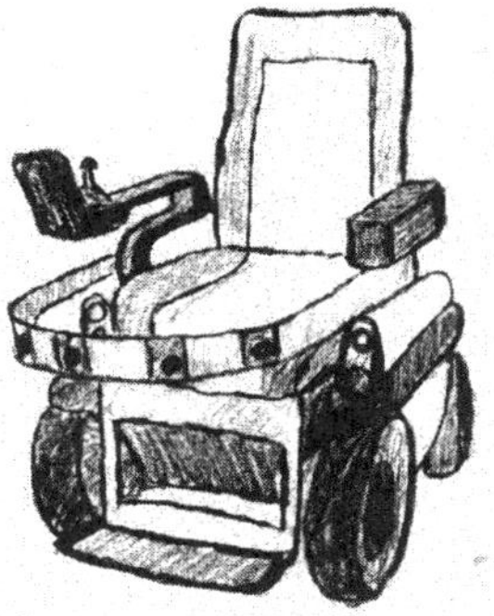

The ultrasonic ring was utilised for obstacle avoidance. This fuction is assisted by the active marking system. The active marker uses a laser source that projects three lines vertical to the drive direction and a ccd camera to detect these lines. By measuring the deviations between the expected line position and the deformed measured lines, the data processing scheme derives the position and shape of obstacles.

5.9 Maid - Mobility Aid for Elderly and Disabled People

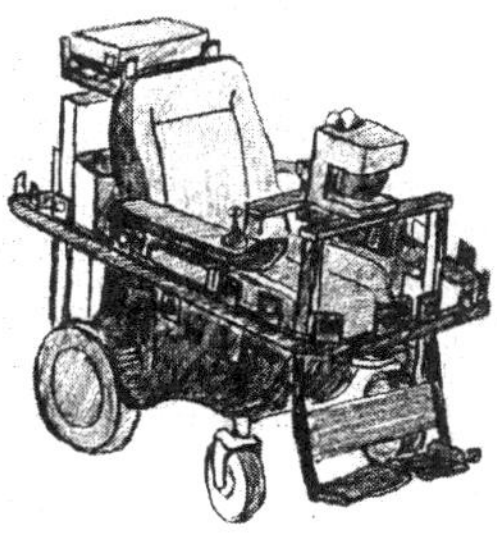

Maid is a development of FAW, Ulm, Germany. Maid is an intelligent robotic wheelchair with primary task to transport elderly persons and persons with mobility impairments. The system is built on a commercial wheelchair (Sprint, Meyra) and is equipped with: encoders, gyroscope, ultrasonic sensor heads, two infrared scanners for short range sensing, and a 2D laser range finder PLS. Two modes of operation exist. The semi-autonomous and the autonomous mode. In the first mode, the user is able to evoke single maneuvers, (like backing up into a room or passing through narrow doorways). This mode was particularly designed in order to allow transportation in narrow, cluttered environments. In the second mode Maid is navigated in an entirely autonomous fashion.

5.10 DX Drive Assist Module

Drive Assist Module is a commercial product of Dynamic Controls Ltd, New Zealand. The module consists of a set of sensors (infrared and ultrasonic sensors). The sensors maybe placed at the specific positions on the wheelchair (on the sides to observe side obstacles or at the rear to prevent collision when moving backwards). The module stops the wheelchair in the case of a potential collision with an obstacle that was detected by the sensors. The module is built to operate in a DX-bus environment. It is a commercial product manufactured and commercialised by Dynamic Controls Ltd, New Zealand. More information maybe found at http://dynamicmobility. co.nz/stagingdcl/dx/auxiliary/dam/dam%5Fintro.htm

5.11 COACH - Computer Assisted Wheelchair for Handicapped People

COACH [11] stands for Computer Assisted Wheelchair for Handicapped People. The project commenced in 1989 through the association of CEA (mobile robotics expert) with POIRIER (wheelchair manufacturer). COACH was officially presented during the ICORR workshop in 1992. A commercial wheelchair from POIRIER equipped with ultrasonic and infrared sensors. Three modes of controlling the system are available. In the direct mode the wheelchair behaves as a standard powered wheelchair. In the filtered mode persons with spasms are aided, as the commands given to the joystick are made smoother and more regular. Also, in that mode, the collision detection facility is efficient in stopping the wheelchair in emergency cases. In the corrected mode, the system may be of assistance in a more specific way. The joystick commands may be corrected by the controller through the use of sensor information. For instance it may ensure that the distance between the wall and the user will be at a maximum allowed predefined value.

5.12 Care-O-bot

Care-O-Bot [22] is a development of Fraunhofer IPA, Stuttgart, Germany. The aim of the robot is to provide help in domestic environments by performing fetch & carry and other supporting tasks. Emphasis in the system was given to the communicational and social integrating activities, like video-phone, automatic emergency calls and interactive communication. The prototype was presented for the first time to the public at the Hannover Fair in April 1998. Further development of the system is conducted based on the results and feedback from customer & supplier's side. The next step will be the integration of a manipulator on the mobile robot.

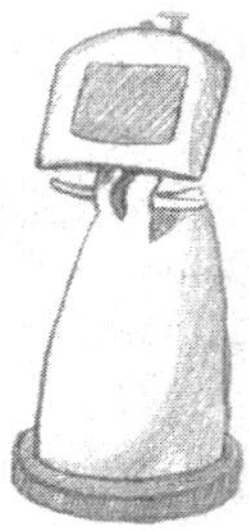

5.13 SENARIO - Sensor Aided Intelligent Wheelchair Navigation System

SENARIO was a three years project started in 1994 aiming the development of an autonomous navigation system as add-on module on a commercially available wheelchair. The project was supported by the TIDE programme of the EC. The project has succeeded in developing all the required technology addressing the full set of problems (global path planning, local path planning - obstacle avoidance, robot localisation, etc.). The system was built on a commercially available wheelchair (Sprint, Meyra). Senario, used ultrasonic sensors placed on the periphery of the wheelchair. A subset of those sensors called the protection sensors were devoted to the safety issues and they were specially designed for those purposes. Protection ultrasonic sensors ensured that the robot will stop before the collision with a near by obstacle. Another set of ultrasonic sensors was devoted to the navigation task. Their readings were the input of the path planning method implementing obstacle avoidance behaviour. The method was based on the potential field principle and introduced a new approach called AKH (see Chapter 8) which incorporated the actual robot shape and dimensions in the calculation of the path. At a higher level of the control loop there was a global path planner that was in close cooperation with local path planner.

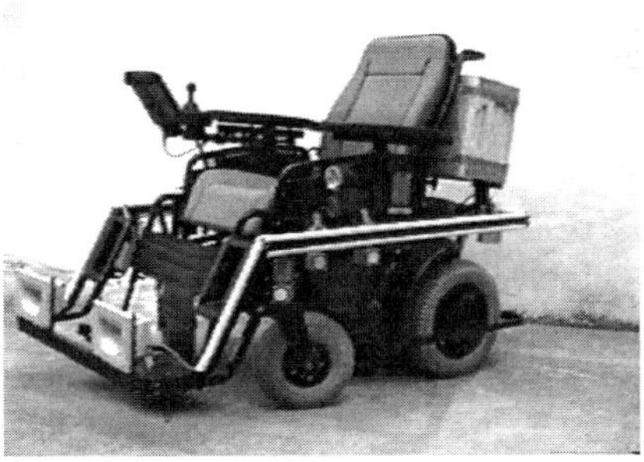

Figure 3. The SENARIO autonomous wheelchair

The system had three modes of operation: a) the manual were the wheelchair was driven like a conventional wheelchair while a protection watchdog was stopping the motion in the case of high risks, b) semi-autonomous mode, in which the system and the user were sharing the control of the robot, and c) fully autonomous mode, in which the system had full control over the robot actions. The user had the choice either to use the on-board speech recognition system or the joystick. The system was able to process and execute high level commands like: 'turn left', 'stop', 'forward', 'increase speed' etc. aiming the driving in semi-autonomous mode, or even global commands like 'go to kitchen', in which the system had to resolve the complete problem on-line. Also the system was enhanced with a 'command anticipation' functionality according to which the user did not needed to take care about the time the command was given, because the system would execute it at the time that the command would be feasible e.g. a turn right command would make the robot to turn on the right at the end of the corridor even if the command was given in the beginning of it. More information about SENARIO may be found in Chapter 5.

5.14 OMNI - Shared Control, Omni Directional Wheelchair

The OMNI project aims at increasing the mobility of a wheelchair in the close confines of a house, as well as exploring strategies for shared control. The user requirements analysis showed that it was necessary to get a high level of versatility and adaptability to meet the widely varying needs of people with motor disabilities. That means, besides the 'normal' function of user-controlled movement several additional modes of operation should be available to the user. A hierarchical approach is used in the wheelchairs control structure.

At the lowest layer it is possible to have direct control of the wheelchair speed and turn rate. Such information could be provided directly from a wheelchair joystick. In the next layer, basic sensors are integrated into the control system to support the user. Thus, for example, sensors can be used for collision avoidance, for safe movements, and to give information about nearby objects that are not in the users field of view. The next layer is built by an environment directed movement of the wheelchair (driving along a wall, driving through a doorway) up to full sensor guidance, e.g. the docking at a station. Special complex manoeuvres like play-back movement (re-driving a recorded path, so as to move from the living area to the bathroom) or back-tracing (inversion of the recent manoeuvres) up to an automated guided movement.This hierarchy also reflects the distribution of efforts between the user and the control system. As the wheelchair becomes more autonomous by using the higher-level control, the burden on the user becomes less. While the functionality increases, safety aspects become more important.

In order to give an adjusted and assistive system to the individual, the functionality has to be easily adaptable to the specific disabilities and needs of the user, that means, the system has to realize a high flexibility to allow transitions between the different layers. Furthermore, this operation on different levels of autonomy ensures that the user never feels patronized by the system; and although much autonomous vehicle and robot technology is used in the system, it doesn't act totally autonomous because the user is always able to interrupt or modify ongoing actions.

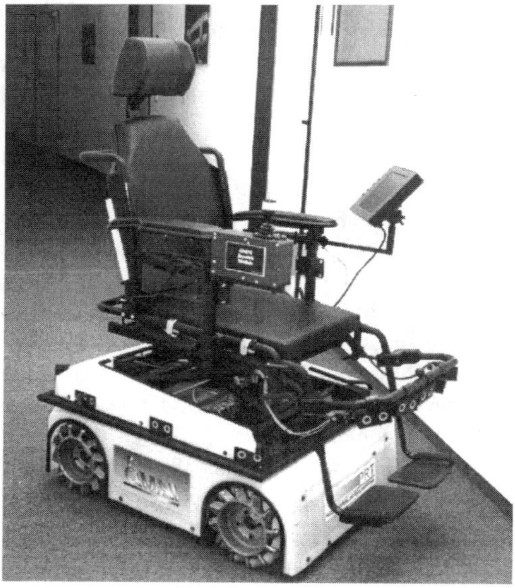

Figure 4. OMNI, A shared control omnidirectional wheelchair

To allow unrestricted wheelchair placement the OMNI wheelchair uses an omni-directional base. Based on previous omni-directional wheel technologies, a pre-prototype was developed using four so-called Mecanum wheels that allow movement with three degrees-of-freedom in a plane. Thus Omni can do any combination of forward, sideways, and rotational movement. The prototype wheelchair had demonstrated the increase of mobility that can be yield by the use of such omnidirectional driving concepts, which allow to move even within packed indoor environments because of a non-restricted positioning capability.

The OMNI Sensor System is based on a proximity sensor array that uses the concept of composite sensors. Each composite sensor is composed of an ultrasonic range-finder and an infrared detector. This particular sensor arrangement is capable to achieve a perception of the explored objects which is not limited to their geometrical properties. The complementary features of reflecting behaviours for ultrasound waves and infrared radiations enable to fuse together the information they supply. This enhances the robustness of obstacle avoidance.

A Human-Machine-Interface provides the user with the means to drive and operate the wheelchair and to have access to external systems such as workstations, communication devices and environmental control systems from a wide variety of input devices. The HMI displays the functionality options of the system (wheelchair and external systems) either textual or pictorial on a screen, activates system functions selected by the user via the input devices, and displays dynamic information from/about the system (like speed or battery power of the wheelchair). The standard input device for driving an omnidirectional wheelchair is a 3-dimensional joystick. However, the user tests have shown that not all persons are able to operate this kind of joystick. Therefore other devices (e.g. switches) can be connected to a standardized interface.

5.15 PAMAID - Navigation for Elderly Frail Visually Impaired Users

PAMAID represents a solution to the navigation problems of elderly frail visually impaired users. The PAMAID project was a 2.5 years project, that started in 1996 and was supported by the Telematics programme of the EC. An elderly person who has good vision can use walking frames or rolators to assist their mobility, likewise a person who is visually impaired can use a blind cane to identify obstacals in their path. Where a person is visually impaired and frail the only solution is to try to use a blind cane (i.e. a guiding tool) from a wheelchair, a strategy difficult to employ effectively since hand movement is needed for the control of both. The alternative, to leave elderly impaired users to sit all day, leads to boredom, muscle wasteage and loss of independance.

PAMAID addresses these difficulties by integrating sensing and control technologies in the structure of a walking frame. An initial version of PAMAID used a wheelchair base to provide active control of the wheels. This had the advantage of allowing the mass of the frame to be compensated, but it was not found to be an intuitive control strategy. The second version of PAMAID used servo-motors to direct the rolator casters. This approach had the advantage of being inherently passive, and provided a more effective interface strategy. The principal sensor on PAMAID was a planar laser range finder. Data from the range finder was processed to identify and classify nearby obstacles. An auxiliary sensor system consisted of an upward directed ultrasound range finder to allow PAMAID to detect the condition when it was pushed under a table. PAMAID had several interface strategies that could be selected by the user. At the lowest level PAMAID simply gives spoken instructions on the location of nearby obstacles e.g. "Obstacle in front". A more advanced interface strategy directs the wheels to prevent the person colliding into walls and navigate them through doors. According to the above two configurations were designed: the active and the passive. The passive configuration provides both physical and navigational support while the user provides the propulsion (figure 5 (b) shows the basic PAMAID arrangement with the ultrasound sensors visible in the front. The laser range-finder is located immediately above the ultrasound sensors), while the active provides also the propulsion to those users require so (figure 5 (a)).

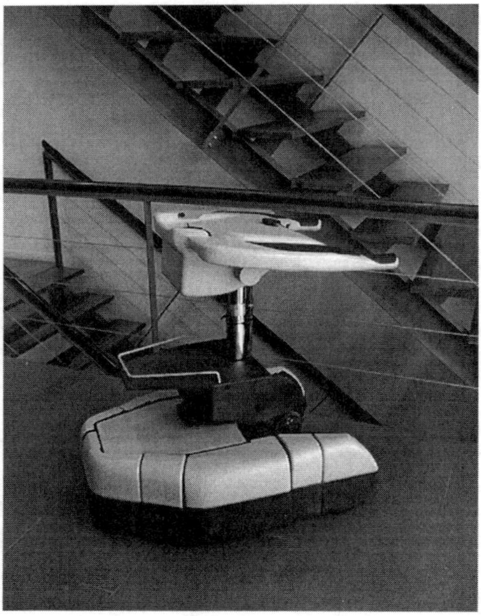

(a)

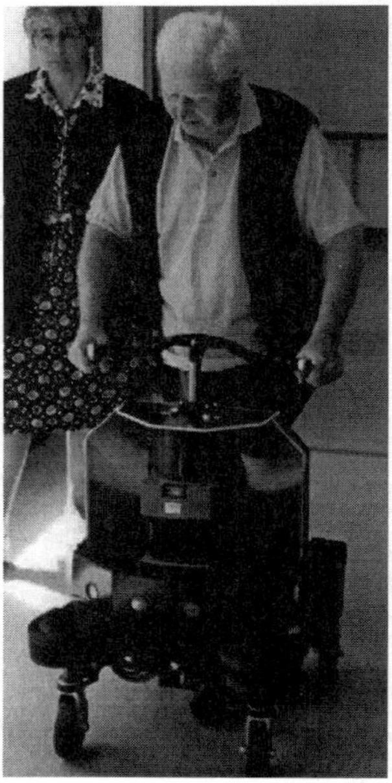

(b)

Figure 5. (a) PAMAID active configuration, (b) PAMAID passive configuration

5.16INDEPENDENCE 3000 IBOT TRANSPORTER

This is an impressive piece of technology developed by Independence Technology, a Johnson & Johnson company. The device is able to negotiate with staircases and uneven terrains. The user pulls the handles of the staircase in order to initiate the climbing up or down motion of the wheelchair. Furthermore the device is able to "stand up" in a two-wheeled configuration, lifting the user to positions that would enable him/her pick up objects from a cupboard or a shelf. The device in either the four-wheeled or two-wheeled configuration is keeping the balance of the system to maintain stability as well as implement the desired motion. The device is heavily equiped with processing power and sensors (gyroscopes). Currently it is under testing in order to get the

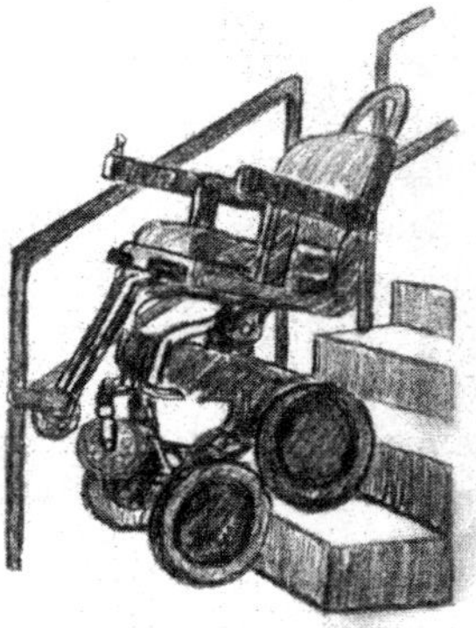

approval required to be commercialised. More information may be found at http://www.indetech.com/productfunction.html

6. Manipulation Assistance for Patients and People with Motor Impairments

There are broadly two approaches to providing someone who has motor difficulties with manipulation assistance. These are to either provide a robot that is directly controlled by the individual requiring each movement of the robotic manipulator to be controlled by a movement of the person, or to provide the robot with sufficient autonomy to achieve the task.

6.1 MANUS

The wheelchair (or mobile robot) mounted MANUS manipulator arm is a good illustration of the first principle, and has been successful applied by people with muscular dystrophy and similar conditions that lead to muscle weakness (figure 5). This principle can be extended so that the person has a physical sense of the environment fed back as forces to the point of interaction.

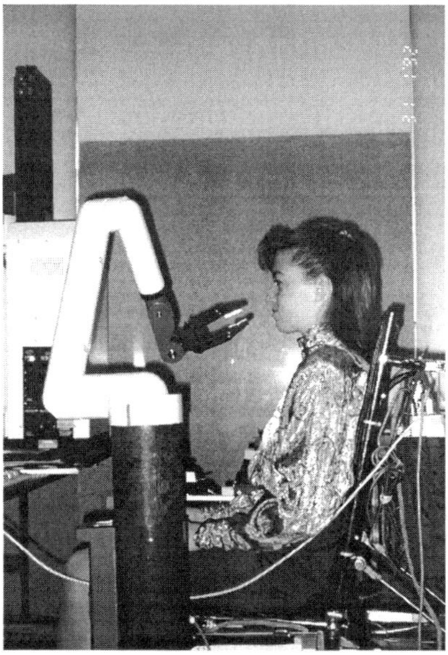

Figure 6. MANUS wheelchair mounted manipulator

The Manus was a collaborative Dutch project started in 1984 and centred at the Institute for Rehabilitation Research (IRV) [5]. Manus built on the conclusions of the Spartacus project by specifying and developing a wheelchair-mounted manipulator. The original Manus manipulator consisted of a 5 degree of freedom arm mounted on a rotating and telescoping base unit which could be attached to a variety of electric wheelchairs. Current versions have a reach of approximately 850 mm and can lift 1.5 kg at full extent.

Today MANUS is 6+2 DOF manipulator. The arm maybe controlled via various input devices like joysticks, chin controllers etc. MANUS has gone through several revisions on both software and hardware. During these years the device has been extensively tested in real-life environments (the first field test lasted over one year). It is currently installed in over 100 units, the most of them being in the Netherlands. More technical information on MANUS maybe found in Chapter 10, section 3. MANUS is manufactured and commercialised by Exact Dynamics B.V. in the Netherlands.

6.2 Handy1

The Handy1 robot illustrates the second concept where the robot interacts with the person but has preprogrammed movements that can be used to assist in rapid completion of the task. Giving the robot autonomy requires either a high level of sensing and intelligence in the robot, or a highly structured environment. Handy is a 5-DOFs arm. The system was designed to aid the severely handicapped to do perform routine tasks such as drinking, washing, cleaning. Mike Topping, at Keele University, initially developed Handy in 1987 in order to assist a 12-year-old boy with cerebral palsy to eat unaided. In 1989 an improvement to the system was made, to create a multi functional system in order to facilitate persons with various disabilities.

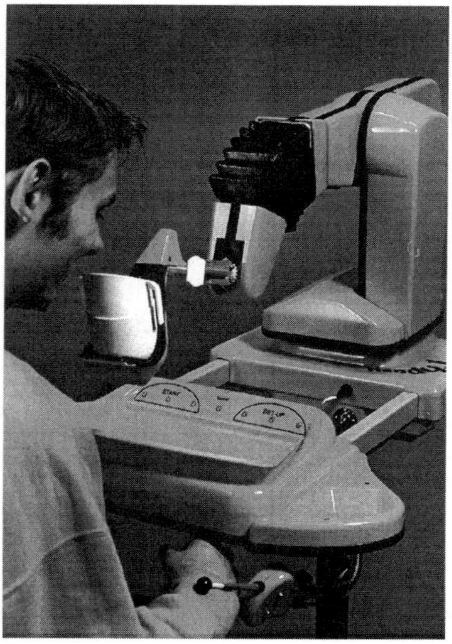

Figure 7. Handy1 assistive robot for drinking and eating

The next version of Handy1 incorporated a switch, by which the user could control the entire system by selecting the desired action from a set of predefined actions stored in the system. There is a simple and effective principle according to which a set of little lamps (each of them representing an action) are illuminated in row. By the use of a single switch (and it may be placed as the user wishes, or may be even operated by the blink of an eye) the user chooses the desired action. The revision project ended in 1992. Since then Handy1 has undergone enormous advancements mainly related to the application spectrum served by the robot. Some of those were achieved within the Robotic Aid to Independent Living (RAIL) project. The aim of the project concentrated on the aesthetic design and the development of trays for applications like drinking, teeth brushing, shaving, game playing etc. as well as technical improvements (calibration, accuracy, pay-load, duty-cycle etc.). Handy1 has achieved appr. 100 installations, mainly in UK. More information on Handy1 maybe found in Chapter 10, section 3. Handy 1 is commercialised and manufactured by Rehab Robotics Ltd. UK.

6.3 RAPTOR - Wheelchair Robotic Assistive Device

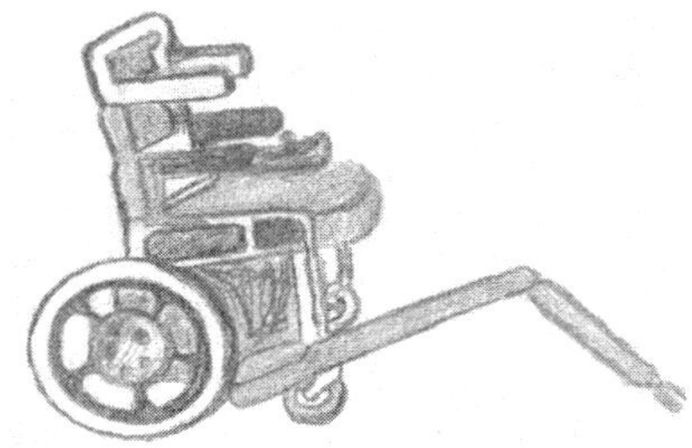

RAPTOR is also a wheelchair attachable manipulator. The aim of the device is to offer the user manipulation abilities in daily activities like fetching objects from the table or the refrigerator, opening doors, operating the light switches etc. RAPTOR is a 4+1 DOF manipulator. The manipulator maybe controlled via the commands given through a joystick, keypad, or sip-and-puff interface. The device has gone through tests in daily life environments. It is manufactured and commercialised by Rehabilitation Technologies Division (RTD) of Applied Resources Corp., USA. The device is commercially available by Applied Resources Corp. and has managed to get the FDA approval. More information on RAPTOR may be found at www.appliedresource.com/RTD/Products/Raptor/index.htm.

6.4 WALKY

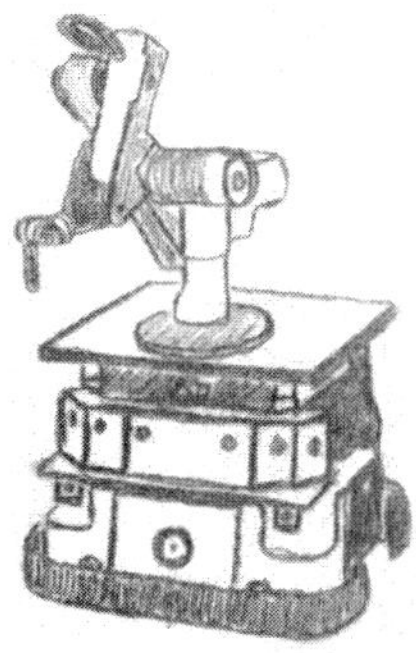

WALKY is a prototype developed by KTH of the Lund University. The system consists of a mobile robot (Labmate of TRC Inc.) and a 5-DOF manipulator (Scorbot ER VII of Eshed Robotic Ltd.) (see drawing besides). The aim was to develop a system aiding people with physical impairments as well as for use in laboratory settings (typically chemical, medical and biological). WALKY is equipped with ultrasonic and infrared sensors for obstacle avoidance and path planning. The user commands the robot from a remote control panel. Path planning, collision avoidance methods and pre-programmed procedures are used as well as direct control in order to grasp objects. The prototype has undergone laboratory tests and limited trials at Rehabcentrum Lund-Orup at Lund University Hospital.

6.5 The Wessex Trolley Mounted Robot

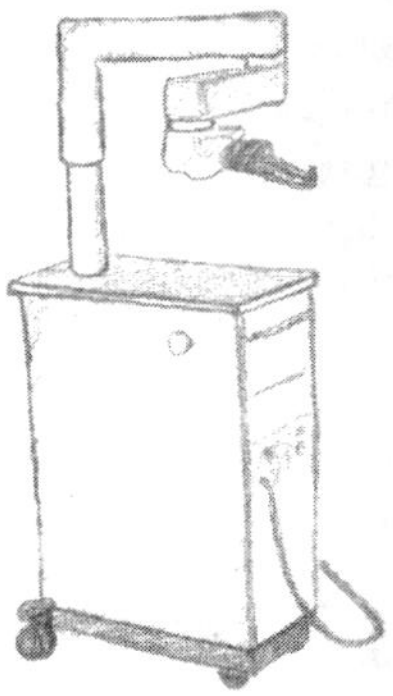

The Wessex arm is the product of the Bath Institute of Medical Engineering of the Bath University, UK. It is a SCARA 4+1 DOFs arm. The aim of the device is to enable users perform daily life tasks. The arm may be controlled directly through an input device (joystick) or can be used at the playback mode (the user selects an action to be performed from a set of pre-taught paths). The device comes along with a workstation. The arm is placed on the top of a trolley that enables easy transportation of the device in domestic environments (see drawing besides). A carer may transport the device at the place that the user likes to operate it. The device was tested at a hospital near by the Bath University. More information on the Wessex arm may be found at www.bath.ac.uk/Centres/BIME/projects/robot/robots.htm.

6.6 The Weston Wheelchair Mounted Robot

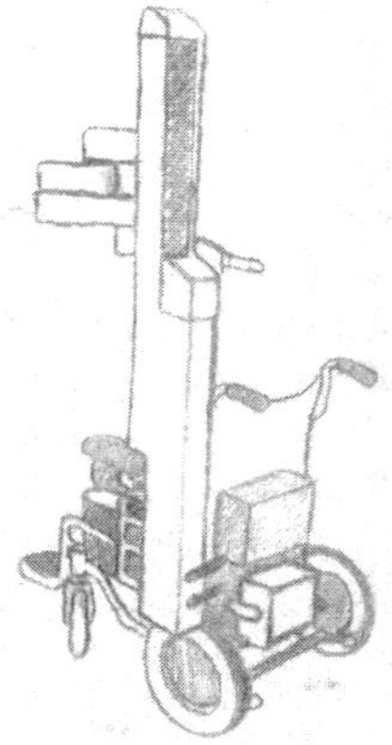

The Weston wheelchair mounted robot, is also a product of research performed by the Bath Institute of Medical Engineering of the Bath University. The design of the trolley mounted Wessex Robot, as well as users feedback lead the research team into the development of a new manipulator. Wessex is a 5+1 DOF manipulator. The Wessex and the Weston robots share components in software (control algorithms) and hardware (the upper part of the arm). Currently the arm is mounted on a trolley in order to demonstrate the functionality and enable user evaluation. The next stage is to develop the mounting system for a wheelchair and enter extensive tests of the device in real-life environments. The drawing besides gives an impression of the system prototype that will be used for the evaluations. More information on the Weston arm may be found at www.bath.ac.uk/Centres/BIME/projects/robot/robots.htm.

6.7 MOVAID

MOVAID seeks a more ambitious solution than Manus, Raptor. Wessex, Weston and Handy1 by providing autonomy in an unstructured environment. It aims to provide severely disabled or bed-ridden persons with tools which will enable them to play a more effective and active role in the everyday domestic activities. These activities are largely of two types: 'chores', which are physically demanding or tedious (e.g. cleaning the house), and more enjoyable activities, such as preparing food in the kitchen. This category of applications need systems which incorporate high levels of autonomy, due to their limited physical capability to interact with the machine.

MOVAID was based on the results of the project *Mobile Robotic Unit for the Assistance of the Disabled* (URMAD) supported by the National Research Council of Italy. URMAID resulted on a 8-DOFs manipulator mounted on a mobile robot. In the TIDE programme of the EU the MOVAID was enhanced by PARTNER, the mobile robot on top of which the manipulator was mounted, and the MARCUS gripper. The result, was an impressive mobile robot high manipulation and mobility features, targeting a broad band of applications.

The MOVAID system comprises of a number of fixed workstations (PCs), located where main activities are carried out at home, such as the kitchen and the bedroom, and a mobile robot able to navigate in the house avoiding unexpected obstacles, to grasp and manipulate common objects and to dock to the fixed workstations for data exchange and power supply. Commands to the robot are given in a high level language through a graphical interface running on the fixed workstation. On the user interface, a continuous visual feed-back from on-board cameras is also shown to the user, allowing him/her not only to monitor what the robot is doing, but also to collaborate with it, by indicating objects and positions on the screen.

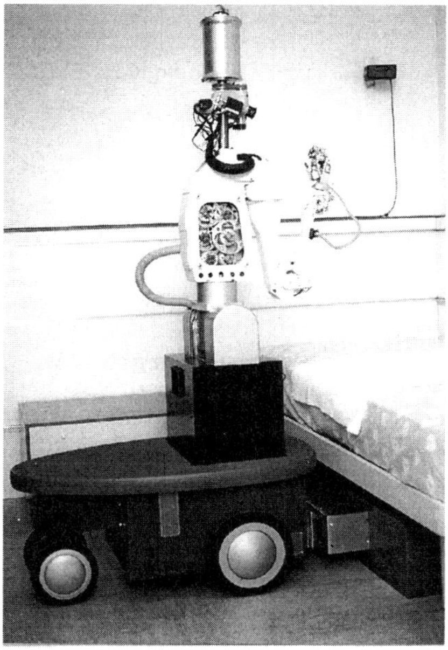

Figure 8. MOVAID showing the URMAD arm

Moreover, in order to allow and to ease the access to standard technological products to disabled and elderly people, interfaces for standard kitchen appliances have been studied, and a prototype of a microwave oven interface, offering the ovens basic functionality, has been developed and tested. A detailed description of MOVAID may be found in Chapter 12.

6.8 The JPL NASA Health Care Robot

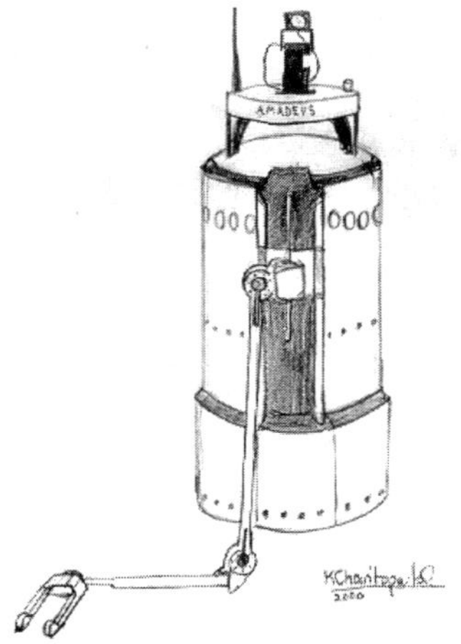

The Health Care Robot [9] is a prototype developed by Jet Propulsion Laboratory of NASA, USA. Like MOVAID, it provides high manipulation capabilities on the top of autonomous navigation in domestic environments. It consists of a mobile robot and a mobile manipulator. It was design to serve and provide assistance to the elderly and the handicapped. The robot is based on a B21 mobile platform manufactured by RWI Inc. It has been equipped with a colour camera mounted on a pan tilt unit, and an array of ultrasound, infrared and contact sensors (integrated in the mobile robot) to enable autonomous navigation capabilities. The arm is of 6-DOFs. The length of the arm (appr. 1m) and its mounting position on the mobile robot has been specifically designed to enable reach of difficult positions (e.g. the in able manipulator to sweep the floor with an elbow-down configuration, e.g. like in the drawing besides). The control station has the ability of interpreting voice, joystick, and mouse commands, and displays real-time images from the robot camera, as well as a schematic map of the robot's environment and the readings of the ultrasound sensors.

6.9 The Technion Nursing Robot

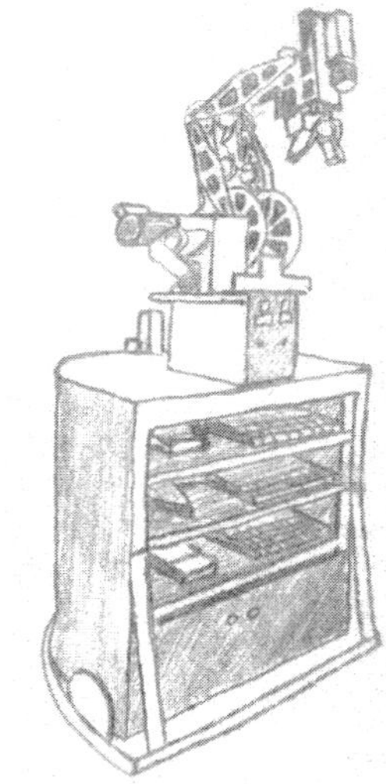

The Nursing Robot is one of the oldest developments in the field performed at Technion, in Israel. The prototype was demonstrated in 1986. The robot could perform actions like, fetching a glass of water, operating electrical appliances or replacing a cassette in a video-recorder. The prototype composed by a mobile robot on the top of which a 5-DOF manipulator was mounted. A 3-DOF gripper was employed at the end point of the manipulator. The mobile robot provides obstacle avoidance behaviour when moving from point-to-point. Ultrasonic sensors and bumpers are used to detect obstacles in the near by area. Light beacons and light detectors are used to localise the robot in the operating environment. The demonstration results of the prototype are impressive given the computational power available (three Singlair Spectrum on-board and an IBM 8086 personal computer off-board) and the complexity of the functionality. For more information see http://www-personal.engin.umich.edu/~johannb/nurserob.htm

6.10 ASIMOV

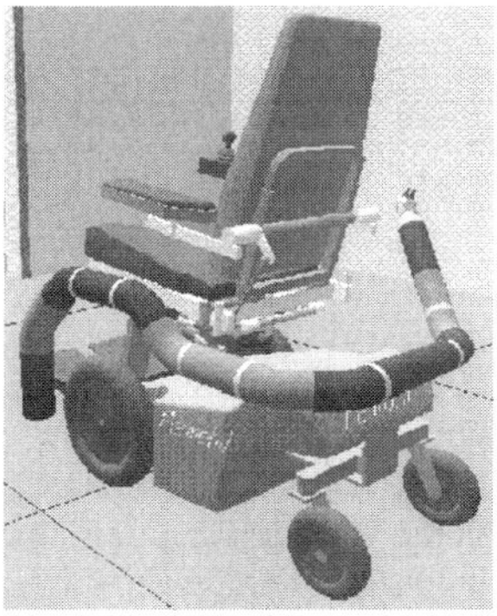

ASIMOV is a very recent development of a highly modular mobile manipulator. The Lund University has mainly performed the development in various projects including the MobiNet project. The manipulator presents high degree of manipulation abilities and can be mounted on powered wheelchairs (see drawing beside). It is ideal for applications were the manipulability is of highest priority while the payload, velocity and acceleration (compared to typical industrial manipulators) is of less importance. The manipulator is consisted of several modules (the number depends on the application and the DOFs that would be required). Each of these modules include in the module body the mechanics and electronics. The modules support the CAN bus concluding to a minimisation of the required cable. The manipulator payload is in appr. 1kg. Light and medium weight materials are used to implement the modules. For more information on ASIMOV, see Chapter 12.

7. Information Structures for Smart Buildings

The level of technology transfer to the building services sector is increasing rapidly. Large buildings are beginning to benefit from large networked control structures for lighting, security and heating ventilation and control systems. Operators are becoming more aware of the benefits of integrated information systems across a facility but at present there are no generic solutions available to locate users in a building and to provide appropriate information for the building users. Emerging technologies are based on industrial standards for network technology. These include Jini, LonWorks, ethernet twisted pair, Bluetooth and other wired and wireless technology. Sending information between these standards is complex although CORBA is a possible protocol to allow this to happen seamlessly (*see* also Chapter 9).

7.1 ARIADNE, a Framework for Hospital and Home Automation

The ARIADNE project directly addresses the access and navigation problems faced by people visiting unfamiliar buildings [10]. The problems of access and navigation have particular relevance for both visitors and building operators. These two distinct sets of users have very different requirements and the ARIADNE project addresses the needs of both groups within the same infrastructure.

For the visitor the problems of ergonomic access and navigation are particularly relevant to people with special needs when faced with poor building design and information support.

- *Physical Access.* The problems of physical access to buildings and ergonomic problems resulting from such things as steps and narrow doors are well known. There is little support for people with visual impairments in most buildings.

- *Navigation.* Navigational information removes the feeling of intimidation felt in unknown environments. The ability to enter a strange building with confidence is the factor that would most greatly affect mobility. This is particularly relevant to a user if there is a large effort penalty in making a wrong turn.
- *Information.* Closely linked to navigation and physical access is the provision of information to a visitor. This may range from locating specific things within a building to providing electronic documentation.

ARIADNE is based on the LonWorks control networks developed originally for process control. The network is based on Neuron Chip nodes, microprocessors running at 10MHZ with a peer to peer twisted pair wires that allow each node to transmit and receive messages at 1.25 Mbit/sec. Software is written in a multiprocess language called Neuron C. Nodes with in the Network can use smart card readers to monitor the movement of people and equipment in the network and, a local object model can be updated. Knowledge of resouces of the building can then be used to assist users navigate through the building, for example spoken commands and intelligent signage can assist a visitor to navigate to the appropriate appointment. Similarly other building users can interrogate the network on the availability of resources such as auditing of equipment or areas of high demand building usage.

Building networks have implications for the control of mobile robots and smart wheelchairs within the building. A major research effort in mobile robots and smart wheelchairs is that of localising the robot within a map, and planning movement to other points within the building. Information contained within the building network is directly usable by the robot. The building can give the robot information about the dimensions of the area in which it is located, and information about what features are in each room within the building. In return the robot can inform the building about changes in the environment, and can provide a range of sensors that the building might not otherwise be able to access.

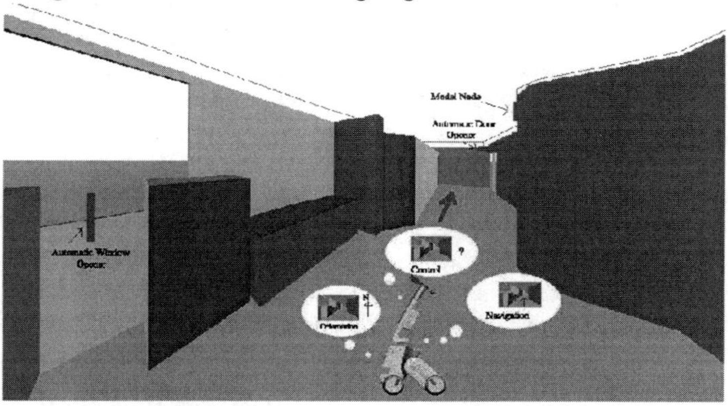

Figure 9. Ariadne, a framework for generalised building communications

8. Conclusions

In this chapter we have given a brief outline on the potential for automation in healthcare and rehabilitation environments by illustrating some emerging technologies. This chapter is by no means comprehensive and focuses primarily on work done in Europe. Japan and the USA also have a strong research interest in this application area. In later chapters of this book further details of the structure of some of the automation described here will be discussed to allow a more indepth analysis of the underlying automation.

This chapter has been necessarily broad discussing a wide range of technologies and application areas. The common area of healthcare is one that is under represented in the general area of research, design and manufacture of high quality automation. As identified earlier this can be attributed to the conservative nature of the industry, the fact that the purchaser is often not the direct or indirect beneficiary of the advantages provided by the automation. It is likewise difficult to establish the benefits of implementing services with the new automation and the return on the investment on the technology.

9. References

[1] Aldon, M. J., Benoit M., Localization system of the hospital transport robot FIRST, *IFAC Conference on Intelligent Autonomous Vehicles*, Helsinki, June 12-14 1995.

[2] Borenstein, J. Levine, S. and Koren, Y., "The NavChair - A New Concept in Intelligent Wheelchair Control for People with Multiple Handicaps", *in the Proceedings of the Fifth Annual Conference on Technology and Persons with Disabilities*, Los Angeles, California, pp.117-124, 1990.

[3] Bourhis G., P.Pino, "Mobile Robotics and Mobility Assistance for People with Motor Impairments: Rational Justification for the VAHM Project", *IEEE Transactions on Rehabilitation Engineering*, Vol. 4, No. 1, Mar. '96

[4] Bourhis G., Y. Agostini, "Man-machine Cooperation for the Control of an Intelligent Powered Wheelchair", *Journal of Intelligent and Robotic Systems*, Vol.22, pp.269-287, 1998

[5] Cinquin P. et al., "Computer Assisted Medical Interventions", IEEE Engineering in Medicine and Biology, 1995, Vol. 14, No. 3, pp. 254, 263

[6] Dario P., E. Guglielmelli, C. Laschi, C. Guadagnini, C. Mulè (SSSA), "Robotic assistants for disabled and elderly people: the URMAD and the MOVAID systems", *27th ISIR - International Symposium on Industrial Robotics*, Milan, Italy, October 6-8, 1996.

[7] Davies B., "Safety of medical robots", *ICAR'93*, Tokyo, Japan, pp. 311-317.

[8] Evans J., B.Krishnamurthy, B.Barrows, T.Skewis, V.Lumelsky, "Handling Real-World Motion Planning: a Hospital Transport Robot". *IEEE Control Systems*, February 1992, Vol. 12, No. 1. pp. 15-18.

[9] Fiorini P., A. Khaled, S. Homoyoun, "Health Care Robotics: A Progress Report", NASA Jet Propulsion Laboratory, California Institute of Technology

[10] Foster G.T., D.E.N. Wenn, F. O'Hart, W.S. Harwin, "Generating virtual environments to allow increased access to the built environment," International Journal of Virtual Reality, Vol.3, No.4, pp. 12-20, 1998

[11] Gelin R., Detriche JM., Lambert JP., Malblanc P., "The Sprint of Coach", Oct. 1993, pp.547-552

[12] Harwin W.S., "Robotic assistance in neuro and motor rehabilitation", European Commission contract KLT/99/02282, Quality of life and management of living resources, 1999.

[13] Harwin W.S., H. Hu, D.P. Stinchcombe, G.T. Foster "An agent based hospital delivery system" *Mobinet workshop in Edinburgh and Santorini* 1998

[14] Johnson M. M. Van der Loos "stroke rehab via steering wheel training" *ICORR99*, Stanford University

[15] Krebs H.I., N. Hogan, M.L. Alisen and B.T. Volpe, "Robot-aided neurorehabilitation" *IEEE T. Rehab engineering*, Vol.6, No.1, pp.75-87, 1998

[16] Kwee H., Duimel J., Smits J., Tuinhof de Moed A., van Woerden J.A. "The Manus wheelchair-borne manipulator: System review and first results", *IARP Proceedings of the 2nd Workshop on Medical and Healthcare Robotics,* pp.385-395,1989

[17] Lauria S., G.T. Foster, W.S. Harwin, O. Habert, "Two Aspects of Multiple Mobile Robots: A Parallel Architecture and an Autonomous Navigation Strategy," *MANSE99* Trinity College Dublin, December 1999

[18] Levine, S., Koren, Y., Borenstein, J. (1990), "NavChair Control System for Automatic Assistive Wheelchair Navigation", *in the Proceedings of the 13th Annual RESNA Conference,* Washington, D.C., 1990

[19] Nisbet, P.D., Odor, J.P., Loudon, I.R. (1988), "The CALL Centre Smart Wheelchair ", *Proc. 1st International Workshop on Robotic Applications in Medical and Health Care,* Ottawa, Canada, 1988, 9.1-9.10

[20] Pierrot F., E. Dombre, E. Decoulange, L. Urbain, P. Caron, S. Boudet, J. Gariepy, J.-L. Megnien, "Hippocrate: a safe robot arm for medical applications with force feedback", Medical Image Analysis (MedIA), *Special Issue on Medical Robotics and Computer Assisted Surgery*, Vol. 3, No.2, pp.1-16, 1999.

[21] Schilling K., "Sensors to Improve the Safety for Wheelchair Users", *Improving the Quality of Life for the European Citizen*, IOS Press 1998, pp.331-335

[22] Schraft R., C.Schaeffer, T.May, "Care-O-bot: The Concept of a System for Assisting Elderly or Disabled Persons in Home Environments", IEEE Conference 1998, pp.2476-2481

Chapter 5

Control Architectures of Intelligent Mobile Robots

by Spyros G. TZAFESTAS, Nikos I. KATEVAS

Mobile Robotics in Healthcare
N. Katevas (Ed.)
IOS Press, 2001

Chapter 5

Control Architectures of Intelligent Mobile Robots

Spyros G. TZAFESTAS, Nikos I. KATEVAS

1. Introduction

The aim of this chapter is to provide an introduction to the control architectures of *intelligent mobile robots* (IMRs) accompanied by a few implementation examples. IMRs constitute a subclass of *intelligent autonomous systems* (IAS) which have attracted over the years a great attention throughout the world with many industrial and every-day human applications [45,50]. Currently the majority of working systems in practice have partial autonomy and a lot of effort is still devoted by research and development groups to further increase the level of autonomy. Compared with other types of robots, IMRs surely have a higher potential to replace the human in industrial and service applications (medical, domestic, etc.) due to their mobility, intelligence, manipulability and dexterity [48].

IMRs possess decision - making capabilities and use multi - sensory information about their internal state and workspace environment to generate and execute plans for performing difficult and complex tasks. System autonomy implies the ability of the robot to support the humans in their work as a human assistant does. To achieve this, the IMR needs an information processing system capable of detailing general task descriptions into sequences of primitive robot movements and handling unexpected uncertainties and / or faults, in addition to the required human-like sensoric and manipulating abilities. Especially in any service IMR system, the basic requirement is the integration of various sensors (vision, haptic, distance, force, etc.) as well as efficient actuators (like arms with dexterous end-effectors and grippers) [47]. In particular, visual sensors in the form of colour and grey scale cameras but also of range sensors are needed for segmentation of the global scene, for shape analysis and 3D shape reconstruction, and for the determination of the position and the size of a-priori unknown objects. Tactile (haptic, touch) sensors are needed for detecting and reacting on contacts and collisions with the environment. To optimize contact points and prevent slipping, IR-light barriers and touch sensors should be used. Dexterous object manipulation needs many degrees of freedom (at least six) for moving the end-effector and/or the grasped object to the desired (arbitrary) position in the IMR work space.

To construct a working-in-practice autonomous IMR, starting from the toy / research level, a modular approach should be followed independently of the particular control architecture that is adopted. Naturally, the basic steps of such a modular approach may be the following:

- Complex task definition.
- Complex task decomposition in simple (generic) tasks.
- Task solving components' development and implementation.
- Integration components' development and implementation.
- System integration.

The structure of the chapter is as follows.

Section 2 discusses the basic functions and the major perceptual tasks of IMRs. Section 3 presents the four classes of generic control IMR architectures, namely: hierarchical, nested, distributed, and behaviour-based architectures. Section 4 gives a short outline of three working IMR research prototypes which have been designed following the hierarchical and/or distributed/behaviour-based architectures, namely the KAMRO/KAMARA [30,21,29], ROMAN [16,15,19,14], and SENARIO [24-26] systems. Finally, Section 5 provides some concluding remarks on future prospects and directions for research.

2. Basic Functions of IMRs

The basic general functions of IMRs are the following :

- Cognition
- Perception
- Planning
- Control
- Sensing
- Actuation

These functions can be interliked in several organized ways depending on the particular architecture adopted and the actual requirements for control action of the IMR. A general architecture for this functional IMR organization is shown in Figure 1.

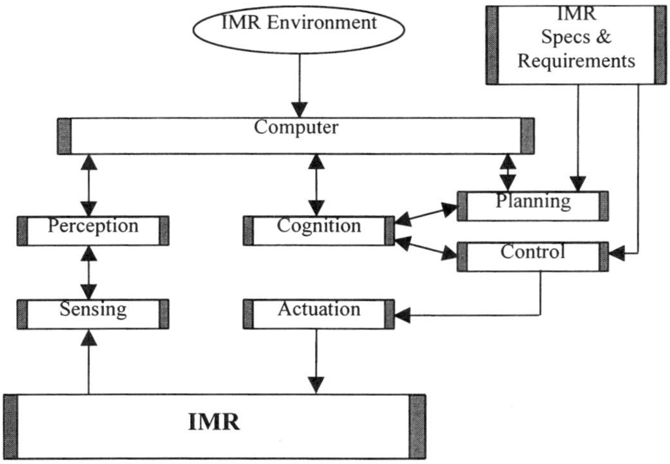

Figure 1. Abstract architecture of IMR organization

The computer of the IMR communicates with the system's environment (world) and performs the functions of *cognition, perception, planning* and *control*. It also sends information to, and receives information via the sensors from, the system under control (the IMR). The perception is needed for organizing a diversified information set from a multiplicity of sensors. A knowledge base and an inference engine are usually employed not only to interpret the results of perception but also to put them in perspective necessary for determining strategies and policies of future operation, as well as to provide all the required information for planning / control processes. The purpose of the planner / controller is to generate proper control sequences required for actuation. The control is executed via the actuation elements. A useful problem solving model used in IMRs is the blackboard model, which is of the distributed type and can integrate several representation schemes, not only complementary, but also as different approaches of the same data.

In IMRs there are four major perceptual tasks, namely : obstacle avoidance, path (road) following, goal identification, and landmark recognition for localization. All these tasks are nontrivial due to the complexity and inhospitability of the real world. Confusing factors are always present. Examples are shadows, reflections, occlusions, and specularities. Also, the complexity of data interpretation is in some way task-dependent. For example, an understanding of the meaning (the semantics) behind what the robot has sensed is in some cases (such as goal recognition and landmark localization) required. In other cases (e.g. obstacle avoidance), the interpretation is less demanding. One can easily verify that most perceptual tasks can be decomposed in two distinct stages : *recognition* and *tracking*. Recognition must rely heavily on expectations produced by internal models of landmarks and how specific sensors would image the object to be recognized. However, once recognized, the a priori models can be set aside in favor of using data from previous sensor data (e.g., earlier video images). Clearly, the goals of an intelligent entity (like the IMR) affect the way it perceives the world. The *action-perception cycle* (Figure 2) depicts the interplay between perception, cognition and motor action. Perception produces cognitive events which drive the motor system to interact with the world so as to generate new perceptual information. Obviously, only the perceptual information needed for conducting relevant motor behaviors must be extracted from the environment. Full-scale scene analysis is unnecessary. The plans (motivations) of an IMR should influence the way in which it perceives the world. Vice-versa the environmental perceptions afforded by the world can modify the plans of an intelligent agent (like an IMR).

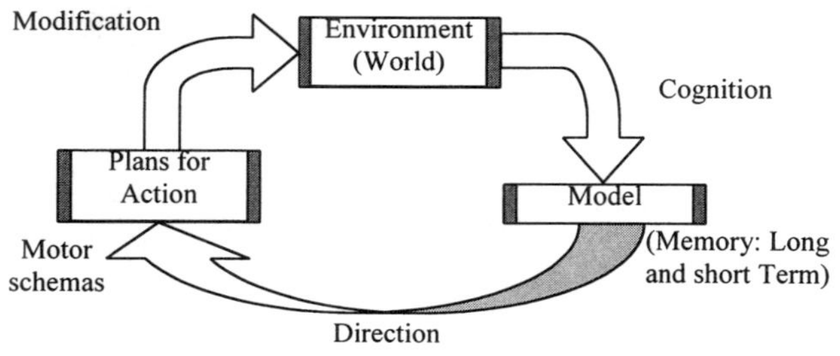

Figure 2. The action-perception cycle

3. Generic Control Architectures of IMRs

Mobile robots are classified as belonging to one of the following distinct classes:

- *Non autonomous mobile robots:* They need a central processor to perform off-line and on-line computations for them.
- *Semi-autonomous mobile robots:* They react independently to dynamic changes in the environment by calculating new path and trajectory segments on line.
- *Autonomous mobile robots:* They need a minimum amount of supervision by a coordinator which varies or they adopt a given plan action based on experience acquired during their entire life cycle.

Obviously, the amount of "intelligence" embodied in the IMR is increasing as we go from non-autonomous to semi-autonomous (partially autonomous) and fully autonomous robots.

Figure 3 illustrates pictorially the degree of autonomy of an IMR as it relates to the amount of knowledge it has for its environment [22].

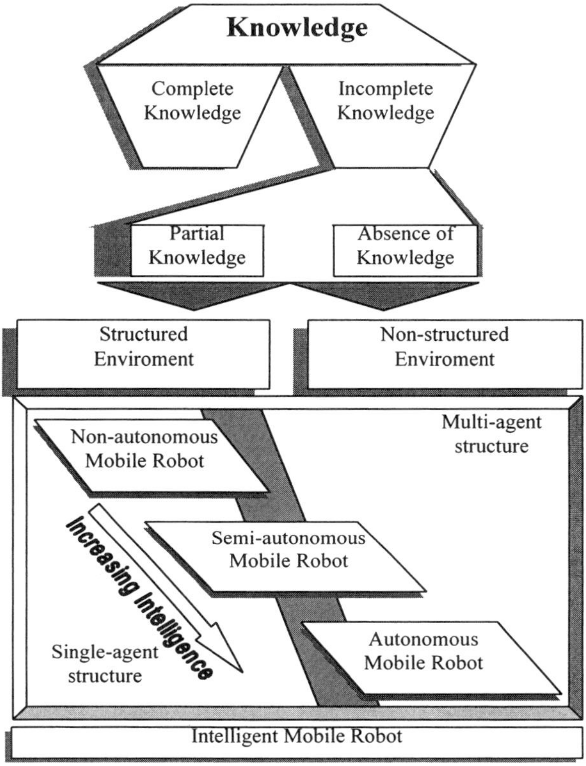

Figure 3. Autonomy degree versus the amount of knowledge in an IMR

When partial or no knowledge is available (non-structured environment) a multi agent structure which possesses no clear grouping of components is more suitable for developing plans and reacting to dynamic changes of a non-structured environment. All the computations must be carried out on-line, and this calls for more processing power and faster algorithms than in a structured environment, where only the operations in the execution stage have to be performed in real time.

Due to the complexity of the control problem of an IMR several organizational and implementation alternatives have been proposed over the years with various capabilities and advantages.

Among them, the following major generic *intelligent control architectures* (ICAs) of IMRs will be discussed here:

- Hierarchical ICA
- Nested ICA
- Distributed ICA
- Behaviour based ICAs

3.1 Hierarchical Intelligent Control Architecture

This architecture (Figure 4) involves three basic levels of control, namely [43,42,58,28]:

- Organization level
- Coordination level
- Execution level

each one of which may contain several layers.

The organization level implements the higher-level functions (e.g. learning, decision making) which imitate functions of human performance and can normally be represented and treated by artificial intelligence techniques.

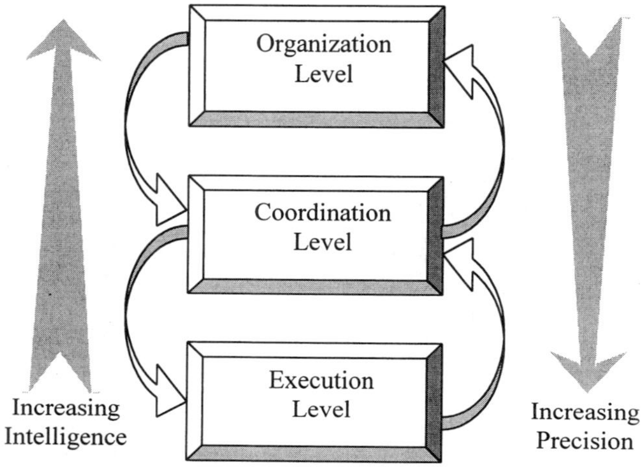

Figure 4. Hierarchical architecture of an IMR

This level receives and interprets feedback information from the lower levels, defines the planning/sequencing and decision making strategies to be executed in real time and processes large amounts of knowledge/information with little or no precision. Here long-term memory exchange is taking place.

The *coordination level* consists of several coordinators (each implemented by a piece of S/W or a dedicated microprocessor) which receive the task(s) from the organization level. All necessary details must be provided so that the chosen task's plan is successfully executed.

The *execution level* involves the actuators, the hardware controllers and the sensing devices (visual, sonar, etc.), and executes the action programs issued by the coordination level.

The control problem of an IMR system consists of two principal sub-problems:

- The logical or operational control sub-problem which deals with the coordination of events under the existence of ordering constraints on event sequences.
- The geometric and dynamic control sub-problem which deals with the determination of the geometric and dynamic parameters of motion such that the underlying geometric and dynamic constraints are satisfied at all times.

The various classes of formal models that are needed for the planning and control of the IMR are embedded in a suitable knowledge base such as the one shown in Figure 5. [22].

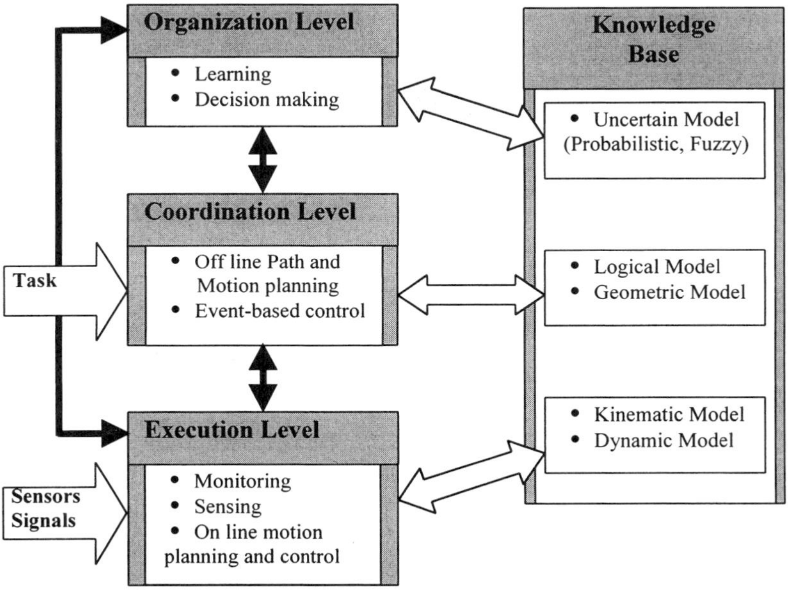

Figure 5. Knowledge base involving the formal models of an IMR

The learning, decision making and planning functions are implemented at the higher levels. Learning and self-planning procedures implemented in an interactive way can be employed to improve the performance of a system designed following this 3-level intelligent control architecture.

3.2 Nested Intelligent Control Architecture

The nested intelligent control architecture (NICA) also called "multiresolutional control architecture" (MCA) was first introduced in the area of computational mathematics as "domain decomposition or multi-grid method" [18,9]. Hierarchical aggregation of linear systems with multiple time scales was considered in [12] and provided a mathematical study of nested hierarchical Markov controllers. In the mobile robotics area it was used by Meystel in [32-34]. One of the common models for IMRs is the commonsense model: Planner-Navigator-Pilot-Execution Controller. The *planner* delivers a rough plan and performs a rough planning of the time-profiles of input variables which are supposed to ensure the desirable output time-profiles. The *navigator* computes a more precise trajectory of motion to be executed, and determines motion compensation and refinement of the initial plan, if required.

The *pilot* develops on-line tracking open-loop control taking into account the deviations from the expected situations that can be observed only in the immediate vicinity.

Finally, the *execution controller* executes the plans and compensations computed by the planner, the navigator and the pilot.

The multi-resolution 6-box (P,K,P/C,S,W,A) control architecture (three levels) is pictorially illustrated in Figure 6, where P stands for perception; K for knowledge representation, interpretation and processing; P/C for planning and control; A for a set of actuators; W for the world (process under control) and S for a set of sensors.

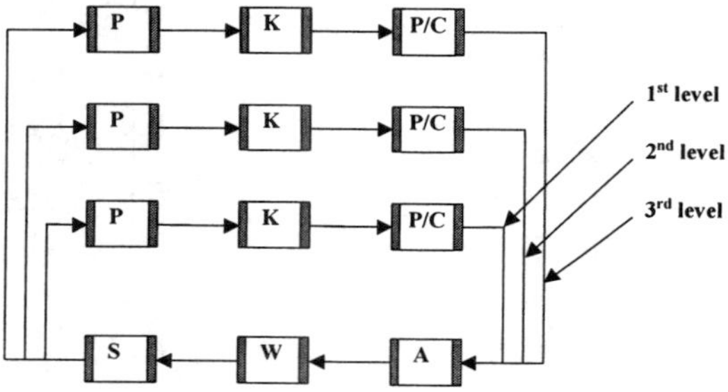

Figure 6. Three level multiresolution architecture (each level has its own feedback loop)

The fundamental properties of MCA are the following:

P1. Computational independence of the resolutional levels.
P2. Each resolution level represents a different domain of the overall system.
P3. Different resolution levels deal with different frequency bands within the overall system.
P4. Loops at different levels are 6-box diagrams nested in each other.
P5. The upper and lower parts of the loop correspond to each other.
P6. The system behaviour is the result of superposition of the behaviours generated by. the actions at each resolution level.
P7. The algorithms of behaviour generation are similar at all levels.
P8. The hierarchy of representation evolves from linguistic at the top to analytical at the bottom.
P9. The subsystems of the representation are relatively independent.

A different self-explanatory pictorial illustration of the multi-resolutional/nested ICA for a mobile robot system consisting of six levels is shown in Figure 7. The six nested hierarchical elements are: high-level planner, navigator, pilot, path monitor, controller, and low-level control system (sensors, actuators).

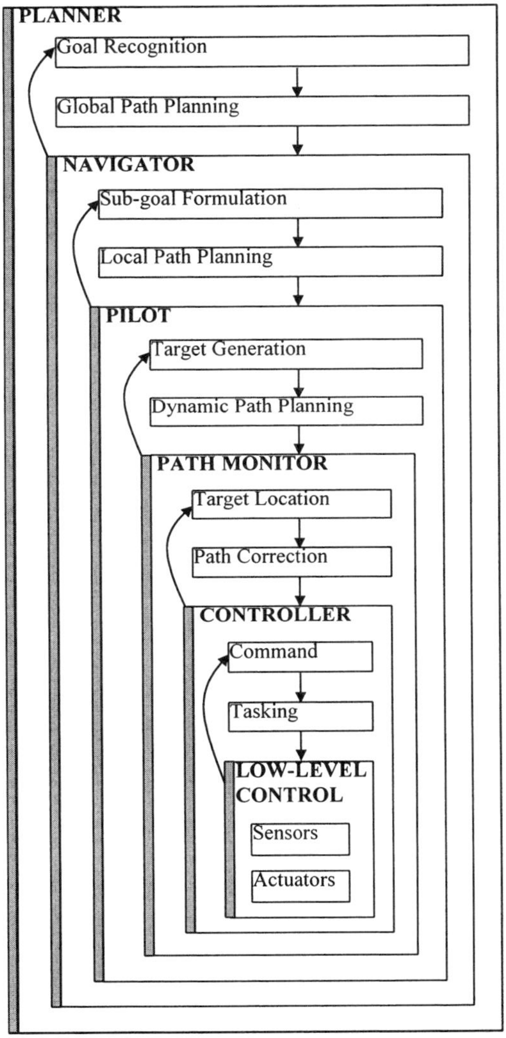

Figure 7. Six-level nested ICA

3.3 Distributed Intelligent Control Architecture

In general, complex systems that involve several executive subsystems (agents) are distinguished in three distinct types:

- *Centralized systems:* All decisions are made by a control mechanism and sent to the executive components.
- *Decentralized systems:* Each executive subsystem makes its own decisions and executes only these decisions.
- *Distributed systems:* Here, the decision is made through a negotiation among the executive subsystems and executed by them.

Using the concept of an *agent*, it is possible to describe and explain both the hierarchical and nested architectures. An agent consists of three parts (Figure 8):

- *Communicator* (for connecting the head to other agents on the same communication level or higher).
- *Head* (for planning and action selection).
- *Body* (for action execution).

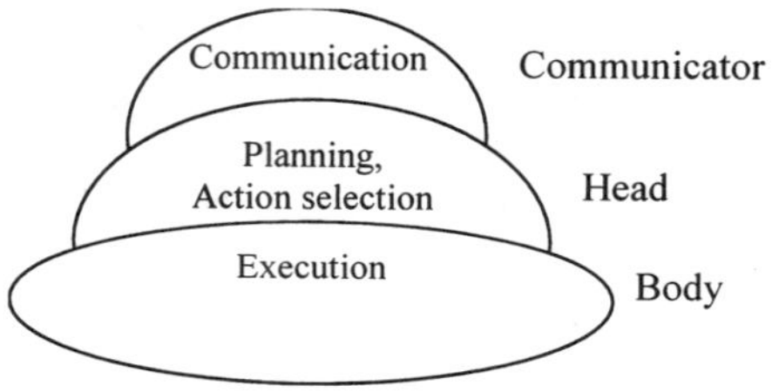

Figure 8. Pictorial representation of the elements of an agent

The planning and action components (heads of agents) as well as the overall agents belong to one of the three classes (types) mentioned before, i.e. [30]:

- *Centralized action selection:* The information is centrally processed by a central decision making component and transformed into action for the agent's body.
- *Decentralized action selection:* The information is processed independently by each decision making component and transformed locally in their own action decision for the agent's body (motor schema).
- *Distributed action selection:* The information is processed by several decision-making components, which communicate and negotiate to arrive at a decision. Then, the information is transformed locally and globally into an action for the agent's body.

From an execution-oriented view point, the above classification allows the description of available ICAs, and also the description of multi-agent systems in a way similar to single-agent systems.

3.4 Behaviour-Based Architectures

The concept of "agent" has contributed to the development of the so-called behaviour-based intelligent control architectures. Though considerably varied, these architectures possess the following common features:

- emphasis is on the importance of coupling sensing and action tightly.
- avoidance of representational symbolic knowledge.
- decomposition into contextually meaningful units (behaviours or situation-action points).

Two very popular behaviour-based architectures are the "subsumption architecture" [10] and the "motor schemas architecture" [5-7]. The subsumption architecture which is based on the *sense-plan-act* paradigm was firstly employed in the autonomous robot Shakey [37].

Subsumption Architecture

In the subsumption architecture the tasks-achieving behaviours are represented as separate layers. Individual layers work on individual goals concurrently and asynchronously. An *augmented finite state machine* (AFSM) is used to represent each behaviour at the lowest level (Figure 9).The AFSM encapsulates a particular behavioural transformation function. Stimulus or response signals can be suppressed or inhibited by other active behaviours. A reset input is used to return the behaviour to its start conditions. Each AFSM performs an action and is responsible for its own perception of the world [5].

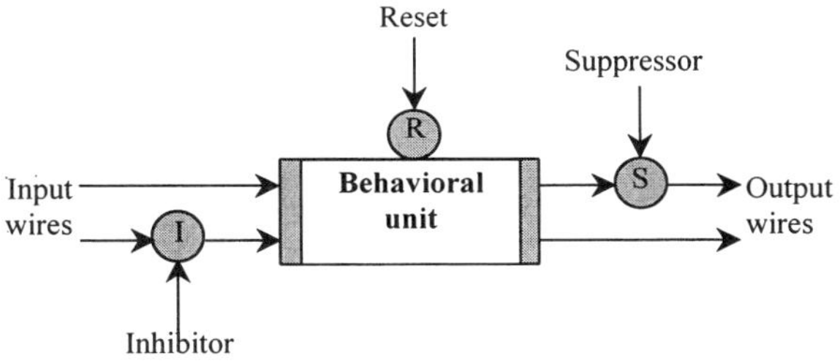

Figure 9. AFSM employed in the subsumption architecture

The reactions are organized in a hierarchy of levels where each level corresponds to a set of possible behaviours. Under the influence of an internal or external stimulation a particular behaviour is required. Then it emits an influx towards the inferior level. At this level, another behaviour arises as a result of simultaneous action of the influx and other stimuli. The process continues until terminal behaviours are activated. The name subsumption arises from the co-ordination process used between the layered behaviours within the architecture. Complex actions subsume simple behaviours. A priority hierarchy fixes the topology. The lower levels in the architecture have no awareness of higher levels. This allows the use of incremental design [44]. That is, higher-level competencies are added on top of an already working control system without any modification of those lower levels. The world itself serves as the primary medium of communication. Actions taken by one behavior result in changes within the world of the robot's relationship to it. New perceptions of those changes communicate those results to the other behaviours.

Motor Schemas Architecture

This architecture was more strongly motivated by biological sciences and uses the theory of schemas, the origin of which goes back to the 18th century (Immanuel Kant). Schemas represent a means by which understanding is able to categorize sensory perception in the process of realising knowledge of experience. The first applications of schema theory include an effort to explain postural control mechanisms in humans, a mechanism for expressing models of memory and learning, a cognitive model of interaction between motor behaviors in the form of schemas interlocking with perception in the context of the perceptual cycle, and a cognitive model which employs contention-scheduling mechanisms as a means for cooperation and competition between behaviours [8,20,36,39,40].

From among the various definitions of the schema concept available in the literature we give here the following representative ones [5]:

- A pattern of action or a pattern for action [36]
- An adaptive controller which is based on an identification procedure for updating the representation of the object under control [3]
- A perceptual entity corresponding to a mental entity [40]
- A functional unit that receives special information, anticipates a possible perceptual content, and matches itself to the perceived information [27].

A convenient working definition is the following [5]: "*A schema is the fundamental entity of behaviour from which complex actions can be constructed, and which consists of the knowledge how to act or perceive, as well as the computational process by which it is enacted*".

Using schemas, robot behaviour can be encoded at a coarser granularity than neural networks while maintaining the features of concurrent cooperative-competitive control involved in neuroscientific models. More specifically, schema theory-based analysis and design of behaviour-based systems possesses the following capabilities:

- It can explain motor behaviour in terms of the concurrent control of several different activities.
- It can store both how to react and how to realise this reaction.
- It can be used as a distributed model of computation.
- It provides a language for connecting action and perception.
- It provides a learning approach via schema elicitation and schema tuning .
- It can explain the intelligence functions of robotic systems.

Motor schema behaviours are relatively large grain abstractions, which can be used in a wide class of cases. Typically, these behaviours have internal parameters which offer extra flexibility in their use. Associated with each motor schema there is an embedded perceptual schema which gives the world specific for that particular behavior and is capable of providing suitable stimuli. Perceptual schemas are defined in a recursive manner. Some examples of motor schemas are the following [5]:

- *Move ahead* (i.e. move in a particular direction).
- *Move to goal* (i.e. move towards a desired goal).
- *Avoid static obstacle* (i.e. move away from passive or non threatening navigational obstacles).
- *Escape* (i.e. move away from the projected intercept point between the robot and an approaching object).
- *Dock* (i.e. approach an object from a desired direction).
- *Avoid past* (i.e. move away from places visited in the past).

The typical design steps for creating a schema-based robot system are the following [4]:

- Represent the problem in terms of the motor behaviours required to achieve the goal(s).
- Decompose the motor behaviour to their most elementary level (in a way similar to biological systems whenever feasible).
- Formulate mathematical models that express the robot's reaction to perceived environmental events.
- Assess by simulation the performance of the behaviour under study in the desired environment.
- Specify the perceptual requirements needed to satisfy the inputs for each motor schema.
- Develop suitable perceptual algorithms for extracting the required data for each behaviour (via action-oriented perception, expectations, and focus-of-attention processes).
- Embody the designed control system into the robot hand.
- Evaluate the overall performance of the system.
- Iterate and modify / improve the behavioural issues as appropriate.

3.5 Other Architectures

Throughout the years a variety of specialised architectures have been used which however may be regarded as variants of the architectures described above.

The Reference Model Architecture

One of the earliest architectures is the so-called *Reference Model Architecture* (RMA) developed at NIST, which has the structure shown in Figure 10 and is suitable for modular expansion [1,2].

The control problem in RMA is decomposed in the following sub-problems:

- Task decomposition
- World modelling
- Sensory processing
- Value judgement

The various control elements are clustered into computational nodes arranged in hierarchical layers, each one of which has a particular function and a specific timing behaviour. The NIST paradigm has been refined many times. Starting with the cerebellar model in the 70's, it was evolved to the RCS-4 (Real-time Control System-4) in the 90's, and was applied to automated manufacturing systems, army field material handling systems, multiple underwater mobile robots, and telerobotic service systems. The main design issues addressed by RMA are the following:

- Real time task and software execution.
- Smart interface/communication methods.
- Information/knowledge base management.
- Optimized allocation of resources.

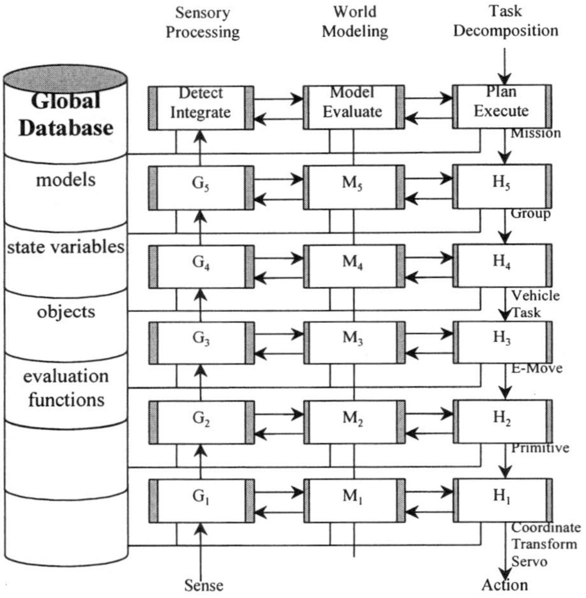

Figure 10. The NIST RMA hierarchical control architecture

The LAAS Architecture

The LAAS generic architecture is depicted in Figure 11 and is structured into three levels corresponding to two decisional levels above the functional level [17,38,11]. General criteria satisfied by this architecture are: reactivity, flexibility, reconfigurability, autonomy, and programmability. The two upper levels are designed following the supervisor/planner paradigm. The highest level employs a temporal planner and the second level receives tasks and transforms them into procedures composed by primitive actions and supervises the execution of these processes while reacting to asynchronous events. At this level, planning performs the refinement on the basis of the available knowledge about the task or the domain. The temporal planner (IxTeT) reasons about the symbolic or numerical relations, and produces the plan in the form of a partially ordered set of tasks in compatibility to the time constraints such that minimal and maximal bounds on the durations of the execution are defined and used for synchronization with external events.

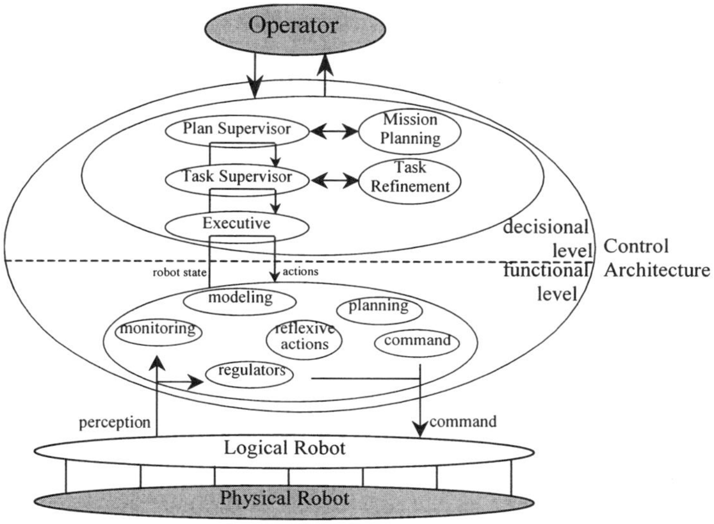

Figure 11. The LAAS hierarchical architecture

The task supervision and task refinement are integrated using a procedural reasoning system (that supports the interaction between decision and reaction) and the role of the execution level is purely reactive without any planning capability. The execution of actions is controlled according to pre-defined schemes selected by taking into account the context. A set of rules is used for the implementation which produces a program to search a decision tree in bounded time.

Other Behaviour-Based Architectures

Although a detailed description of behaviour-based architectures is outside the scope of this chapter, it may be helpful for the reader to list a few other architectures besides the "subsumption" and "schema" architectures.

DAMN architecture: This architecture: Distributed Architecture for Mobile Navigation [41] involves asynchronous behaviours each producing outputs as a collection of votes over a range of responses. These votes can be cast for each behaviour in several ways, e.g. by various statistical distributions over a repertory of responses. DAMN works following the multiple winner-take-all strategy in which the response(s) with the largest number of votes is (are) selected for adoption.

Action-Selection architecture: This architecture [31] employs a dynamic mechanism for behaviour selection and has some similarities with the "Motor schemas" architecture [5]. It does not use a predefined priority-based strategy (as in the subsumption architecture) but a set of competence modules (behaviours) that have corresponding activation levels which constitute the basis for run-time arbitration. The activation level for each competence module is influenced by the current state, higher-level goals, and inhibition from conflicting modules. The activation levels decay with time. The module with the highest activation level is selected for execution among all modules the preconditions of which are satisfied.

Other behaviour-based architectures include: the *circuit architecture,* (an early reactive architecture that uses the arbitration with abstraction coordination method) [23], the *colony architecture* [13] which uses simpler coordination strategies (i.e. suppression only) and allows a more flexible specification of behavioural relations, and the *skill network architecture* (an architecture originally developed for graphical animation rather than robotics) [60]. Currently this architecture is used to model not only graphical creatures' responses to their fictional environments but also their dynamics. It can work with a variety of computing elements such as sensing agents, skill agents, and goal agents.

4. Examples of IMR Prototypes and Control Architectures

The control architectures presented in Section 3 were adopted–in one or the other form–for designing and building several integrated research prototypes. The architecture most commonly used in the hierarchical ICA, of course with differences in the actual implementation of each hierarchical level [46,21]. Here three IMR examples will be briefly presented which will illustrate many of the concepts, issues and tools involved.

4.1 The KAMRO IMR/KAMARA Architecture

The KAMRO (Karlsruhe Autonomous Intelligent Mobile Robot) system is a mobile robot equipped with two PUMA-260 robots in a hanging configuration [21]. The overall system consists of three principal subsystems, namely the vehicle, the robots and the sensory system. The vehicle has four wheels of the MECANUM type allowing x-y motion and rotation on the spot (omnidirectional vehicle) [35,59]. The navigation of the IMR is performed via ultrasonic range finders and a vision system involving hand-eye cameras and one overhead camera. The original hierarchical control architecture [21,54] of the KAMRO system has been replaced by a distributed control architecture of the type described in Section 3.3. [30]. This architecture was named KAMARA (Karlsruhe Multi-Agent Robot Architecture) and is capable of overcoming coordination problems produced, for example, by the independent task execution of the two arms.

The original KAMRO agent control architecture is shown in Figure 12.

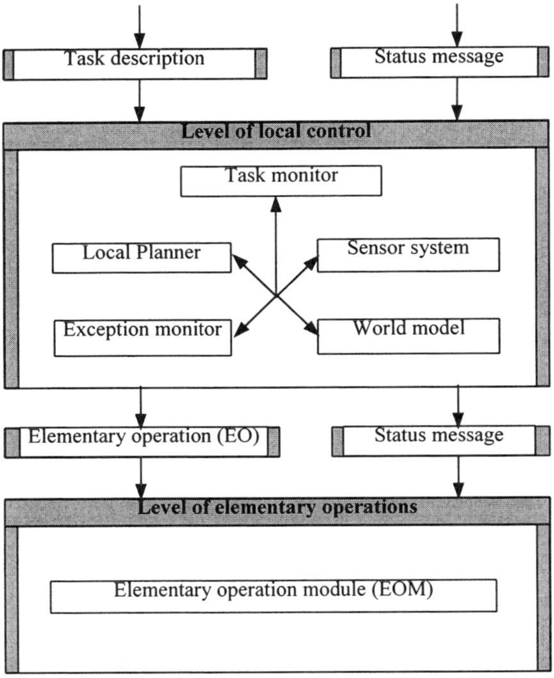

Figure 12. The KAMRO hierarchical agent control architecture

The task sequence (action plan) is derived from a computer-aided planning system [21] by decomposing the task-oriented instructions into sequences of elementary instructions. The cope with any erroneous situations that may occur, the execution of the action plan is adapted to the actual state of the world through sensor controlled plans and sensor guided actions [21]. Each active component (agent) is provided with a set of elementary operations (EO) which cannot be decomposed any further and are executed by elementary operation models (EOM). Each EOM is dedicated to a particular EO and comprises the expert knowledge needed to execute this EO. The EO specifies the desired goal, and the EOM determines how this goal should be actually achieved via complex sensor guided tasks and suitable reaction to unpredicted events within a certain repertory. The local planner handles the exceptions (errors) by modifying the initial plan on the basis of the sensory information received. The task monitor supervises and coordinates the activation of the overall system. The exception monitor is activated whenever an EOM cannot correctly execute an EO. The world model is actually a database in which all information about the agent(s) and the overall robotic system is stored. The navigation EOs are: MOVE, and DOCK/UNDOCK. The assembly EOs are: CALIBRATE, TRANSFER (gross motion of the end effector) and CONFIGURATE (manipulation of the angular position of the arm joints). The process and processor management is performed by the specialized operating system HEROS (Hierarchically

Extendable Real Time Operating System) which employs a message-passing mechanism. The task specification in the latest version of KAMRO is accomplished through a natural language system called KANTRA [29]. The user can tell the robot which action has to perform with which object, for example "Grasp the yellow screw driver". Here, perception and action are separated.

The communication mechanism used for all agent and for task distribution or task allocation is the so-called Blackboard (BB) mechanism [30,52]. Among the early BB-based systems it is useful to mention here the speech recognition system (Hearsay II) and the system HASP which was used for the interpretation of continuous sonar signals. A BB consists of two main parts (i) *knowledge sources* (KS) each one of which contains some part of the knowledge about the system (empirical, statistical, fuzzy etc.), and (ii) *control mechanism* which leaves the KSs to respond dynamically and opportunistically to the changes of the BB and are self activating. The communication and interaction of the KSs is possible only implicitly via the BB.

In the distributed KAMRO control system [30], the communication of each robot is the head of an agent, and so more than one robots may cooperate to perform complex tasks like carrying a large object or loaning one manipulator arm to a second KAMRO robot. (Figure 13)

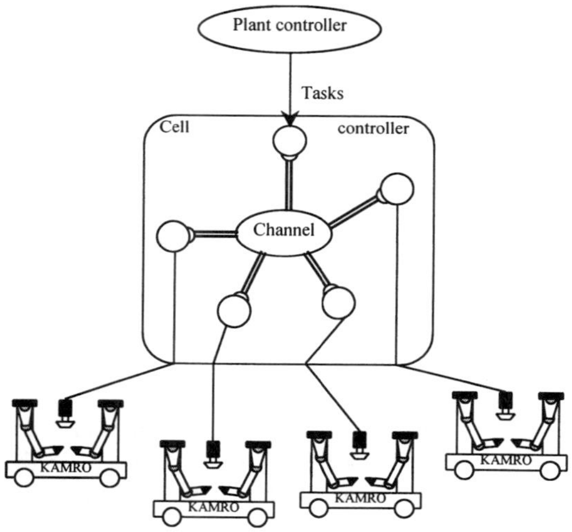

Figure 13. Distributed control of a family of KAMRO robots

Due to the distributed control architecture the following cooperation forms were implemented:

- Independent task execution.
- Asynchronous communication (teams).
- Synchronous communication (special agents).

The number or the type of agents in a team may change during the task execution, i.e. the agent teams are dynamic. For example to exchange an obstacle between the two arms of a KAMRO robot, the camera and an arm must form a team to perform the task. However, for a regrasping operation to change the gripping configuration of an object, the team must be formed by the two arms. In this case the communication between agents is asynchronous. But, when two arms grasp a large/heavy object by closing a kinematic chain, asynchronous communication is not sufficient. In this case the utilization of special executive agents with synchronous communication are needed [30].

In the KAMARA architecture the system agents perform the following operations:

- *Two-arm manipulator:* PICK and PLACE.
- *Manager:* Task decomposition into its executable parts.
- *Database:* Provides the agents with world state information.
- *Overhead camera:* Determines the position of obstacles in the work space.
- *Arm camera:* Determines exact relative object positions based on absolute position estimation.
- *State Controller:* It is responsible for the BB structure and the state of the other system components.

The KAMARA system uses a communication/cooperation mechanism that guarantees dead-lock freeness for the following dead-lock situations:

- Dead-locks caused by agent bodies/external resources.
- Dead-locks caused by special agents.
- Dead-locks caused by agent teams.

In KAMARA, a mission is appended to the mission set by the overhead camera requesting the blocking component to leave the scene. If the state controller finds that a mission cannot be realized by the system itself, it sends the mission to the planning component which invites other systems to be involved in the solution process.

4.2 The ROMAN IMR

The ROMAN service IMR was designed and built in the Technical University of Munich [16,15,19,14] and consists of the following components (Figure 14):

- *Mobile platform:* A 3-wheel (diameter 0.2m) omnidirectional platform (0.63m width × 0.64m depth × 1.85m height) equipped with a multi-sensoric system (a laser-based angle measurement system and an eye-safe laser beam for scanning the workspace in an horizontal plane and measuring the azimuth angle).
- *Robotic arm:* An anthropomorphic manipulator (max range 0.8m, max payload 1.5kg) for carrying out service tasks.
- *Task planner and coordinator:* The planner enables ROMAN to autonomously perform typical tasks such as finding its way to the goal position, opening the doors or handling the desired objects.
- *Vision system:* The camera is mounted on a tilt-unit to allow object recognition over the entire workspace. Two object recognition techniques are used to handle a variety

of objects in health care services (a feature based method for recognizing extended objects, and an appearance-based method for small-object recognition.

- *Human-robot interface (HRI):* For natural voice/speech based dialogue between the human (user) and the robot.

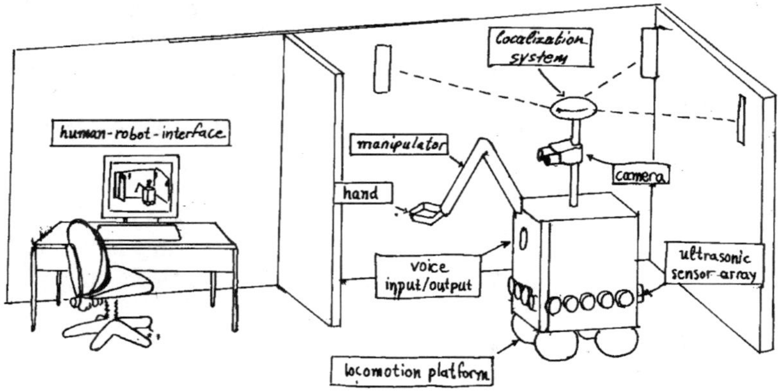

Figure 14. The ROMAN IMR (on-board components and HRI)

The navigation of the platform is helped via a localization system that provides platform position and orientation data in real time. An ultrasonic sensor array helps to detect any obstacle(s) and works with the motion platform controller to avoid collisions with the obstacles.

The 6-DOF robotic arm of ROMAN is suitable for manipulating/handling light-weight geometrically simple objects (e.g. dishes, glasses, bottles, journals, etc.). The control, strategy for motion coordination of the robotic arm and the mobile platform of ROMAN is shown in Figure 15.

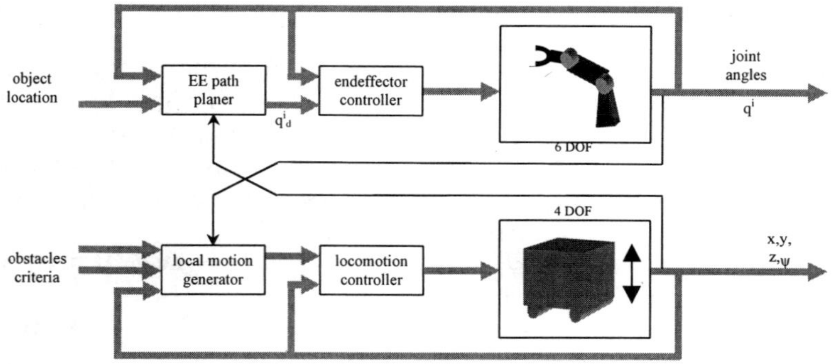

Figure 15. Coordinated control loops of ROMAN's platform and arm

The overall processing and control architecture of ROMAN is shown in Figure 16, and is implemented on a VME bus-based multiprocessor system, communicating with the outside world via an Ethernet link (10 M bit/sec).

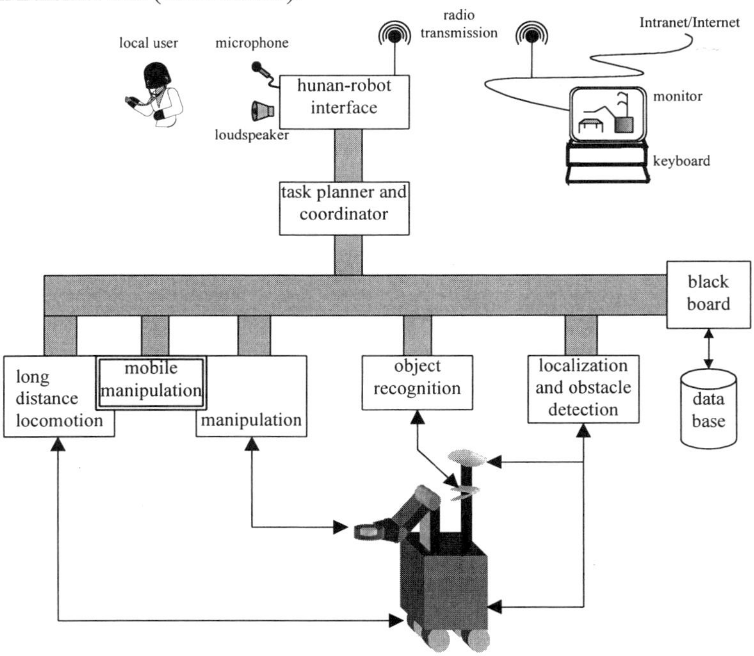

Figure 16. ROMAN's hierarchical processing and control architecture

A multi-modal human-robot interface (HRI) is used for commanding and monitoring task specification and task execution (Figure 17). It involves a *command generator* (to convert user inputs into robot commands), and a *knowledge base* (to store operator knowledge and environmental information).

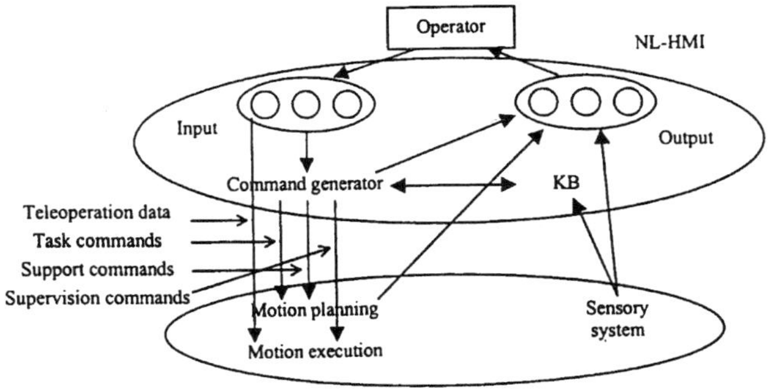

Figure 17. Structure of ROMAN's multi-modal natural language HRI (NL-HRI)

The commands are distinguished according to level of abstraction in the following types:

- *Task commands:* Service task-specific actions compatible with ROMAN's anatomical and planning capabilities.
- *Support commands:* Operator's responses to requests from motion planning during task execution.
- *Supervision commands:* They are initiated by the operator during task execution and interrupt immediately the operation currently performed. A special command language and command interpretation are used [16].

When receiving a natural language command from the user, ROMAN's interface Converts the voice signal into an executable robot command, and splits up it via the task planner into a sequence of typical subtasks such as "open door", "pass door", or "travel along corridor", etc. These typical tasks are then executed by either the expert for long distance (e.g. room to room) or by the mobile manipulation expert. The task planner also coordinates the experts during task execution (Figure 16). For example, during the "open door" task execution, the object recognition expert is connected with the expert for mobile manipulation to locate the door handle.

Examples of how ROMAN works to execute typical service commands are the following [14,15]:

Example of the Command "*Clean the table*"

Since the data base involves more than one table, ROMAN asks which table is to be cleaned. After the specification of the desired table by the user (via natural language or mouse clicking), ROMAN decomposes the command into a sequence of subtasks, plans a suitable path to the table, and starts moving. If a closed door exists on its way, ROMAN opens it (via a standard opening maneuver of its manipulator) and passes it. If an obstacle is encountered on its way, ROMAN slows down and performs an obstacle avoidance maneuver, if possible. Upon arriving at the desired table, ROMAN looks for specified objects. In Figure 18, a bottle exists on the table which is grasped by ROMAN and put into the refrigerator.

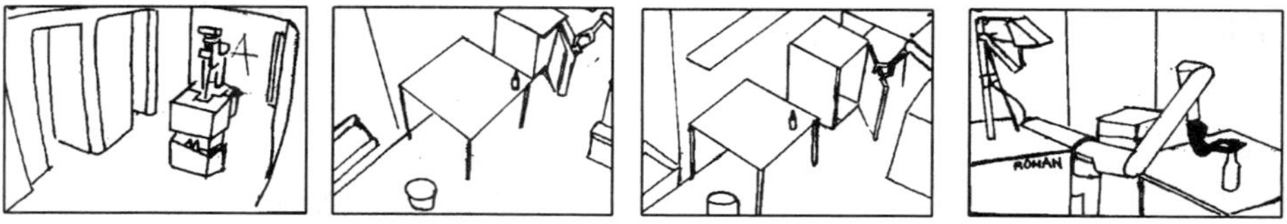

(a) (b) (c) (d)

Figure 18. ROMAN at work: (a) passing a corridor, (b) opening a refrigerator, (c) virtual work space, (d) grasping a bottle from the table

Example of the Command "*Bring me the box*"

Since the object location is not given, ROMAN asks the operator to specify it. After receiving the object location ROMAN generates a locomotion path and approaches the goal with the help of the self-localization unit. If an obstacle is detected on its way, ROMAN performs an evasive maneuver or asks the operator to clean the way. When approaching a door, ROMAN works as before. That is, if the door is closed, ROMAN opens it and continues moving to approach the drawer. Then ROMAN determines the drawer's position (via the object recognition unit), opens the drawer, takes out the box, carries the box back, and hands it to the user.

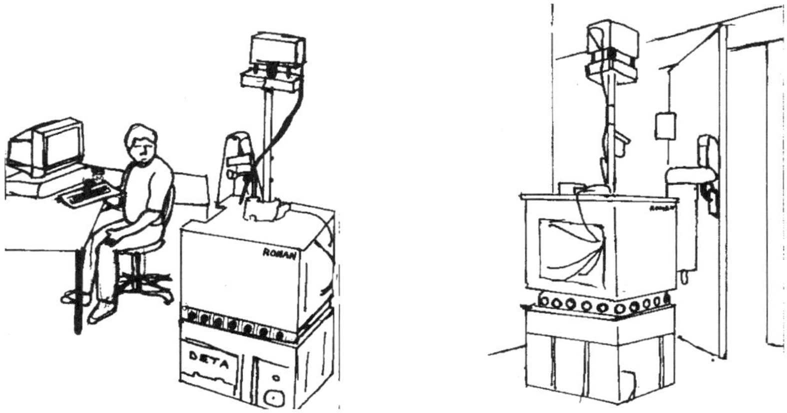

Figure 19. ROMAN at work: (a) user at HRI and ROMAN, (b) door opening

4.3 The SENARIO IMR Wheelchair

This IMR wheelchair prototype (Figure 20) was developed by a Consortium within the frame of the EU project SENARIO: Sensor-Aided Intelligent Navigation System for Powered Wheelchairs [25,26].

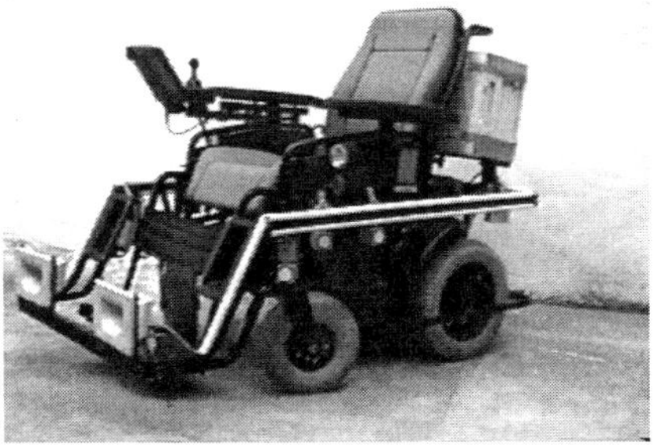

Figure 20. The SENARIO wheelchair IMR

The architecture of the SENARIO IMR is shown in Figure 21. Two functional alternatives are possible in SENARIO: (i) *Semi-autonomous*, and (ii) *Fully autonomous*.

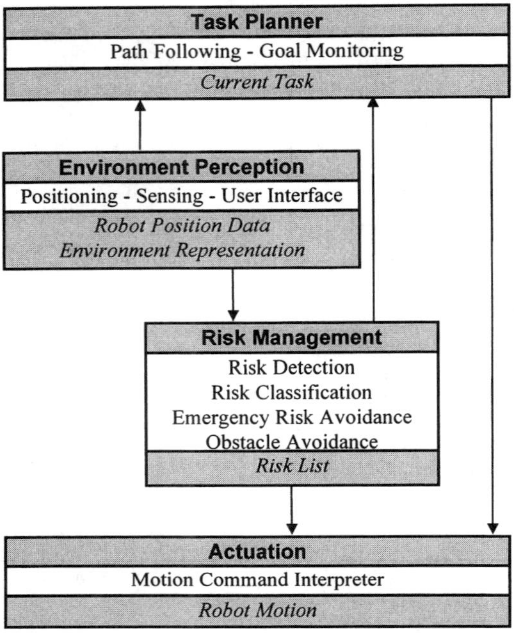

Figure 21. The SENARIO virtually centralized hierarchical control architecture

The autonomous behavior actions are divided into the following four processes shown in Figure 21:

- *Task planning,* which schedules the execution of all the other processes and is responsible for overall system control. The planning, path following, and goal monitoring procedures reside in the task planner. Task planning is on the top of the control hierarchy of the robot.
- *Environment Perception,* where a set of sensors is used to track the interactions of the robot with its environment. Sensor data processing, environment features extraction, and positioning, as well as user input, are grouped together as environment perception processes.
- *Risk Management,* which is responsible for both risk detection and avoidance. This process uses the output of environment perception to detect potential risks and determine their importance. It then computes the necessary sequence of actions for risk avoidance.
- *Actuation,* which handles the interface with the robot actuators.

This organization is an instance of a *centralized control scheme,* because Task Planning assumes the responsibility for the coordination of all the other processes in the system *(organization level).* However, some of the processes can override Task Planning and can communicate with each other directly, in cases of emergency. This option offers a distributed alternative to the centralization organisation. This hybrid solution is called *virtually centralized control* [24]. Virtually centralized control combines the reactivity of the distributed approach, along with the high-level control features of the centralized one.

In *Semi-Autonomous* mode, the system accepts commands to move on a direction, or to take an action (e.g., go ahead, tern left, stop, etc.) The system realizes the instructed action, while preventing risk conditions and avoiding obstacles during execution. Each time a risk is detected, SENARIO informs the user and takes appropriate corrective measures to preserve safety and continues with the execution of the instruction. In Semi-Autonomous mode, the user can override system actions, e.g., approach closer to a wall than the system's alarm distance. In these cases the system applies minimum speed limit in all instructed commands. In any case, if SENARIO detects an emergency situation, it stops moving and asks for user instruction to recover. So, the responsibility of actions is shared between the system and the user. This mode requires *Risk Detection* and *Risk Avoidance* functionality.

Fully Autonomous mode is a superset of Semi-Autonomous mode. The system accepts all the commands of Semi-Autonomous mode, along with "go to goal" commands. For example, the user can issue commands such as "go to living room". In this case, the system locates itself and then the target position in the environment map. It then plans and executes a path to the specified destination, avoiding all obstacles and risks on the way. During goal execution the user can interfere with the system, as in Semi-Autonomous mode, or he/she can specify a new destination at any point of the goals set. In this mode, the system takes full responsibility for execution. Full autonomy requires *Path Planning,* along with *Risk Detection* and *Risk Avoidance* functionality.

Each process of the system consists of a series of executive tasks. These are specialized procedures computing the parameters that characterize each process. In particular the task planner monitors the overall system functionality through the *Path Following* and *Goal Monitoring* tasks. The Task Planner computes the *current task* of the robot based on the Risk Management and Environment Perception outputs. Environment Perception consists of the *Positioning, Sensing,* and *User Interfacing* executive tasks. Similarly, Risk Management is split into *Risk Detection, Risk Classification, Emergency Risk Avoidance,* and *Obstacle Avoidance* tasks.

The Positioning task is responsible for reporting the robot's position, whenever it is asked to report, while running individually in its loop. As a task belonging to Environment Perception, it employs sensors and processes their information. We refer to the output of this task as the *position estimation* of the robot or, equivalently, as the *robot position data.*

Supplementary to the action of Positioning is the Sensing task. Both tasks employ sensors, and occasionally, share the same environmental information. We refer to the output of the sensing task as the *environment representation.* SENARIO supports multiple environment representations ranging from simple combinations of sensor data to occupancy grid representations for the environment.

Risk Detection has the responsibility to detect both *external risks* threatening the robot and originating from the environment and *risks internal* to the control system, such as malfunctions. The detection and reaction methods to these risks are different. The former, allows the subsequent use of Risk Classification, while the latter is implemented by low-level, robust, reliable and fast components, that do not require additional processing and that directly react on the actuators through emergency lines.

Risk Classification uses a default set of criteria for classifying risks according to their emergency. All the risks identified during the detection process the classified, according to the criteria used in the risk classification task. The outcome of these tasks is a *risk list* sorted in decreasing order of emergency. This risk list is further processed, either by Task Planning, or by Risk Avoidance (emergency risk avoidance task), or directly by the Actuation processes, thus supporting the virtually centralized control scheme specified above.

Obstacle Avoidance accepts input from three processes: Environment Perception (positioning-position estimation, and sensing-environment representation), Risk Detection (risk classification-risk list) and Task Planning (current target position or direction).

The task needs only one of the three input sources in order to maintain reliable operation: the environment representation. Any additional information is affecting the robot route according to the needs of either task planning or risk detection with varying priority. This scheme is another instance of virtually centralized control, due to the fact that either Risk Avoidance or Task Planning has absolute control of the system, but there is a *supervised distribution of control* [24] among the subsystems based on dynamic priority ordering.

Summarizing the interactions between Risk Detection and Risk Avoidance, the difference between emergency risk avoidance and obstacle avoidance tasks should be noticed. Emergency risk avoidance is triggered by an emergency risk situation (i.e., a risk with a highest emergency classification in the risk list), while obstacle avoidance covers the rest of the cases. Obstacle Avoidance uses a local path planning module.

Actuation realizes the commands of the rest of the supervised distributed control scheme described above. It consists of a Motion Command Interpreter task, which receives commands by the Risk Management and Task Planner tasks in a common format, and translates these instructions into motion commands for the actuators. The output of the Actuation task is identical to the output of the overall system and is referred to as the *Robot Motion.*

Implementation

SENARIO was implemented and tested on the wheelchair of Figure 20, a commercial powered wheelchair. In the following, the configuration used for testing, and the results obtained are described.

Sensing Task: The Sensing task uses a combination of sensing principles (ultrasound, infrared light, etc.). The wheelchair is equipped with proximity (ultrasonic) and positioning (encoders-infrared scanners) sensors. A minimum number of sensors was used to achieve the required functionality in order to keep the tradeoff between functionality and cost in balance. Specifically, there are thirteen ultrasonic sensors in total, supplied by Microsonic GmbH - Dortmund. The ultrasonic sensors are divided into two clusters: navigation and protection.

The difference in the two sensors' clusters is that protection sensors supply human protection functionality, working in fail-safe mode. Both protection and navigation sensors cover a range of 250cm, while the robot dimensions are 132cm in length and 82cm in width. The ultrasonics sensors are placed on the robot as shown in Figure 22. The letter "n" denotes the navigation sensors, while "p" denotes the protection ones. The angular range of each sensor is indicated by the corresponding letters at the end of the range arrows.

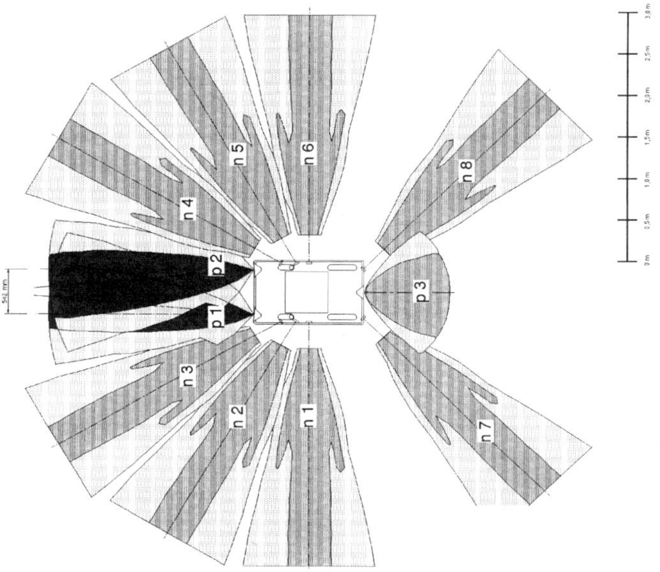

Figure 22. Field of view of navigation and protection ultrasonic sensors

Man-Machine Interface: The user interface supports speech recognition using an automatic speech recognition module. The module can record and interpret user commands, providing the appropriate control signals to the Task Planner. The emphasis is on user dependent speech recognition, to avoid accidental command initiation, due to other people talking nearby. During this phase, the speech recognition unit maps the acoustic signal (voiceprints) in its input, to a set of commands for the Actuation onto the range finder position in less than one minute.

The system was tested in several environments with complexity below and above average, involving points in adjacent rooms acting in real time, and showed a successful performance. All tests were performed with an average speed of 0.2m/sec.

A representative set of actions of the SENARIO system is shown in Figure 23.

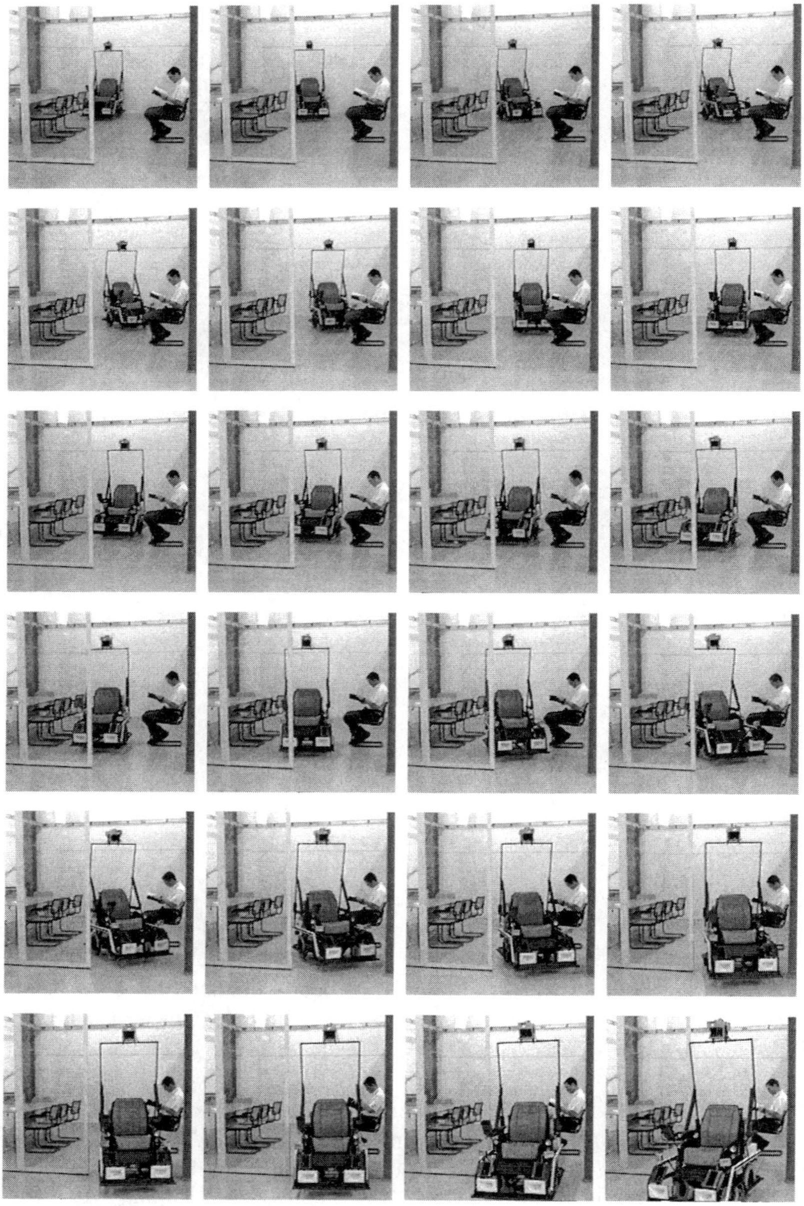

Figure 23. The SENARIO robotic wheelchair at work: From Start position, avoiding furniture on the right, avoiding the person seating on the chair on the left, locating the door besides the glass wall, passing through the door, and finally existing the room

Mobile Robotics in Healthcare, N.Katevas (Ed.)

5. Conclusions

This chapter was devoted to the basic IMR area of control architectures. Over the history of intelligent robotic systems, in particular mobile robotic systems, a number of architectures have been developed and implemented. Here, we have classified them in some major categories and presented their main characteristic features. In all cases, the functions of cognition, perception, planning, sensing, actuation and control are accommodated in one or the other way actually implementing the action-perception cycle. It was explained how the degree of autonomy of IMRs relates to the available and used amount of knowledge about the robotic environment.

The classification of IMR architectures in hierarchical, nested, distributed and behavior-based covers all systems available in the literature and built by various groups, with the last category overlapping and crossing all the others. The concept of agent as used in IMRs was briefly discussed. The agent concept plays a predominant role in the distributed behavior-based control architectures.

Three representative IMR research prototypes have been discussed in this chapter, which illustrate many of the issues involved and show three different philosophies of design. These prototypes, and many others not presented here for lack of space, prove that with the methodologies and technologies currently available it is possible to construct semi-autonomous/autonomous mobile robots equipped with robotic arms/manipulators which are able to perform difficult human like tasks for service, industrial and domestic applications.

However, much room for further work and developments exist for the following issues:

- Reduce command to action time (e.g. faster task/path planning and inverse kinematics/dynamics algorithms are needed).
- Cover more practical cases of environmental uncertainties (e.g. rapidly moving obstacles) and risks.
- Embed in IMR systems more robust and fault tolerant control/computing algorithms, hardware and software.
- Design mobile vehicles/platforms with more flexible motion/maneuvering capabilities (e.g. more work on specialized wheels with high maneuverability/stability is needed).
- Design smart user-robot interfaces suitable for special type of users (e.g. in wheelchair IMRs, the user has disabilities of various types and degrees).
- Last but not least, work is needed for designing fail-safe multi-mobile robot systems for several types of industrial and service operations.

6. References

[1] Albus J. and Quintero R., "Towards a Reference Model Architecture for Real-Time Intelligent Control Systems (ARTICS)", *Robotics and Manufacturing (ASME)*, 1990, New York, Vol. 3.

[2] Albus J., "System Description and Design Architecture for Multiple Autonomous Undersea Vehicles", *NIST Tech. Note 1251*, Washington, DC, Sept. 1988.
[3] Arbib M.A., "Perceptual Structures and Distributed Motor Control", Handbook of Physiology - The Nervous System II: Motor Control, Brooks V.B. (ed.), American Physiological Society, Bethesda, MD, 1981, pp. 1449-1480.
[4] Arbib M.A., "Schema Theory", The Encyclop. of Artificial Intelligence, S. Sharipo (ed.), Wiley, New York 1992, pp. 1427-1443.
[5] Arkin R.C., "Behavior-Based Robotics", The MIT Press, Cambridge, (Mass), London 1998.
[6] Arkin R.C., "Cooperation without Communication: Multi-Agent Schema Based Robot Navigation", *J. of Robotic Systems*, 1992, Vol. 9, No. 2, pp. 351-364.
[7] Arkin R.C., "Motor Schema-Based Mobile Robot Navigation", *Int. J. of Robotics Research*, 1989, Vol. 8, No. 4, pp. 92-112.
[8] Bartlett F.C., "Remembering: A Study in Experimental and Social Psychology", London, Cambridge University Press, 1932.
[9] Brandt, Ron D. and Amit D., "Multi-Level Approaches to Discrete States and Stochastic Problems", *Multigrid Methods II* (LNM 1228), Hackbush W. and Trottenberg U. (eds.), Springer-Verlag, Berlin 1986.
[10] Brooks R., "Intelligence Without Reason", *AI Memo* No. 1293, MIT, AI Lab., 1991.
[11] Chatila R., Alami R. and Haruelle H., "Integrated Planning and Execution Control of Autonomous Robot Actions", *Proc. IEEE Int. Conf. on Robotics and Automation (ICRA '92)*, Nice, France 1992.
[12] Coderch M., Willsky A., Sastry S. and Castanon D., "Hierarchical Aggregation of Linear Systems with Multiple Time Scales", *IEEE Trans. on Automatic Control*, 1983, Vol. AC-28, No. 11, pp. 1017-1029.
[13] Connel J., "A Colony Architecture for an Artificial Creature", Tech. Report No. 1151, AI Lab., MIT, August 1989.
[14] Ettelt, Furtwängler R., Hanebeck U.D. and Schmidt G., "Design Issues of a Semi-Autonomous Robotic Assistant for the Health Care Environment", *J. Intell. & Robotic Systems*, 1998, Vol. 22, No. 3-4, pp. 191-209.
[15] Fischer and Schmidt G., "Multi-Modal Human-Robot Interface for Interaction with a Remotely Operating Mobile Service Robot", *Proc. 6th Intl. Workshop on Robotics in Alpe-Adria-Danube Region (RAAD '97)*, Cassino, Italy 1997, pp. 559-564; Also: *Advanced Robotics*, 1998, Vol. 12, No. 4, pp. 397-409.
[16] Fischer, Buss M. and Schmidt G., "Hierarchical Supervisory Control of Service Robot Using Human-Robot Interface", *Proc. Intl. Conf. on Intelligent Robots and Systems (IROS '96)*, Osaka, Japan 1996, pp. 1408-1416.
[17] Giralt G., Chatila R. and Vaisset M., "An Integrated Navigation and Motion Control System for Autonomous Multisensory Mobile Robots", *Proc. First Intl. Symp. on Robotics Research*, Brady M. and Paul R. (eds.), MIT, Cambridge, Mass., 1983.
[18] Hackbush W., *Multi-grid Methods and Applications*, Springer-Verlag, Berlin 1982.
[19] Hanebeck U.D. and Schmidt G., "A New High Performance Multisonar System for Fast Mobile Robot Applications", *Proc. Intelligent Robots and Systems (IROS '94)*, Elsevier Science, Amsterdam 1995, pp. 1-14.

[20] Head H. and Holmes G., "Sensory Disturbances from Cerebral Lesions", *Brain*, 1911, Vol. 34, pp. 102.

[21] Hörmann, Huggel Th. and Meier W., "A Concept for an Intelligent and Fault-Tolerant Robot System", *J. Intell. & Robotic Systems*, 1988, Vol. 1, No. 3, pp. 259-286.

[22] Jacak W., *Intelligent Robotic Systems: Design, Planning and Control*, Kluwer/Plenum, New York/Boston, 1999.

[23] Kaelbling L. and Rosenschein S.," Action and Planning in Embedded Agents", In: Maes P. (ed.), *Designing Autonomous Agents*, MIT Press, Cambridge, Mass., 1991, pp. 35-48.

[24] Katevas N. and Tzafestas S.G., "Analysis of the Risk Detection and Avoidance Architecture for Indoor Autonomous Mobile Robots", *Proc. First ECPD International Conference on Advanced Robotics and Intelligent Automation*, Athens, Greece, 1995, pp. 464-470.

[25] Katevas N. et al., "SENARIO - The Autonomous Mobile Robotics Technology for the Locomotion Handicap: Operational & Technical Issues", *Proc. 2nd TIDE Congress: The European Context for Assistive Technology*, Paris, France, IOS Press 1995, pp. 371-374.

[26] Katevas N.I., Sgouros N.-M., Tzafestas S.G., Papakonstantinou G., Beatie G., Bishop P., Tsanakas P., and Koutsouris D.G., "The Autonomous Mobile Robot Senario: A Sensor-Aided Intelligent Navigation System for Powered Wheelchairs", *IEEE Robotics and Automation Magaz.*, 1997, Vol. 4, No. 4, pp. 60-70.

[27] Koy-Oberthur R., "Perception by Sensorimotor Coordination in Sensory Substitution for the Blind", Visuomotor Coordination: Amphibians, Comparisons, Models and Robots (eds.) Ewert J.P. and Arbib Plenum M.A., New York 1989, pp. 397-418.

[28] Kusiak, *Intelligent Manufacturing Systems*, Prentice Hall, 1990.

[29] Laengle T., Lueth T., Hezzog G., Stopp E. and Kamstrup G., "KANTRA: A Natural Language Interface for Intelligent Robots", Intelligent Autonomous Systems IAS-4, IOS Press, 1995, pp. 365-372.

[30] Laengle T., Lueth T.C., Rembold U. and Woern H., "A Distributed Control Architecture for Autonomous Mobile Robots: Implementation of the Karlsruhe Multi-Agent Robot Architecture", *Advanced Robotics*, 1998, Vol. 12, No. 4, pp. 411-431.

[31] Maes P., "The Dynamics of Action Selection", *Proc. 11th Int. Joint Conf. on Artificial Intelligence (IJCAI '89)*, Detroit, MI, 1989, pp. 991-997.

[32] Meystel (ed.), "Intelligent Control in Robotics" (Special Issue), *J. Intell. & Robotic Systems*, 1989, Vol. 2, No. 2-3.

[33] Meystel, "Autonomous Mobile Robots: Vehicles with Cognitive Control", *World Scientific*, Singapore, 1991.

[34] Meystel, "Cognitive Controller for Autonomous Systems", *IEEE Workshop on Intelligent Control*, RPI, Troy, New York 1985.

[35] Muir P.F. and Neuman C.P., "Kinematic Modeling for Feeding Control of an Omnidirectional Wheeled Mobile Robot", *Proc. Intl. Conf. on Robotics and Automation (ICRA '87)*, 1987, pp. 1772-1778.

[36] Neisser U., *Cognition and Reality: Principles and Implications of Cognitive Psychology*, W.H. Freeman, San Francisco 1976.

[37] Nilsson N., "Shakey the Robot", *Tech. Note 323*, AI Center, SRI International, Menlo Park, CA 1984.

[38] Noreils F. and Chatila R., "Plan Execution Monitoring and Control Architecture for Mobile Robots", *IEEE Trans. Robotics and Automation,* 1995, Vol. 11, No. 2, pp. 255-266.

[39] Norman D. and Shallice T., "Attention to Action: Willed and Automatic Control of Behavior", *Consciousness and Self-Regulation: Advances in Research and Theory*, Vol. 4, R. Davidson, G. Schwartz and D. Shapiro(eds.), Plenum Press, New York, 1986, pp. 1-17.

[40] Piaget J., *Biology and Knowledge: An Essay on the Relations Between Organic Regulations and Cognitive Processes*, Univ. of Chicago Press 1971.

[41] Rosenblatt J. and Payton D., "A Fine-Grained Alternative to the subsumption Architecture for Mobile Robot Control", *Proc. Int. Joint Conf. on Neural Networks*, June 1989, pp. 317-323.

[42] Saridis G.N., "Analytic Formulation of the IPDI for Intelligent Machines", *Automatica*, 1989, Vol. 25, No. 3, pp. 461-467.

[43] Saridis G.N., "Intelligent Robotic Control", *IEEE Trans Autom. Control*, May 1983, Vol. AC-28, No. 5

[44] Tzafestas E.S. , Tzafestas S.G., "Incremental Design of a Flexible Robotic Assembly Cell Using Reactive Robots", Artificial Intelligence in Industrial Decision Making, Control and Automation, Tzafestas S.G. and Verbruggen H.B. (eds.), Kluwer, Dordrecht / Boston, 1995, pp. 555-571.

[45] Tzafestas S.G. (ed.), Advances in Intelligent Autonomous Systems, Kluwer, Dordrecht/Boston 1999.

[46] Tzafestas S.G. (ed.), Intelligent Robotic Systems, Marcel Dekker, New York 1991.

[47] Tzafestas S.G. (Guest ed.), "Autonomous Mobile Robots in Health Care Services" (Special Issue), 1998, *J. Intell. & Robotic Systems*, Vol. 22, Nos. 3-4.

[48] Tzafestas S.G. (Guest ed.), "Intelligent Mobile Robots" (Special Issue*), Advanced Robotics (The Intl. Journal of Robotics Society of Japan)*, 1998, Vol. 12, No. 4.

[49] Tzafestas S.G. and Tzafestas E.S., "Human-Machine Interaction in Intelligent Robotic Systems: A Unifying Consideration with Implementation Examples", *Proc. IMACS Intl. Symp. on Mathematical Modeling (MATHMOD '2000)*, Vienna, February 2-4 2000.

[50] Tzafestas S.G. and Tzafestas E.S., "Intelligent Industrial and Service Robotic Systems: Architectural", *Artificial Intelligence and Prototyping Issues, Systems Analysis-Modeling-Simulation*, 1999, Vol. 35, pp. 131-173.

[51] Tzafestas S.G. and Tzafestas E.S., "Learning, Reasoning and Problem Solving in Robotics", In: *Handbook of Industrial Robotics* (Ch. 20), Nof S.Y. (ed), John Wiley, New York 1999.

[52] Tzafestas S.G. and Tzafestas E.S., "The Blackboard Architecture in Knowledge-Based Robotic Systems", Expert Systems and Robotics, Jordanides T. and Torby B. (eds), Springer, 1991, (Series F), Vol. 71, pp. 285-317.

[53] Tzafestas S.G., "Integrated Sensor-Based Intelligent Robot System", *IEEE Control Systems Magaz.*, 1988, pp. 61-72.

[54] Tzafestas S.G., "Intelligent Robotic Systems: Overview and Integrated Examples", *Robotics: Applied Mathematics and Computational Aspects*, Warwick K. (ed), Clarendon Press, Oxford 1993.

[55] Tzafestas S.G., Koutsouris D.G. and Katevas N.I. (eds), *Mobile Robotics for Health Care Services (Proc. 1st MobiNet Symp.)*, Athens, Greece, May 1997.

[56] Valavanis K. and Yuan P.H., "Hardware and Software for Intelligent Robotic Systems", *J. Intell. & Robotic Systems*, 1988, Vol. 1, No. 4, pp. 343-373.

[57] Valavanis K., "Architectural Models for Intelligent Machines", *Proc. 25th IEEE Conf. on Decision and Control*, Dec. 1986, Vol. 2, pp. 1231-1236.

[58] Valavanis K.P. and Saridis G.N., *Intelligent Robotic Systems: Theory, Design and Applications*, Kluwer, Boston/Dordrecht 1992.

[59] Watanabe K., Shiraishi Y., Tzafestas S.G., Tang J. and Fukuda T., "Feedback Control of an Omnidirectional Autonomous Platform for Mobile Service Robots", *J. Intel. & Robotic Systems*, 1998, Vol. 22, No. 3-4, pp. 315-330.

[60] Zeltzer D. and Johnson M., "Motor Planning: An Architecture for Specifying and Controlling the Behavior of Virtual Actors", *J. Visualization and Computer Animation*, 1991, Vol. 2, pp. 74-80.

Chapter 6

Tackling Control Systems Complexity

by Ricardo SANZ, Miguel SEGARRA, Fernando MATIA, Angel de ANTONIO

Mobile Robotics in Healthcare
N. Katevas (Ed.)
IOS Press, 2001

Chapter 6

Tackling Control Systems Complexity

Ricardo SANZ, Miguel SEGARRA, Fernando MATIA, Angel de ANTONIO

1. Introduction

Control systems complexity is increasing due to the need of performing tasks of higher difficulty. Complex controllers incorporate advanced sensors and actuators but most of the functionality is built using software technologies. In the case of intelligent control systems, as those used in advanced mobile robotics or strategic process control, the need of complex information processing lead to the use of heterogeneous software technologies to provide the needed functionality: digital signal processing, neural networks, fuzzy systems, communications, expert systems, artificial vision, etc. Development life cycles for these systems are not linear at all, with a high amount of prototyping and exploratory programming. New methods are needed to cope with the inherent difficulties in handling this type of system construction. Some ideas from advanced software engineering can be used to tackle this control systems complexity.

When control system developers try to build a large and complex controller like the controller shown in Figure 1, they must confront a lot of problems. Some of them are classical control or robotics problems (path following, task planning, etc.) but there are many problems that are —traditionally— out of scope of classical control engineers. These problems are related with the implementation process of the controller and have a strong relation with software systems construction.

Controllers that manage huge amounts of control loops, advanced sensors, large plants, complex algorithms, etc. are *software intensive* systems that are difficult to build due to the large collection of requirements that are requested from implementers which are very difficult to meet: real-time behavior, distribution, heterogeneity, intelligence, etc.

How many programmers do you know that are capable of dealing with five hundred KLOC applications? Efforts in the software engineering community have been done to cope with the issues of large software systems development that are of special importance for control systems engineers.

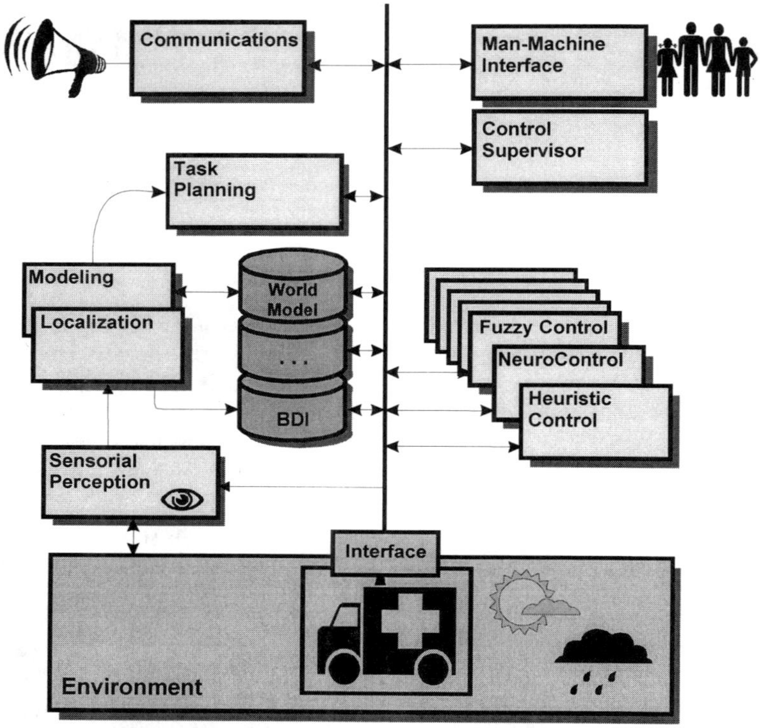

Figure 1. Mobile robot systems are one of the best examples of complex control applications. They are characterized by the coexistence of multiple computational models to support task heterogeneity under the uncertain conditions forced by real environments

Control software complexity is increasing due to several reasons, the principal being the increased functionality of modern controllers. Systems are designed to reach targets never thought for an automatic system. Mars Sojourner's are now real and this type of robotic systems will be increasingly common in next years [17]. Control engineers must tackle a problem that has its origin in the way software is done: as software complexity increases, construction difficulty and risk of failure increases in non-linear proportions. Even if we can afford the cost, we cannot afford the risk. It is not admissible to have software systems in control of platforms with persons on-board that are not safe enough.

If we want our systems to be deployed and used by common persons they must achieve engineering objectives beyond functionality: safety, cost, usability, etc. Have you recently evaluated the development cost of your latest mobile robot? It is not a matter of what is the cost of a prototype, it will be always high for prototypes, but what is the cost of an intelligent machine? Intelligent machines of the future can be as Moravec's universal robots, but in many cases they will not be based on static designs replicated by millions to pay development costs. They will be designed and built almost in a one-by-one basis, because requirements for intelligent machines tend to be too specific to be generalized. The classic GOFAI approach to general intelligence has fallen short of results when dealing with real world problems.

What we need are approaches to intelligent controller design and construction that are both tailorable, safe, maintainable and cost effective. Modular designs have been the key to these issues in other areas of engineering. In our business this means the identification of control-oriented information processing modular functions; the implementation of reusable modules; the design of product architectures; the construction of integration middleware; the reusability of designs; etc. Some insights, ideas and developments are presented in this chapter and we hope they can contribute to enhance the design and construction of complex intelligent controllers.

2. Systems Complexity

As Wilson points out in his tour-de-force [25], complexity is the main matter of research nowadays. Impressive success of mathematical physics has created a solid support for reductionism approaches to science; but while reductionism works quite well for analytical approaches to simple entities, it does not work so well to complex entities or synthesis approaches.

Engineering is the art of synthesis, exploiting knowledge to build new futures. In control systems engineering we are confronting now problems that touch the border of deep complexity. Cell biologists know quite well the behavior of DNA, membrane proteins or any other component of the cell, but they do not expect to be capable of building new cells in a short future.

Control systems complexity is increasing in a steep way, and while we are far from cell complexity, we are touching, however, the issues and nuances of complex systems synthesis. Requirements for control systems are progressively complex. Mobile robotics has demonstrated during years that a simple problem like —going from here to there— can be real hard when done in real settings. Modern plant controllers are far from single loop PID control systems. They have thousands of multivariable loops, with auto-tuning or adaptive functions; integrated in plant-wide systems; with fault tolerance and reconfiguration features. Advanced intelligent systems are fusing multi-sensorial information and they also fuse multi-policy actions. The number of tasks, actions or functions in a single controller is getting vary large. And they are built with software.

Complex controllers are, perhaps, the most complex software systems ever built. As Douglas says [10], complexity is the main substance of software.

2.1 Plant Complexity

The main reason for making complex control systems is that the plants that we want to control are complex themselves. Examples can be found everywhere, from the small (like a double pendulum) to the large (like a country-wide electricity distribution network). Controller complexity is only a manifestation of the law of *requisite variety* of Ashby [3]. Paraphrasing his words, we can say that we need controller variety to destroy plant variety, i.e. we need a complex controller behavior to simplify plant behavior and make it attain to our specifications (220 V and 50 Hz, for example).

The nature of plant complexity is elusive, however, as is the proper interpretation of the term *complexity* itself. We are witnessing a process of creation of a collection of new disciplines that uses the generic name of *theories of complexity* (see [14],[9]), but each one of these disciplines is only related with a small point in the complexity landscape, for example in the case of Kaufman's theory, it is the *origins or order* in biological, ecological or economic systems.

Lets try to define more clearly what a *complex system* is. Complexity in plants under control is appreciated in a heterogeneous collection of systems with quite different structures and properties. Paradigmatic examples of complex systems are:

- Chemical plants can contain up to fifty thousand measured variables with thousand of control loops distributed across several control locations.
- National infrastructures (air traffic, communications, electricity, etc.) are composed by collections of semi-autonomous entities that interact to reach individual objectives without falling into a collapse due to selfishness of behaviors.
- Non-linear systems are very difficult to control because in many cases non-linear interactions can lead to chaotic behavior.
- Fault tolerant control systems are examples of systems where the most part of them are devoted to handle the uncertainty inherent to failures.

First of all, we must have a clear idea that *complexity* is an epistemological issue, i.e. it is in the eye of the beholder —or his mind— more than in the system perceived as complex itself. What is not so clear is if it is also an ontological issue. We perceive complexity in things when we try to manage them in our minds, so complexity is related with the mechanisms of representation that we use to manage knowledge about systems. But in some sense, this perception of complexity is based on what is perceived from the system. In control systems engineering it is interesting to differentiate between three main types of complexity in the system itself and its interaction with the environment:

- *Primary complexity* refers to the complexity derived from size. A plant with one hundred variables is more complex than a plant with one variable.
- *Secondary complexity* is the complexity originated due to interactions (relations, dependencies, etc.) between the component of a system. Non-linearities, reaction couplings, etc. are examples of such couplings.*Tertiary complexity* is the complexity due to uncertainty. Uncertainty that comes in several forms: imprecision of the models of plants that we use, uncertainty in the perception of

the state of the plants or the environment, uncertainty in the control strategies to follow, etc.

In the study of autonomous systems it is sometimes confusing the meaning of the concept of autonomy. From our point of view it means *capable of doing a task without external help*, so in the analysis of these systems a clear distinction must be done between three types of entities:

- The *environment*; the collection of non-controlled systems and conditions that constitute the framework for robot activity.
- The *task* to do; i.e. what we want to be changed in the environment.
- The *system*, the robot we build and program to do the task.

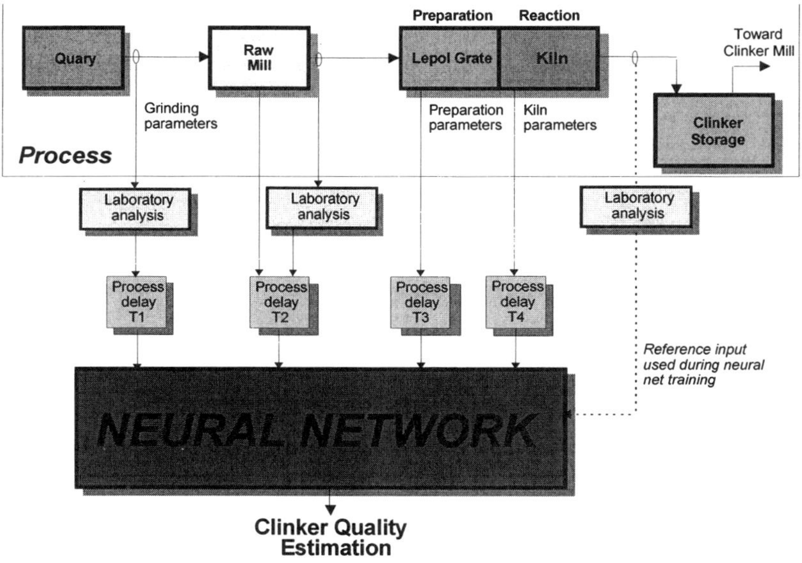

Figure 2. Complexity lurks everywhere. Even the apparently simple task of perception *can be very hard indeed. For example, on-line clinker quality determination in a cement kiln is a basic perceptual activity for a kiln controller but it is very difficult to perform. Among the best approaches tried so far is the use of complex neural networks as clinker quality estimators*

The objective for control systems design is the design and implementation of robotic minds to let robots perform their tasks. Intelligent control systems are control systems that enable its hosts to do their tasks under the presence of uncertainty. So the focus of *intelligence* is uncertainty management. This uncertainty manifests itself in all the three components mentioned:

- *Uncertainty in the environment*, as happens in the real world is what makes completely different the work of a real-world robot from the work of a toy-world robot (like robotic football, for example).

- *Uncertainty in the task*, because we want our robots to do tasks that are imprecisely defined, like going from a place to other without specifying the whole path.
- *Uncertainty in the robot system itself*, in the form of non complete models of bodily capabilities, tolerance to physical failures or overcoming sensor limitations using sensor fusion.

In relation with the type of plants under control in this book (i.e. mobile robotics), we can say that primary and secondary complexities are not very high (at least in relation with the mobile robot itself). Modern computers and controllers can cope easily with these issues.

Tertiary complexity, on the other hand, is a real complex issue here. There exists a lot of uncertainty in the perception of the state of the environment and also in the control law; in fact due to the uncertainty in the environment, that limits controller designability.

2.2 Control Systems Complexity

Complex controllers are a difficult entity to define because there are so many aspects that make controllers complex: non-linearity, fault tolerance, large scale, etc. In this paper we will focus in the software complexity aspect of a controller for an intelligent autonomous system.

Autonomy, as stated before, is in some sense tolerance to uncertainty and from this point of view, what the robot needs to be autonomous is capability to exploit all the available information to perform the task commissioned to it. This information comes from three sources:

- *A-priori* information put into the robot's memory in advance.
- *Sensed* information about the environment and about the robot itself.
- Learned information *created* by the robot using the information gained from its activity.

In conventional control systems a priori information is based on mathematical models of the plant under control. This information is the best one when it is well designed, i.e. when the models fit enough the plant, but in some cases, it is not possible to get good mathematical models simple enough to be used in the implementation of classical controllers. In these cases, control has been usually performed directly by humans. Intelligent control technologies [11], [24] are the main technology used to overcome this problem.

Complex controllers do use expert system technology to incorporate human knowledge, fuzzy technology to handle uncertain knowledge, neural networks to build models based on raw plant data (a form of system identification), genetic algorithms explore alternatives, etc. This means a heterogeneous collection of software technologies that require specific implementation processes and tools.

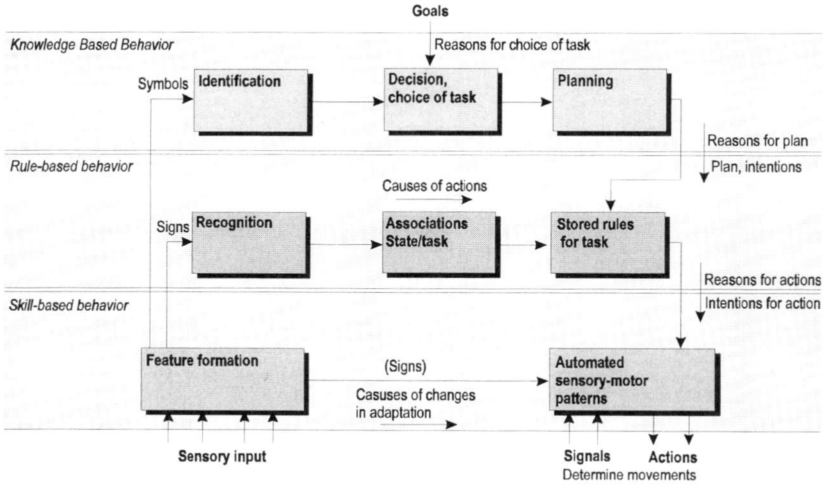

Figure 3. Rasmussen's model of cognitive control is a conceptual example of the high level control functions performed by humans in charge of technical systems

2.3 Software Complexity

Software Complexity is a measure of the efforts spent in a system. These are used during the system's lifecycle in its development, debugging and maintenance and also in its utilization. Complexity measures are useful to discern difficult-to-built systems from those that are not and to rank competitive architectures for their construction. These measures should also provide guidance for planning and scheduling and for personnel assignment to each step of the development process.

Software Complexity, as presented above, is a measure of the entropy of a system in terms of amount of work. Nevertheless, complexity measures do not allow us to separate the different aspects that make up the system's overall complexity. Take for instance an application based on the client-server model. When several system architects are asked to build the application, all of them would agree that its design should inspired in the client-server model but each one will split the system into different modules and different assignments of functionality. Why is this so? The answer to this question is simple, when the number of variables is too high the system architects simply cannot handle all of them in their own minds and subjective abstractions are made to simplify the problem.

The most common approach, as stated above, is *reductionism*. Split the problem into pieces that can be handled by the intellect of the architects. Nevertheless, this approach proves insufficient in a broad range of applications. Software Complexity depends not only on the size of the problem but also on its *intrinsic*. The problem *domain* is as important as its size. It is necessary then to consider the problem domain before making any assessment in order to solve it. This point of view is not reductionism, you need to visualize the whole system to make the correct decisions. These decisions will be embodied in the final system and will show up in its characteristics: performance, maintainability, availability, safety, security, etc.

Regarding *mobile robotics for healthcare* there are two issues that must be considered first when thinking about the complexity of the envisaged system: safety and reliability. The system that does not meet those conditions may cause injuries or death. Damage to equipment or environmental harm should also be considered. Software must be reliable; it should conform to its specification. Notice that the system must be safe even if it is not reliable. If these two qualities are the best assets a system of this kind can have then the metrics used to evaluate its complexity must be related to them. Take for instance the selection of the development language. Software Complexity will depend on characteristics of the selected language such us facilities for fault tolerance programming. If we select a language that doesn't allow the developers to cleanly deal with fault or failure we will be making some kind of *software asset-stripping* on the qualities the system should have.

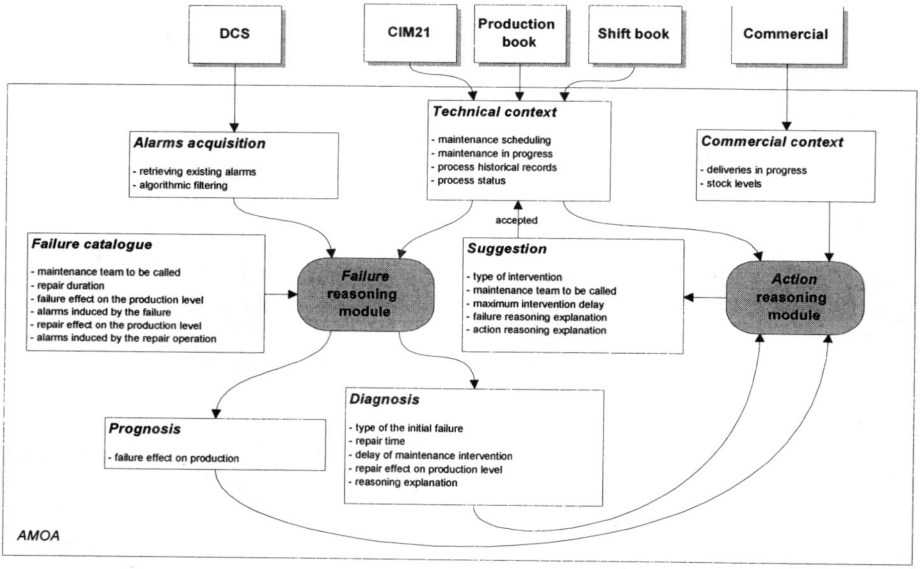

Figure 4. The AMOA expert system was designed to provide plant-wide alarm management for the strategic control of cement plants. It was integrated with an heterogeneous collection of systems like Distributed Control Systems (DCS), process databases (CIM/21), human shift coordination systems, production control and commercial exploitation packages

Unfortunately, software complexity metrics does not easily allow us to compare different programming languages. Further they are more often than not language dependent and the complexity rules for each language are different. This assert is also applicable at different levels to other elements involved in the development of the system such as the election of a suitable architecture or the most efficient compiler for the purpose at hand.

Metrics for safety and reliability are needed when talking about control systems that interact with human beings. The aim of these metrics should be considered as the degree to which characteristics that affect safety or reliability are present. From this point of view the system must be kept simple. Disappointingly, the decomposition of a system into parts introduces a new level of complexity. This new form of complexity is derived from the interconnection of the separated modules. The types and sequencing of the communication protocols must be thoroughly specified and checks for structure and protocol consistency must be established.

Given these constraints, software is a delicate piece of a safety critical system. Safety and reliability must be taken into account in all steps of the development lifecycle. A systematic approach to system safety requirements must be made inside the framework of a methodology for software safety (NASA Software Safety Standard NSS1740.13).

3. Complex Controller Construction

In the development of any system, and specifically in the development of complex intelligent autonomous systems, two *architectures* are defined:

1. The *architecture of the final* system, i.e. the structure that will provide the final functionality (for example see Figure 1). Most of the chapters in this book deal with this type of architecture, because it is —obviously— of maximal importance for the objectives of the development.
2. The *architecture of the construction process*, or as is most commonly known in software engineering, *the process*. This express how a collection of interacting actors perform tasks and coordinate their activities in order to achieve a final result: a working system.

While product architecture is of extreme importance for autonomous intelligent systems, the technology is established enough to start thinking in real applications of the technology outside laboratories and this means that some effort should be put in the engineering aspects of autonomous systems construction.

3.1 Architecture Based Development

Modern control systems are digital almost entirely. Complex controllers in continuous process plants are software intensive systems with millions of lines of code. The more abstract view of a system –its core design– receives the name of architecture of the system. Software architecture is emerging as a new sub-discipline inside the software engineering discipline.

Software system architecture is of increasing importance as the size and life span of the system increase, because it is the main ingredient of system integrity. As Brooks remarked in *The Mythical Man·Month*, conceptual integrity is the single, most important property of a computing system with some future (i.e. that will be maintained in operation after its development) [6]. In opinion of Clements, there are three reasons why the architecture of a system is a valuable informational resource [8]:

- It serves for *mutual communication*. Software architecture represents a common high-level abstraction of the system that most, if not all, of the system's stakeholders can use as a basis for creating mutual understanding, forming consensus, and communicating with each other.
- It captures *early design decisions*. Software architecture represents the embodiment of the earliest set of design decisions about a system, and these early bindings carry weight far out of proportion to their individual gravity with respect to the system's remaining development, its service in deployment, and its maintenance life.
- It is a *transferable abstraction of a system*. Software architecture embodies a relatively small, intellectually graspable model for how the system is structured and how its components work together; this model is transferable across systems; in particular, it can be applied to other systems exhibiting similar requirements, and can promote large scale reuse.

The architecture of a complex software system is so important that a software engineering movement is promoting the use of it as the backbone of all system developments. This software methodology is called architecture-based development.

Why we should care about architecture based development? Even when the field is not mature enough to have a consensus form, there are some promises it offers based on early experience [8]:

- Systems can be built in a rapid, cost-effective manner by importing (or generating) large externally developed components.
- It is possible to predict certain qualities about a system by studying its architecture, even in the absence of detailed design and code.
- Entire product lines can be developed by sharing a common architecture. Large-scale reuse is possible through architectural-level planning.
- The functionality of a component can be separated from its component interconnection mechanisms for good reasons.
- Less is more: it pays to restrict the vocabulary of design alternatives.

Effort has also been done in developing generic architectures for systems in a specific domain. For example, software architectures for avionics, for medical equipment, for banking systems, etc. This type of architecture receives the name of *Domain Specific Software Architecture* (DSSA).

If you are questioning the need or suitability of DSSAs, we can use the words of Kazman to argue in favour of them. DSSAs serve:

- To *build better*: tools, specification languages, domain- specific reusable components, application frameworks, product families; and
- To *understand better*. Software problems are very complex. A DSSA is ready–made, reusable domain analysis and problem decomposition.

3.2 Pattern Based Design of Control Systems

The *increasing precision with decreasing intelligence* (IPDI) principle proposed by Saridis is sometimes considered a *feature of intelligent systems* but it can only be considered a feature in the sense of *documented bug*. It is not intelligent at all to have *decreasing intelligence* in any sense. The supposed principle is only a demonstration of how to overcome the problem of reduced information-processing capability.

IPDI does not talk about how intelligent systems should be, but how they are when computing resources are scarce. At most it can be considered as a *design pattern* that solves – partially– the problem of lack of computing power needed for fast, intelligent performance. An example of the evolution of this problem –specifically in relation with artificial vision for mobile robotics can be found in [17].

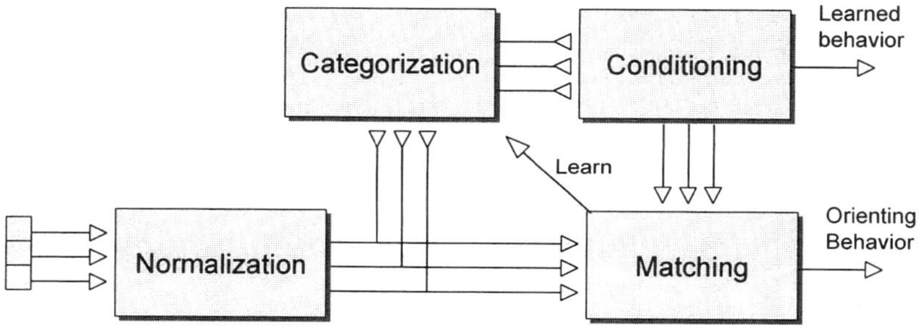

Figure 5. Interaction between normalization, categorization, matching and conditioned expectations as proposed in [9]. It can be considered a design pattern for behavior learning in behavior based creatures

4. A Methodology for Tackling Controller Complexity

4.1 The Need of a Methodological Approach

The search of quality and cost/time reduction leads to the definition of coherent methodologies for system development. What we need is a body of methods, rules and postulates (a procedure) to build complex controllers. Finding the *correct procedure* to build complex process control systems is almost a no hope task. Heterogeneity in process problems leads to a high degree of variety in application structure and technology. Some of the reasons for the complexity of the search of a methodology are:

1. Use of heterogeneous software technologies and heterogeneous platforms.
2. Need of integration with legacy systems.

3. Non deterministic[1] computational methods; and in particular artificial intelligence inference-based technologies, which are mostly unpredictable.
4. Knowledge based processing. Knowledge extraction, representation, sharing and coherence problems.
5. Application structure dynamics.
6. Exploratory programming.
7. High level of novelty. Most systems are of the one-of-a-kind type.
8. Strong coupling between development phases: inherent life-cycle feedback.
9. Postponed specifications and designs.
10. Complex non-hierarchical development teams.
11. Multidisciplinarity of the expertise needed.

Even when the ultimate methodology is not achievable, at the end, what is really needed, is a basic *software* methodology coupled with some *control* submethodologies. The complexity of the tasks the complete methodology must address is enormous:

- *Software development methodologies*: There is a need for a global application design, process, distributed system construction, real-time, artificial intelligence, validation and verification, product line management, etc.
- *Control systems methodologies*: The heterogeneity of elementary controllers lead to specific (sub)methodologies for all them. Classical controllers, expert systems (knowledge management), fuzzy controllers (uncertainty representation), neural networks (topology, laws), genetic algorithms, learning, heterogeneous system performance (stability, etc.).

Classical software methodologies offer good alternatives as starting points for a more suitable one for our domain (a *domain specific methodology* address problems in a focused domain). Some examples of useful methodologies (they offer some ideas valuable for an integrated control methodology) are:

- Shlaer-Mellor, Booch, OMT, Objectory: Generic object oriented methodologies.
- ROOM, OCTOPUS: Real time distributed systems.
- ODM, FODA: Domain analysis.
- KADS: Knowledge acquisition and elicitation.
- HINT: Heterogeneous control systems.
- AOM: Agent oriented methodology.

Each one has it niches, strengths and weaknesses, focusing on specific aspects of the development process or the target system. They are commented below only as a sample of the methodological hodgepodge that managers have available throughout the world of

[1] Non-deterministic in the restricted sense of not having a usable model to make correct estimates of computation time and outcome.

information systems development. There are –literally– thousands of methodologies out there. A question arises: Do we need another one?

4.2 A Global Application Model

Authors' research group has been working on architectures for complex controllers for years, and our objective was to develop a comprehensive technology for such controllers. This technology reference model is called the Integrated Control Architecture [22] or ICa for short. The three main components for ICa are:

1. A collection of reusable entities in a framework for component development: *ICa Generic Agents*.
2. An integrative infrastructure: *ICa Glue*.
3. A development methodology and reference model based on modular composition of systems: *ICa Methodology*.

This separation matches the description made by Rossak [18] about the elements for building integrated systems: *basic technologies*, *integration technologies* and *integration architectures*.

The basic model we follow is an agency model [5]. ICa models control systems as a collection of interacting autonomous agents. Agent is a carelessly overloaded word, which has been used to refer to a collection of quite different approaches in software construction. Our vision is more generic than most of them, viewing agents as mere *active objects* [7]. The use of the term by many people in the "agent" community is somewhat biased towards their specific interests[2]. In fact we think that control systems are the natural example of agent based systems in opposition to opinions of agent gurus. The flexibility requirement posed by Jennings [13] (*responsiveness*, *pro-activeness* and *sociality*) is obvious in control systems:

- Controllers are *responsive*: This is, in fact, the nature of control systems. A control system that is not responsive is an open-loop controller that has a little use in industry today. Feedback is *the word* in control systems engineering.
- Controllers are *pro-active*: Considering this aspect different form *responsiveness* is a mistake. Pro-activity and responsiveness are two sides of the same coin. When an agent is pro-active (it can initiate activities directed by goals) it is because it is responsive to changes in the environment. An agent that is pro-active without connection to the world, is a solipsist agent of little interest (except from the philosophical point of view).
- Controllers are *social*: Pieces of control systems interact to reach a global objective, but each one is only trying to reach its own objectives. Take a look for example at a typical DCS (distributed control system). Examples of agents there are: intelligent

---

[2] There is even a definition of agent as *a piece of code in Java that is self-contained and can be executed on remote virtual machines.*

sensors, programmable logic controllers, process controllers, human operators, etc. All of them have their own goals and, by interaction, reach global control objectives for the plant.

The conclusion is that the agent paradigm and the control paradigm fit perfectly. That's the reason why this is the natural model for complex control systems construction (controllers are software intensive systems). Other examples of agent based industrial control systems are [12] and [23].

4.3 A Development Methodology

The ICa development methodology is based on domain engineering concepts. The very basic idea is *progressive domain focalization* [20]. We do not make a strong difference between domain engineering and application engineering because we consider application engineering as sub-domain engineering, i.e. components that have been built or tailored for a specific application can also be reused, at least in any domain that is included in the previous one. This forces developers to *think generic* even when building application specific things.

ICa methodology proposes a base list of activities:

- *(Sub)Domain analysis*. To provide support for cohesion in different control systems, sub-domain analysis must be fused with the domain analysis previously done. This phase should include classical requirements engineering phases.
- *Control tasks identification*. Related with domain analysis, but focused in control aspects more that plant behavioral aspects that are mostly addressed in the domain analysis phase. Identification of individual or group control tasks.
- *Control technology selection*. Identification of the more suitable technologies for solving control tasks.
- *Controller architecture design*. Base architecture definition based on domain architectures. Control task partition and grouping following compositional criteria (speed, technology, layering, etc.). This means agency design if using ICa.
- *Detailed controller design*. Depending on the degree of reusability of controller assets, the need of redesigning and re-implementing controllers will be diverse.
- *Controller implementation*. Construction of isolated control modules, based on true reuse and parameterization or complete reconstruction of the controller. This means agent implementation if using ICa.
- *Integration*. Following architectural guidelines. Middleware support simplifies this process.
- *Test and validation*. System testing, verification and validation.
- *Maintenance*. Classical maintenance (defect correction, new functionality, keep working) and controller maintenance: retuning, continuous learning, knowledge enhancement, etc., which obviously includes controller monitorization.
- *Make it generic*: Obtaining reusable assets from application specific developments. Reengineering of specific components.
- *Asset base maintenance*. Incorporation of new assets into asset base. Reengineering of obsolete assets.

5. Examples

In this section we will comment some examples of complex control systems addressing some of the mentioned issues. We will present some complex control systems with different degrees of reusability and a more deep comment of one of them: a system for risk management in a chemical plant.

5.1 Real Time Control Systems (RCS)

The Real-time Control System (RCS) architecture proposed by Albus [1] defines a generic design for a hierarchical control system. It is not specifically tailored as an intelligent controller and hence his value: intelligence appears from what the system does, not from the type of technology employed. The RCS architecture consists of a hierarchically layered collection of processing modules connected by a network of communications links.

The four basic types of modules that compose RCS-based systems are:

- *Behavior Generating* modules that contain the task knowledge i.e. they are responsible of systems activity.
- *World Modeling* modules that model the state space of the problem domain.
- *Sensory Processing* modules that process data from visual, auditory, tactile, proprioceptive, taste, or smell sensors.
- *Value Judgment* modules that contain algorithms for computing cost, risk, and benefit, for evaluating states and situations, for estimating the reliability of state estimations, and for assigning cost-benefit values to objects and events.

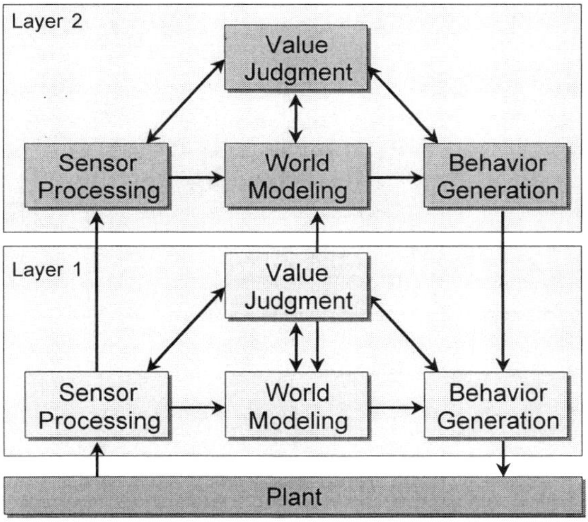

Figure 6. RCS provides a framework for the development of layered control systems based on the use of a pattern for a control layer with four roles: sensor processing, world modeling, behavior generation and value judgment

The main contribution from RCS is that it was one of the very first attempts to provide a reusable design for a wide domain. This design is based on the use of a central pattern for a control layer with the four mentioned roles: sensor processing, world modeling, behavior generation and value judgment.

5.2 AFREB

The extended AFREB architecture is an example control scheme used for autonomous robot navigation. It is an hybrid architecture which needs an off-line path planner that, using a static map of the environment, sets the controller path reference, while, under it, a reactive control system performs the task, by processing a high amount of on-line sensor information for on-line obstacle avoidance. On the other hand, and at the same time, it is a good example of the use of intelligent control algorithms for reactive navigation.

The intelligent control module is composed of three internal layers. At the bottom, several low-level controllers are able to implement behaviours, such as turn, go back, follow a path, follow the contour of an obstacle, and follow a corridor. They don't use maps of the environment, but sensor information as data source. PID or fuzzy control are adequate to implement these basic behaviours.

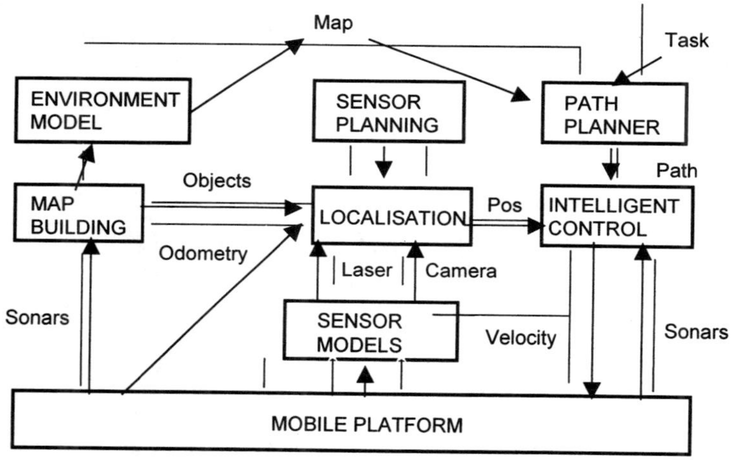

Figure 7. AFREB architecture components: intelligent control perception and planning

Over it, a decision system is used to reach the target, following a path or a corridor, and using collision avoidance algorithms. The previous primitive behaviours are fused to complete the desired task, originating an emergent behaviour. The decision system must determine the most adequate values for the behaviour weights used to fuse them. A path planner for trajectory generation is used to set the reference for this level. The higher level is a co-operative planner that allows to change between the two decison systems, depending on the environment characteristics.

Different perception modules allow to supply better information to the control module, by reducing uncertainty in sensor data, position estimation and information about the environment. These three topics are respectively addressed by combining sensor models with sensor data, and using probabilistic techniques.

5.3 RiskMan

RiskMan is an application for *global risk management* in a chemical plant (*see* Figure 8). The scope of activity was:

- *Risk reduction*: enhancing practices for minimizing the hazards.
- *Risk prevention*: by means of on-line fault detection and isolation.
- *Risk control*: by means of emergency management in accordance with safety regulations, operating policies and constraints of the plant.

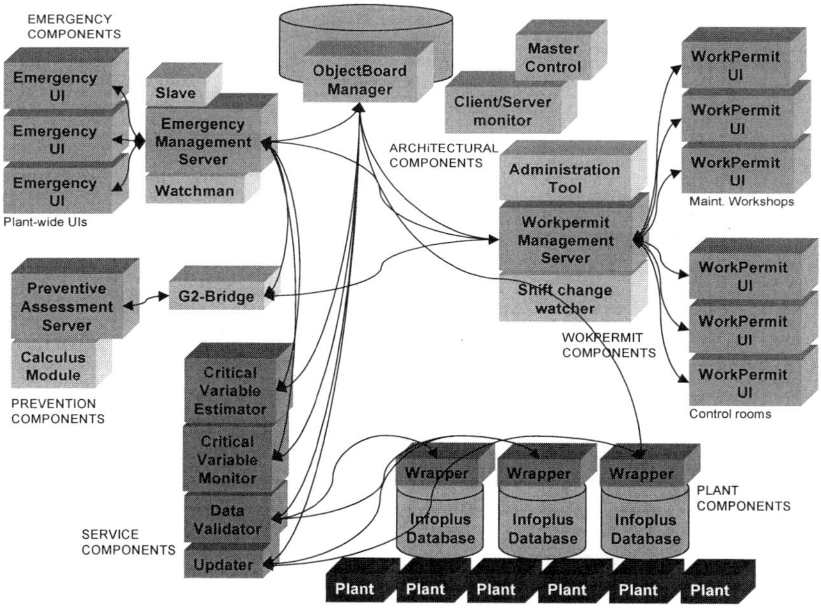

Figure 8. Components and some of the interactions between them in RiskMan. The system was designed for semi-autonomous behavior, monitoring nine plants in a chemical complex using an heterogeneous collection of intelligent control technologies

The RiskMan application was developed around three subsystems that were devised for the three main different tasks (risk reduction, risk prevention and risk control):

- A *workpermit management system*, to handle all works that were performed in plant. This subsystem tried to minimize the risk of each work by itself (by automatic handling of work-specific safety measures), the risk of each work in a specific plant condition (workpermit emission was done taking into account plant state) and inter-work interactions.
- A *preventive system* was built to identify faults and plant state deviations from safety conditions.
- An *emergency management system* was built to help people handle emergencies when happening. The system was designed to disseminate real-time information about emergency situation, coordinate the activities of persons, interact with external entities and made predictions about emergency evolution.

The application was built using the ICa framework and was composed by ICa agents, legacy applications, wrappers, helper components and independent non-agentified components.

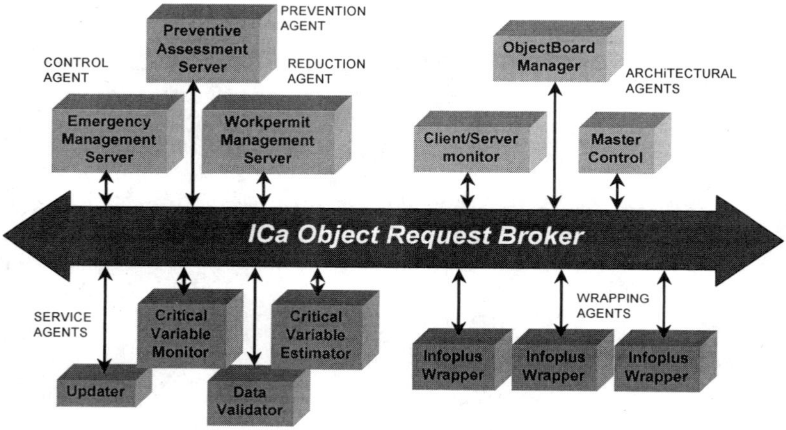

Figure 9. RiskMan is an application for plant-wide risk control (prevention, reduction and management) in a petrochemical complex. It uses heterogeneous technologies as expert systems, fuzzy filters and neural network models to serve as a strategic decision support system for plant personnel. Agent interaction is done through the ICa object request broker. Non-agentified components (as user interfaces) and helper applications interact using specific integration mechanisms and have been suppressed from the figure

6. Conclusions

The design of complex controllers is more an art than a technique, because due to the large collection of factors to take into account and the spectrum of technologies used, no proper design procedure exist so far. The main guideline we have when designing the architecture of an artificial mind is a collection of aesthetic clues.

It may sound strange to claim for the use of aesthetics in engineering design, but it is not nonsense. Aesthetics in design lead us to designs where we feel beauty and in our case this is mainly *technical beauty*. Examples of these beauty properties are classic objectives of system development, and have their biggest manifestation in software construction because software is so soft that it is a good matter for art:

- *Simplicity*: The property of being simple affects understandability and so any global property related with human's mental model of the system.
- *Equilibrium*: Equilibrated systems tend to present less problems related with bottlenecks and support better a process of refactoring.
- *Modularity*: The property of being part-replaceable is important for factors as easy of construction, maintenance or fault isolation.

Other properties also present esthetical characteristics but they are, however, harder to perceive and evaluate. Examples are:

- *Evolvability*: Intelligent systems development is evolutionary by nature and designs must be devised to support this type of development.
- *Maintainability*: As problems appear and new requirements are expressed, the system will be modified. It should be designed with this perspective in mind. As complexity increases, the longevity of the system increases also. Complex systems tend to survive and maintenance will be inevitable.
- *Constructability*: The easiness of putting parts together to compose the system is critical for real-world applications. If autonomous robotic systems are going to be out of laboratories development costs must be lowered.

All of these properties —and many others— express non-functional requirements and when the complexity of a system increases, the relative importance of non-functional requirements increases in relation with functional ones.

As Hexmoor pointed out [15] in relation with GLAIR, *smarts are in the architecture*. This means that the architecture of a system is perhaps the single most important factor that affects global performance —intelligence— of the system. This is the base design of an intelligent being, and this has been perceived by researchers for years. In the early times of AI, the search was for architectures for general intelligence (GPS, STRIPS, SOAR, etc.), after that work other types of solutions were sought, like behavior-based systems [6][2] or BDI architectures (beliefs, desires & intentions) [16]. More interesting are those approaches that try to serve as generalized foundations for wide domains, like RCS [1] or ICa [21].

From our point of view, generalized architectural designs that are of any value for the future of the discipline, must take into account the variability of requirements posed to intelligent autonomous entities and be flexible enough to serve as a basis for any type of system in a broad domain. This can only be achieved with a progressive foundation, where limiting design decisions are done for specific domains, keeping core issues reusability at hand.

More knowledge on complex software system construction is needed by the autonomous controller community. The opposite is also true. Software engineers need the insights and systemic views from our discipline because we are building the most complex software systems ever done. While the money can be in the development of Microsoft Windows applications to serve big corporation purposes, the fun is in making autonomous systems. They are the bearers of intelligence.

7. References

[1] Albus J.S., "A reference model architecture for intelligent systems design", Antsaklis P., Passino K. (eds.), *An Introduction to Intelligent and Autonomous Control*, Kluwer Academic Publishers, Boston MA 1992, pp. 57–64.

[2] Arkin R. C., " Behavior-Based Robot Navigation for Extended Domains", *Adaptive Behavior,* 1992, Vol. 1, No. 2, pp.201-225.

[3] Ashby W.R., *An Introduction to Cybernetics,* Chapman & Hall. London, 1957.

[4] Balkenius C., "Natural Intelligence in Artificial Creatures". *PhD Thesis*. Lund University, Lund 1995.

[5] Bradsaw K., *Software Agents,* MIT Press 1998.

[6] Brooks R. A.,. "Intelligence without representation". *Artificial Intelligence*, 1987, 47:139–159.

[7] Brugali D., "From Objects to Agents: Software Reuse for Distributed Systems", *PhD thesis*, Politecnico di Torino.

[8] Clements P. C., "Coming Attractions in Software Architecture", *Technical Report CMU/SEI-96-TR-008,* January 1996.

[9] Cowan G. A., Pines D., Meltzer D. (Eds.), Complexity. Metaphors, Models and Reality, Addison-Wesley, Reading MA., 1994.

[10] Douglass B.P., "Doing Hard Time. Developing Real-Time Systems with UML, Objects, Frameworks and Patterns", Addison-Wesley, Reading MA 1999.

[11] Gupta M.M. and Sinha N.K., *Intelligent Control Systems,* IEEE Press, 1996.

[12] Iglesias C.A., González J.C. ,Velasco J.R., "A Fuzzy-neural Multiagent System for Optimisation of a Roll-mill Application".

[13] Jennings N.R., Sycara K., and Wooldridge M., "A Roadmap of Agent Research and Development", *Autnonomous Agents and Multiagent Systems*, 1998, 1: pp. 7-38.

[14] Kaufmann, S. A., The Origins of Order: Self Organization and Selection in Evolution, Oxford University Press 1993.

[15] Lammens J., Hexmoor H., Shapiro S., "Of elephants and men", *NATO ASI Series on biology and technology of intelligent autonomous agents,* Springer-Verlag 1995.

[16] Ming R., Integrated System for Intelligent Control, Springer-Verlag, Berlin, 1992.

[17] Moravec H.P., Robot: from Mere Machine to Transcendent Mind, Oxford University Press, Oxford 1999.

[18] Rossak W., Ng P., "Some thought on systems integration: A conceptual framework". *International Journal on Systems Integration*, 1991, Vol. 1 No. 1, pp. 97– 114.

[19] Sanz R., "Agents for Complex Control Systems", Samad T. , Weyrauch J. (Eds.), Automation, Control, and Complexity: New Developments and Directions. John Wiley and Sons, 1999.

[20] Sanz R., Alarcón I., Segarra M. J., de Antonio A., and Clavijo J. A., "Progressive domain focalization in intelligent control systems". *Control Engineering Practice*, 1999a, Vol. 7 No. 5, pp.665–671.

[21] Sanz R., Matía F., and Puente E. A., "The ICa approach to intelligent autonomous systems", Tzafestas S. (ed.), Advances in Autonomous Intelligent Systems, chapter 4, pp. 71–92, Kluwer Academic Publishers, Dordrecht, NL. 1999c.

[22] Sanz R., Segarra M. J., de Antonio A., Clavijo J. A., "ICa: Middleware for intelligent process control", *Proceedings of IEEE ISIC/ISAS 99*, Cambridge, MA 1999d.

[23] Wang, H. and Wang, C., "Intelligent agents in the nuclear industry", *Computer,* 1997, Vol. 30, No. 11, pp.28–34.

[24] White D.A. ,Sofge D.A. (Eds), Handbook of Intelligent Control, Van Nostrand-Reinhold 1992.

[25] Wilson E.O., Consilience: the Unity of Knowledge, Alfred A.Knopf, New York 1998.

Chapter 7

Mobile Robot Kinematics and Control

by Ulrich BORGOLTE, Nikos KATEVAS

Mobile Robotics in Healthcare
N. Katevas (Ed.)
IOS Press, 2001

Chapter 7

Mobile Robot Kinematics and Control

Ulrich BORGOLTE, Nikos KATEVAS

1. Introduction

This chapter introduces the basic concepts of mobile robotics. By way of introduction, a survey on the current state of the art is given, followed by application areas of mobile robots, and different implementation approaches for specific problems. Furthermore, sections both on wheeled mobile systems as well as on so-called walking machines are included.

Within the section on wheeled robots, different wheel configurations are discussed with regard to their advantages and disadvantages. Furthermore, co-ordinate systems, transformation matrices, and velocity calculations/Jacobians are addressed. The section on walking machines handles different models of walking, leg configurations, as well as possible fields of application of these systems. Different kinds of gait and static/dynamic stability are also discussed.

Again, the section on control of mobile robots deals with wheel driven systems. Without going further into the concepts of control technology (this can be looked up in corresponding text books and is beyond the scope of this book), different control architectures are discussed, in particular for the lower level of control (motor control). The effects of mutual influencing in over-determined systems as well as resulting measures for the reduction of these effects are handled in a section on system coupling.

The chapter does a turn from the technical details to the application areas of mobile robots. In the first instance, different application scenarios are described, and current application fields are outlined. With respect to the specific situation in health care applications, suggestions for safety treatment are given.

The chapter closes with a suggestion for the practical selection of a mobile robot which can serve in the healthcare sector.

2. History of Mobile Robots

There are two lines of predecessors to mobile robots: devices with mechanical 'program' (artificial animals), and remotely controlled vehicles. Both lack the basic requirements of robots: a re-configurable program structure, and some kind of independence from human intervention. First devices of mobile robots, but without autonomy, are based on ELSI by W. Grey Walter in England. They are driven by simple reactive behaviour via environmental conditions.

Looking at the development of mobile robotics, there is an obvious close coupling with advances in computer hardware, software methods, and artificial intelligence. A short overview on the history of *autonomous mobile robots* (AMRs) might read like this (without any claim of completeness) [12]:

- *Shakey by Stanford Research Institute, early 1960s*. Equipped with TV camera and a tactile sensor. Radio link to off-board mainframe computer. World representation by means of a grid model and a property list model. Localisation by dead reckoning only.
- *JPL AMR by Jet Propulsion Laboratory, early 1970s*. Car-like base, equipped with stereo TV cameras, laser range-finder, tactile sensors, and proximity sensors. Manipulator on-board. On-board minicomputer and cable link to off-board computer. Localisation by dead reckoning (gyroscope, optical encoders). Ability of analysing simples scenes and path planning.
- *Stanford Cart by Stanford University Artificial Intelligence Laboratory, 1973-81*. Equipped with a sliding camera for stereo imaging. Ability of path planning with optimising strategies.
- *CMU AMR by Carnegie-Mellon University, 1981-84*. Omnidirectional (3 degrees of freedom - DOF) steering. Equipped with movable TV camera, short range infrared and long range ultrasonic sensors, and contact switches. Several on-board processors. Hierarchical control structure with planning, execution, and actuation.
- *Hilare by Institut National des Sciences Appliques, France, 1978*. Tricycle drive. Equipped with infrared triangulation system, video camera, telemetry laser, and ultrasonic proximity sensors. Link to off-board mainframe. Ability for absolute positioning by active beacons.
- *Meldog by Mechanical Engineering Laboratory of MITI, Japan, 1979-83*. Tricycle base. Equipped with ultrasonic sensors. Ability of obstacle avoidance. Used as a guidance 'dog' for blind people. Connected to the user by a wire link, getting commands from the user, sending alarm signals to the user.
- *Robart-I by Naval Postgraduate School, 1982*. Tricycle drive. Equipped with ultrasonic sensors, near-infrared proximity detector, tactile feelers, and bumper switches. No planning capabilities, but total autonomy and collision avoidance. Used to randomly move around, sensing for fire, smoke, flooding, toxic gas, etc.
- *SCIMR by University of Pennsylvania Moore School of Electrical Engineering, 1981*. Differential drive. Equipped with rotatable ultrasonic transducer. Three interconnected microprocessors. Graph representation of hallways, with intersections as nodes, and hallways as edges. Wall following ability. Total autonomy.

- *FMS by Komatsu Ltd and others, since early 1980s*. Industrial transporting device. Different steering techniques. In general, no intelligent functions. Application of state-of-the-art algorithms and sensors.

Apart from the mainstream in mobile robot research, there is a good tradition in biologically inspired developments. Especially to overcome problems with uneven terrain and environments not designed for wheeled vehicles, walking robots are one possible alternative (caterpillar drives are another one):

- *Walking Horse by General Electric, 1968*. Four legs, each with 3 DOF. Provided with simple force feedback. Master/slave architecture.
- *Hexapod by Ohio State University, 1976-77*. Six legs. Equipped with two stereo cameras. Master/slave architecture. Possesses the ability to keep the motion of the body uniform by activating complex leg motions.
- *Quadruped Stair Climber*, Tokyo Institute of Technology, 1979. Similar to Walking Horse.

The devices listed so far are all earth-bound. Furthermore, most of them are intended for industrial or at least indoor usage. Despite the fact that this is also the background for health care service applications, a few more research areas on mobile robots should be mentioned:

- *Underwater AMRs, Airborne AMRs, Autonomous Cars*. There is a huge number of mobile robots for specialised application areas. Nearly any known vehicle has been used as a base for autonomous mobility. To mention just a few, there are ships, submarines, cars, planes, helicopters, and missiles.

3. Wheeled Robots

Despite the fact that a lot of research has been done on different mobility concepts, most mobile robots are wheeled ones. This is due to the fact that they are best suited for standard applications. The mechanical complexity is relatively low, the same holds for energy consumption. When used on even terrain, they can achieve high speeds while moving very smooth.

3.1 Mobility Configurations

Looking at wheeled mobile robot architectures, there are some standard configurations that fit best for most application areas [1][2][4]. The basic distinction is made with the manoeuvrability of the robots, i.e. if they are able to move freely on the ground, or if they have restricted capabilities. In the latter case, in general it is more complicated to reach the goal position and orientation.

2 DOF

The advantage of a mobile robot with two degrees of freedom is the need for only two motors (nevertheless, some systems are employing more than two motors, e.g. for redundancy). In most cases, standard hardware can be used (especially wheels). The most important disadvantage is, that in general shunting is necessary to reach a desired position/orientation. This can be a major drawback if the environment is very tight. The most common configurations are

- *Differential drive* with two parallel, unsteered drive wheels. For stability reasons, castor wheels (from one up to four) are mounted in front and/or back. Incremental encoders are mounted onto the drive motors, counting the wheel revolutions. Dead reckoning is simple through geometric equations.
- *Tricycle drive* with two parallel, unsteered back wheels and one steered front wheel (or vice versa). The steered wheel may be driven or the unsteered wheels (in the latter case, it's a differential drive with additional steering). An incremental encoder is used for sensing the rotation of the steered wheel, and an absolute encoder for the steering angle. Alternatively, differential odometry of the rear axle is done like before. If only one unsteered back wheel is used, the configuration turns to a bicycle drive.
- *Ackermann steering*: car-like steering. This is a good choice for outdoor applications because of its ground clearance, traction, and fairly accurate odometry (by elimination of geometrically induced tire slippage).
- *Synchro drive*. Three or more driven and steered wheels are used, which are coupled mechanically or electrically. Their rotation is always in the same direction, and they are driving with the same speed. With this, all wheels generate equal and parallel force vectors. For linear motions, this concept obtains reduced slippage and therefore improved accuracy of odometry. Problems occur when driving sharp turns, as the wheels have to drive different radii in this case.

3 DOF

The general advantages of 3-DOF mobile robots are the disadvantages of 2-DOF ones and vice versa. Therefore, 3-DOF robots are characterised by best manoeuvrability, no shunting is necessary for them when driving in free space (nevertheless, in cluttered areas shunting can still be inevitable). On the other hand, at least three motors are needed to achieve the desired mobility:

- *Omnidirectional drives* with three or four omnidirectional, unsteered wheels, e.g. Mecanum wheels. Advantage is that no steering of wheels is necessary. Disadvantages are bad odometry, and restriction to indoor-applications. If more than three wheels are used, system coupling (see 5.2) is necessary.
- *Multi-degree-of-freedom drives.* Multiple drive and steering motors are used, thus introducing redundancy. Examples are steered differential drive wheels, or a n-wheel (n>2) design with all wheels driven and steered. The disadvantage of this concept is that in general, more than the minimum number of motors (3) is required.

3.2 Kinematics

Definition of a *wheeled mobile robot* [14]:

"A robot capable of locomotion on a surface solely through the actuation of wheel assemblies mounted on the robot and in contact with the surface. A wheel assembly is a device which provides or allows relative motion between its mount and a surface on which it is intended to have a single point of rolling contact."

For the scope of this book, some simplifying assumptions will be made. They don't affect the understanding of mobile robots in health care applications, as they just restrict the theoretical possibilities to the practical conditions:

- the robot is built up from rigid mechanisms,
- the robot contains a maximum of one steering link per wheel,
- all steering axes are perpendicular to the floor,
- the surface is a smooth plane,
- no translational slip occurs between the wheel and the floor,
- the wheel is able to turn about a vertical axis through the point of contact with the floor (friction does not prevent this).

The kinematic modelling of mobile robots is based on a methodology developed by Muir and Newman [14]. There is a number of differences with kinematics of manipulator arms:

- In general, at least three wheels are in contact with the ground the robot is moving on (there are experimental robots with two or just one wheel on the floor, but they are not included in our discussion). This forms a multiple closed link-chain.
- A wheel is able to turn and translate with respect to the contact point between it and the surface it is moving on. This is called a *pseudo joint* and described as a *higher order pair*.
- Some of the wheels may not be actuated, and some degrees of freedom may not be actuated on some of the wheels.
- In general, it is not necessary to measure position, speed, and acceleration of each degree of freedom of each wheel.

These peculiarities of mobile robots induce the distinction between internal and external kinematics. The former is related to the relationships between linkages within the robot. It describes the steering of the robot. The latter is related to the relationships between robot and environment. It describes the trajectory of the robot.

Coordinate frames

To describe the kinematics of serial link manipulators, the Denavit-Hartenberg convention normally is used. But this convention leads to ambiguous transformation matrices when applied to wheeled robots. This is because there is no distinguished joint ordering in wheeled robots. The Sheth-Uicker convention overcomes this problem.

Definition:

*"A **pair** is a joint between the surfaces of two rigid bodies that keeps them in contact and relatively movable. A **lower pair** is defined by a surface contact, a **higher pair** is defined by point, line, or curve contact. A **planar pair** is a lower pair that keeps the surfaces of two rigid bodies together, allowing two independent translational motions in the plane, and a rotary motion around the axis that is perpendicular to the plane."*

Each wheel is modelled as a planar pair at the point of contact with the ground. A conventional wheel is reduced to two degrees of freedom, as the x component of wheel velocity is set to zero to eliminate sideways slip. Links of a wheeled robot are the floor, the robot body, and the steering links. These links are connected by three joints: the wheel, the steering axis, and the mid-point of the robot. The latter one is no physical joint, but defines a relationship between the body of the robot and the floor. Coordinate frames are assigned at both ends of each link.

Transformation matrices and velocity

To obtain the position of a coordinate frame with respect to a second one, homogeneous transforms are used [15]. This holds both for manipulator robotics as for mobile robotics. A homogeneous transformation matrix can be defined as the (4×4) matrix ${}^{Z}\mathbf{T}_{B}$ having the property of transforming a vector from one coordinate frame to another by means of performing translation and rotation simultaneously. It is composed from a (3×3) rotation matrix $\mathbf{R}$ that defines the orientations with respect to orthogonal unit vectors $\mathbf{i}$, $\mathbf{j}$, $\mathbf{k}$, and a position vector $\mathbf{p}$, defining the translation with respect to the reference frame:

$$
{}^{Z}\mathbf{T}_{B} = \begin{pmatrix} i_x & j_x & k_x & p_x \\ i_y & j_y & k_y & p_y \\ i_z & j_z & k_z & p_z \\ 0 & 0 & 0 & 1 \end{pmatrix} = \begin{pmatrix} \mathbf{i} & \mathbf{j} & \mathbf{k} & \mathbf{p} \\ 0 & 0 & 0 & 1 \end{pmatrix} = \begin{pmatrix} \mathbf{R} & \mathbf{p} \\ \mathbf{0} & 1 \end{pmatrix}
$$

If only a translation is applied, the rotation matrix $\mathbf{R}$ is the (3×3) identity matrix $\mathbf{I}$. For mobile robots only moving on a plane, rotation is solely possible about the z axes. This makes transformation matrices much simpler:

$$
\mathbf{Rot}(\mathbf{z},\phi) = \begin{pmatrix} \cos\phi & -\sin\phi & 0 & 0 \\ \sin\phi & \cos\phi & 0 & 0 \\ 0 & 0 & 1 & 0 \\ 0 & 0 & 0 & 1 \end{pmatrix}
$$

Transformation between any two coordinate frames is simply the multiplication of intermediate frames. With this, the position of the robot body frame is known from the positions of the wheels with respect to the robot body and with respect to the fixed floor frame. The former positions can be measured easily and very precisely by means of encoders (see chapter12), the latter ones are much more difficult to obtain (see chapter 13).

Not only the position, but also the velocity of a mobile robot is of interest. The most straightforward way to calculate it is differentiation of the position transformations. A problem arises when using mechanisms not only containing lower pairs, but also higher pairs. It is not allowed to differentiate transformation equations for higher pair mechanisms. In [11], a velocity cascade algorithm was introduced to overcome this problem. This algorithm calculates velocities in terms of the multiplication of transforms.

As for manipulation robots, a methodology for dealing with position and velocity by means of *Jacobian* has been developed [14]. The Jacobian is developed by differentiating the transform equation of the mobile system. A pseudo-velocity vector for each wheel contains components of linear velocities of the wheel in x- and y-direction with respect to the floor, angular velocity around the contact point, and angular velocity of the steering link around the hip joint. As typical (conventional) wheels have less than four wheel variables, there is a mapping from the physical velocity vector to the pseudo velocity vector with a wheel matrix. The physical wheel Jacobian is derived in a similar way. The number of degrees of freedom of a wheel is determined by the rank of the physical Jacobian.

In most cases, the velocity of the robot body with respect to the fixed floor frame is of interest.

4. Walking Robots

Despite the fact that motion of most of the highly developed animals is by means of legs, walking robots are experimental platforms only at the time being. Especially the mechanical complexity of legged robots prevents application in standard environments. Nevertheless, there are possible application areas for legged mobile robots: rough outdoor environments, stairs, heaps of rubble.

4.1 Mobility Configurations

Although there are many possible leg configurations, only systems with two, three, four, or six legs are of general interest. Mobile robots with one leg have been studied in detail, but as the only way to move for them is hopping, possible application areas are very rare. Especially in health care services, there is actually no demand for them. For this reason, we will concentrate on the configurations mentioned before [10][11][19].

To be helpful in everyday tasks, a system should be *statically stable*. This condition keeps, if the centre of gravity always lies within the polygon defined by the contact points of the feet actually on the floor. This can be achieved only if at any time at least three feet are in contact with the floor. Therefore, a robot must have at least four legs for statically stable walking. If the feet don't have contact *points*, but *lines* or *planes* of contact, this might not be true. In this case, a statically stable robot with only two legs is possible. As this kind of robots suffer from some drawbacks in everyday tasks, we will only deal with robots having contact points or at least very small contact areas with respect to their body size.

While moving, it is not possible to guarantee static stability of a walking robot with only two or three legs at any time. Even for robots with four or six legs, design and gait need a careful layout to obtain continuous static stability. Nevertheless, if a robot is not statically stable, but if it does not fall over, it is called *dynamically stable.*

4.2 Gait

Legs are very different from continuous motion elements like wheels. Legs need to be lifted from and returned to the ground. A *gait* describes the phases of leg motion to accomplish a motion of the body. *A gait of an articulated living creature or a walking machine is the corporate motion of the legs, which can be defined as the time and the location of the placing and lifting of each foot, coordinated with the motion of the body in its six degrees of freedom, in order to move the body from one place to another* [18].

Gait analysis

A repetitive pattern of foot placement is called a *regular gait*. Though non-repetitive patterns are possible, they are only used in situations where regular gaits are temporarily not applicable (e.g. on uneven terrain). In gait analysis, the feet of a walking machine are modelled as two-state devices: a foot is either on or off the ground (on-state, off-state). This reduces the complexity of the continuous process of motion. With this supposition, recording of gaits can easily be done by

- diagram of feet in on-state at state changes (footfall diagram),
- continuous diagram of feet in on-state (gait diagram),
- matrix of feet positions at certain times within a cycle.

Diagrams enable to record even complicated gaits, e.g. where legs are in off-state for a longer period of time. A well-known animal gait is the four-leg trot. It is characterised by simultaneous motion of the opposite feet (left-front and right-back resp. right-front and left-back). Using the foot numbering from figure 1a (where the direction of motion is towards the feet 1 and 2), the trot gait can be noted 1-3,2-4, where '-' denotes a simultaneous motion, and ',' a sequential motion. Figure 1b shows a footfall diagram, where 'X' denotes foot in on-state. Figure 1c shows a gait diagram, where a bar denotes foot in on-state. Figure 1d shows a gait matrix, where '0' denotes foot in on-state.

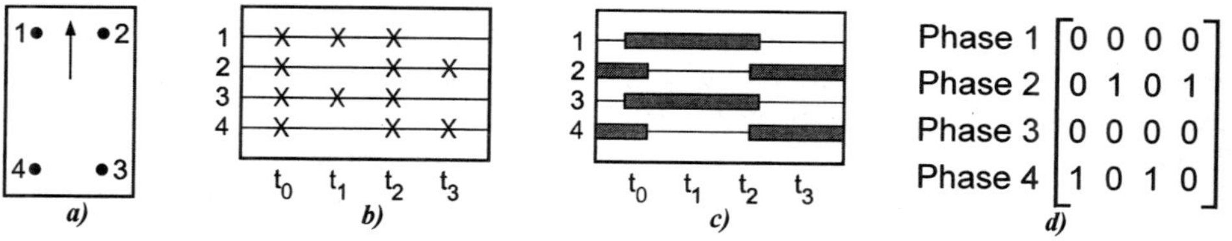

Figure 1. Gait diagrams

Some more terms are needed to describe a certain gait in more detail. The basic cycle of a gait is called a *stride*. It describes the complete cycle from one occurrence of a leg motion to its repetition. The *duty factor* of a foot is defined as that fraction of a stride during which the foot is in on-state. The minimum duty factor for statically stable walking is 3 divided by the number of legs (3 is the minimum number of feet in on-state to assure static stability). Two feet which are almost in the same state are called a *pair*. The *relative phase* of a pair is defined as that proportion of a stride between the two feet in off-state touching the ground. A *symmetrical gait* is characterised as a gait where the feet of a pair have equal duty factors and a relative phase of less than half a stride. A *walking gait* is one where at least one foot is on the ground at any time. If there are periods when all feet are in off-state, it is a *running gait*.

With this, the trot gait from figure 1 is a symmetrical walking gait.

Dynamic stability

When using robots with three or less legs, or when a gait is chosen that does not ensure static mobility at every time, measures for dynamic stability are necessary. These have to prevent the body of the robot from falling over. The behaviour of a walking robot can be expressed by a sequence of states, and controlled by finite automata (state machines). A simple example is that of a one-leg hopping machine. There are five states of a hopping machine:

- thrust (leg is on the ground, compressed),
- unloading (leg is extending),
- flight (leg is fully extended and leaves the ground),
- landing (leg is touching the ground),
- compression (leg is on the ground, shortening).

Depending on sensor measurements, time and parameters of the transitions between states need to be chosen.

Drawbacks of robots without static stability are a higher energy consumption for achieving dynamic stability, and the need of additional *stabilising* motions (in addition to *productive* motions) to prevent the body from falling over.

5. Mobile Robot Control Methods

As mentioned before, walking robots are not applicable in health care services at the time being. Therefore, the rest of the chapter will concentrate on wheeled robots. Task of mobile robot control is to keep the robot on a given trajectory with a given velocity. In order to achieve good results, the dynamic behaviour of the system needs to be taken into account.

5.1 Low Level Control

Different levels of control apply to complex systems such as mobile robots. On the lowest level, speed or torque of each single motor needs to be controlled. The next level coordinates the single actions of the motors to achieve a desired motion. Next, the given trajectory must be tracked and deviations must be reduced to a minimum [1][3]. First of all, a kinematic modelling needs to be done.

Kinematic modelling of non-holonomic mobile robots

Considering the kinematic constraints applied on mobile robots, we concentrate on a specific family of mobile robots with non-holonomically constrained kinematic configurations. For this family of robots first we will analyse the so-called *bicycle kinematic model* [8]. In [9], the definitions of holonomic and non-holonomic constraints are given.

- *Bicycle model*
  In Figure 2, the bicycle model is shown. For the analysis purposes we named *steering wheels* denoted by s_i the steerable wheels of a mobile robot, and *powered wheels*, denoted by p_i the wheels where power is transmitted (*i* denotes either an index indicating the numbered wheels of a robot or the configuration index, as appropriate). A wheel can meet both definitions, thus can be both a powered and a steering wheel. The notion of steering and powered wheels could be expanded so to include other means used for mobile robot move (e.g. chains), but under special considerations. Under the assumption of ideal terrain traction and non-antagonistic wheels action, it can be proved [7] that all powered wheels are contributing to one equivalent powered wheel denoted by *p,* and all steering wheels to one equivalent steering wheel denoted by *s*.

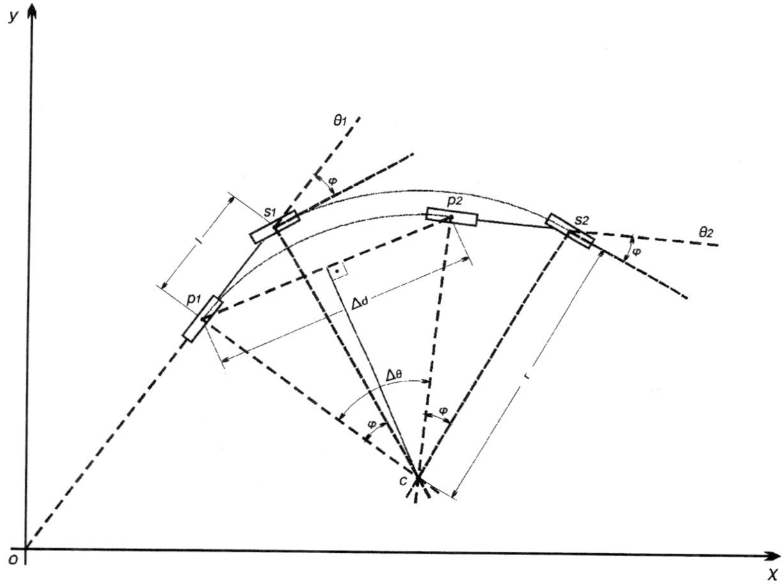

Figure 2. The bicycle kinematic model

P_i, S_i denotes the position of powered and steering wheel respectively w.r.t. XYO - i is the robot configuration index,
τ_p, τ_s denote the path followed by the powered and steering wheel respectively,
l is the wheelbase, the constant distance between the center of powered to center of steering wheel,
φ denotes the robot's steering angle,
r the radius of the circle drawn by p_i wheel,
ϑ_1 the robot orientation at configuration q_1,
ϑ_2 the robot orientation at configuration q_2,
$\Delta\vartheta$ the difference of orientation ϑ_1 and ϑ_2 (the deviation in ϑ from q_1 to q_2)
Δd Euclidean distance of P_1 and P_2.

In Figure 2, the bicycle model of *p-s* is shown. The figure shows two robots' configurations w.r.t. the world coordinate frame XYO. The local robot coordinate system is attached to the center of the powered wheel at point *P*, while the y-axis is identical to the p-s axis. A robot's configuration is denoted by the triple (x,y,ϑ), where $(x,y) \in R^2$ are the coordinates of *P* w.r.t. XYO, and $\vartheta \in [0,2\pi]$ is the directed angle between the X axis of the world coordinating frame and the *p-s* axis of the bicycle model.

Stable kinematic behaviour implies non-antagonistic action of the model wheels. In order to have stable kinematic behaviour and under the assumptions of i) ideal friction conditions, and ii) constant l - but not necessarily constant robot dimensions and shape - , the paths of powered and steering wheel should be compatible, thus they should follow tracks of circles of a common center. This point is named *instantaneous rotation point* and it is denoted by *C*. *C* is defined as the intersection of steering and powered wheels axis of rotation. It is obvious that the position of *C* w.r.t XYO is a function of the steering angle φ and it is correlated to l.

For the bicycle model one can notice two special motion cases:

I. *Rotation by the p wheel center*: An arbitrarily selected configuration q_i, and the previous configuration q_{i-1} which both belong on a path τ, have identical x and y, but different orientations ϑ.

$$\forall\, q_i, q_{i-1} \in \tau, \quad x_i = x_{i-1}, \quad y_i = y_{i-1}, \quad \vartheta_i \neq \vartheta_{i-1}$$

II. *Translation on the p-s axis:* An arbitrarily selected configuration q_i, and the previous configuration q_{i-1} which both belong on a path τ, have identical orientations ϑ but differ in position (different *x,y* pairs).

$$\forall\, q_i, q_{i-1} \in \tau, \quad (x_i, y_i) \neq (x_{i-1}, y_{i-1}), \quad \vartheta_i = \vartheta_{i-1}$$

In the general case the robot reference point P moves on a circular track with center the instantaneous rotation point C. Rotation by the p wheel center occurs when $\varphi = \pi/2$. In that case $C \equiv P$. Translation on the p-s axis occurs when $\varphi = 0$. In this case the instantaneous rotation point C trends to the infinity as the axis of rotation of s and p wheels become parallel to each other. In this general case point P describes a curve tangent to the p-s axis, thus the motion of the robot is constrained by:

$$-\dot{x}\sin\vartheta + \dot{y}\cos\vartheta = 0$$

It has been proved [9] that this equation is non-integrable and hence it is by definition a non-holonomic constraint.

Furthermore, geometrically resolving the triangle P_1CP_2, and triangle P_1CS_1 we get:

$$\left.\begin{aligned} \sin\left(\frac{\Delta\vartheta}{2}\right) &= \frac{\Delta d/2}{r} \\ \tan\varphi &= \frac{l}{r} \end{aligned}\right\} \Rightarrow \tan\varphi = \frac{2l\sin\left(\frac{\Delta\vartheta}{2}\right)}{\Delta d}$$

This equation gives the relation of the steering angle φ, the deviation of robot's orientation $\Delta\vartheta$ and the distance covered Δd. Given φ, $\Delta\vartheta$ and Δd, the last two equations correlate the next robot configuration with the current robot configuration.

The analysis following is considering a special case that may be resolved by the application of the general bicycle model described above.

- *Tricycle.*

There are two equivalent configurations of tricycles:

- with powered and steered front wheel
- with two independently powered back wheels and unsteered front wheel (if neglecting wheel slippage).

There is a common description as two-wheel configuration. The driving system of a tricycle is well known as *differential drive* (figure 3). Looking on very small changes in position, dead reckoning is possible by using simple geometric equations to compute the current position relative to a known starting position. Suppose a sampling interval j and pulse increments ${}^{W}v_x(t$ and r_j for left wheel and right wheel encoder:

$$c_m = \pi D_n / (iC_e)$$

where

c_m conversion factor from encoder pulses into linear wheel displacement,

D_n nominal wheel diameter (in mm),

C_e encoder resolution (in pulses per revolution),
i gear ratio.

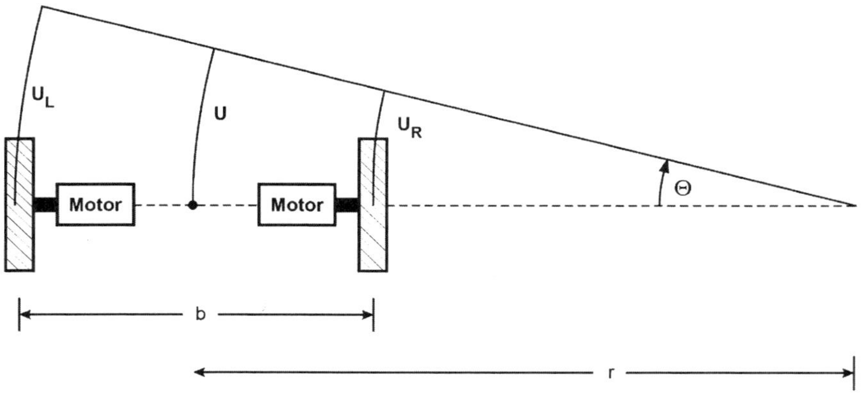

Figure 3. Differential steering

The incremental travel distances for the left and right wheel at interval i are given by

$$\Delta U_{Lj} = c_m N_{Lj}$$
$$\Delta U_{Rj} = c_m N_{Rj}$$

and the incremental linear displacement of the centerpoint C, denoted ΔU_j, is given by

$$\Delta U_j = (\Delta U_{Rj} + \Delta U_{Lj})/2 .$$

The incremental change of orientation is given by

$$\Delta\Theta_j = (\Delta U_R - \Delta U_L)/b$$

where b is the wheelbase, measured as the distance between the two contact points between the motorised wheels and the floor.

The radius r_j of the turn driven is given by

$$r_j = \Delta U_j / \Delta\Theta_j .$$

The new relative orientation Θ_j at interval j can be computed from the orientation at previous interval $j-1$ by

$$\Theta_j = \Theta_{j-1} + \Delta\Theta_j$$

and the relative position of the centerpoint C in world coordinates x, y from

$$x_j = x_{j-1} + \Delta U_j \cos\Theta_j$$
$$y_j = y_{j-1} + \Delta U_j \sin\Theta_j$$

where

x_j, y_j relative position of the centerpoint C at interval j.

To obtain a (small) movement of the system with an orientation change Θ and a travel distance U, the wheels have to move

$$U_L = U + \Theta b/2$$
$$U_R = U - \Theta b/2 .$$

Kinematic modelling of an omnidirectional mobile robot

For the following considerations, we will concentrate on Mecanum wheels [14]. Using an appropriate configuration of these wheels, a minimum of three wheels is necessary but also sufficient to move with three degrees of freedom. For stability reasons, a four wheel design is used in most applications. This introduces over-determination into the system. To prevent wheel slippage on the floor, system coupling has to be applied (see section 5.2).

- *Coordinate system assignments*
  The assignment of coordinate systems is illustrated in figure 4. The Sheth-Uicker convention is applied. A stationary floor coordinate system W serves as the absolute reference coordinate frame for robot motions. The floor coordinate system is assigned with the z-axis orthogonal to the surface of travel. The robot coordinate system R is assigned to the geometric center of the robot body, with the z-axis orthogonal to the surface of travel.

In figure 4, those rollers can be seen which are in contact with the floor. That is, the robot is seen from the bottom.

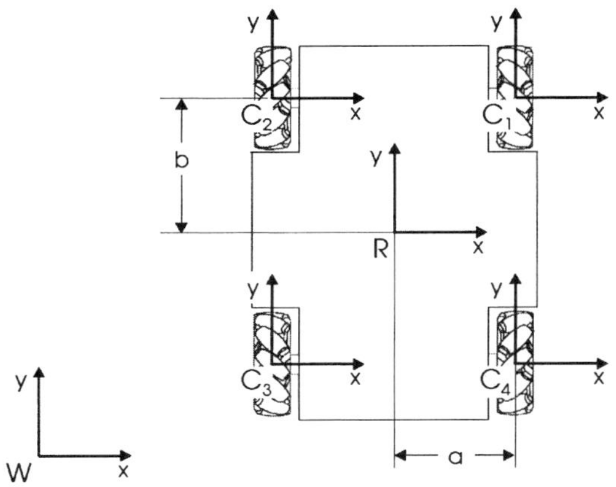

Figure 4. Coordinate system assignments

- *Transformation matrices*

A Mecanum wheel driven mobile robot is characterised by two translational velocities ${}^{W}v_x(t)$ and ${}^{W}v_y(t)$, and a rotational velocity ${}^{W}\omega_z(t)$ with respect to the world coordinate system W. The coordinate system $\overline{R}$ is stationary with respect to W. At the instant of observation, it is located at the same point as R. ${}^{\overline{R}}v_x(t)$, ${}^{\overline{R}}v_y(t)$, and ${}^{\overline{R}}\omega_z(t)$ are the velocity components of $\overline{R}$. The relation between velocities in $\overline{R}$ and R is given by

$$\begin{pmatrix} {}^{W}v_x \\ {}^{W}v_y \\ {}^{W}\omega_z \end{pmatrix} = \begin{pmatrix} \cos\varphi & -\sin\varphi & 0 \\ \sin\varphi & \cos\varphi & 0 \\ 0 & 0 & 1 \end{pmatrix} \begin{pmatrix} {}^{\overline{R}}v_x \\ {}^{\overline{R}}v_y \\ {}^{\overline{R}}\omega_z \end{pmatrix}$$

At every point of contact between wheel i and floor, there is a coordinate frame $C_i(i=1,2,3,4)$. As for R, for every C_i there is a $\overline{C_i}$ located at the same point as C_i and that is stationary with respect to W at the instant of observation. With this, the velocities of the wheels can be determined independently of their position. The velocity vector $\dot{\mathbf{q}}_i$ of wheel i in $\overline{C_i}$ is given by the components ω_{ix} (rotation around the hub), ω_{ir} (rotation of the rollers), and ω_{iz} (rotation of the wheel around the point of contact). With this, the velocity vector with respect to $\overline{C_i}$ is given by

$$\begin{pmatrix} {}^{\overline{C}_i}v_x \\ {}^{\overline{C}_i}v_y \\ {}^{\overline{C}_i}\omega_z \end{pmatrix} = \begin{pmatrix} 0 & r_i \sin\eta_i & 0 \\ R_i & -r_i\cos\eta_i & 0 \\ 0 & 0 & 1 \end{pmatrix} \begin{pmatrix} \omega_{ix} \\ \omega_{ir} \\ \omega_{iz} \end{pmatrix}$$

with wheel radius R_i, roller radius r_i, and roller angle η_i.

- *Wheel Jacobian matrices*

The robot velocity ${}^{\overline{R}}\dot{\mathbf{p}}$ consists of translational velocities ${}^{\overline{R}}v_x$ and ${}^{\overline{R}}v_y$, and a rotational velocity ${}^{\overline{R}}\omega_z$. It is given by

$$\begin{pmatrix} {}^{\overline{R}}v_x \\ {}^{\overline{R}}v_y \\ {}^{\overline{R}}\omega_z \end{pmatrix} = \begin{pmatrix} \cos{}^R\theta_{C_i} & -\sin{}^R\theta_{C_i} & {}^Rd_{C_iy} \\ \sin{}^R\theta_{C_i} & -\cos{}^R\theta_{C_i} & -{}^Rd_{C_ix} \\ 0 & 0 & 1 \end{pmatrix} \begin{pmatrix} {}^{\overline{C}_i}v_x \\ {}^{\overline{C}_i}v_y \\ {}^{\overline{C}_i}\omega_z \end{pmatrix}$$

where ${}^R\theta_{C_i}$ denotes the orientation of C_i with respect to R. ${}^Rd_{C_ix}$ and ${}^Rd_{C_iy}$ denoting the translation of C_i with respect to R. With this, the Jacobi matrix $\mathbf{J}_i$ of wheel i describes the robot velocity ${}^{\overline{R}}\dot{\mathbf{p}}$ as a linear combination of the wheel velocities $\dot{\mathbf{q}}_i$:

$${}^{\overline{R}}\dot{\mathbf{p}} = \mathbf{J}_i\dot{\mathbf{q}}_i$$

with

$$\mathbf{J}_i = \begin{pmatrix} -R_i\sin{}^R\theta_{C_i} & r_i\sin\left({}^R\theta_{C_i}+\eta_i\right) & {}^Rd_{C_iy} \\ R_i\cos{}^R\theta_{C_i} & -r_i\cos\left({}^R\theta_{C_i}+\eta_i\right) & -{}^Rd_{C_ix} \\ 0 & 0 & 1 \end{pmatrix}$$

If the wheels are identical (except for the orientation of the rollers), all radii are equal: $R_i = R$ and $r_i = r$, $(i = 1,2,3,4)$. Using the configuration from figure 4, ${}^R\theta_{C_i} = 0$, $|\,{}^Rd_{C_ix}\,| = a$, $|\,{}^Rd_{C_iy}\,| = b$, $\eta_1 = \eta_3 = -45°$, and $\eta_2 = \eta_4 = 45°$. With this, the equations of motion for each wheel are:

$$\mathbf{J}_1 = \begin{pmatrix} 0 & -r\frac{\sqrt{2}}{2} & b \\ R & -r\frac{\sqrt{2}}{2} & -a \\ 0 & 0 & 1 \end{pmatrix} \qquad \mathbf{J}_2 = \begin{pmatrix} 0 & r\frac{\sqrt{2}}{2} & b \\ R & -r\frac{\sqrt{2}}{2} & a \\ 0 & 0 & 1 \end{pmatrix}$$

$$\mathbf{J}_3 = \begin{pmatrix} 0 & -r\frac{\sqrt{2}}{2} & -b \\ R & -r\frac{\sqrt{2}}{2} & a \\ 0 & 0 & 1 \end{pmatrix} \qquad \mathbf{J}_4 = \begin{pmatrix} 0 & r\frac{\sqrt{2}}{2} & -b \\ R & -r\frac{\sqrt{2}}{2} & -a \\ 0 & 0 & 1 \end{pmatrix}$$

The motion of the robot results from the simultaneous motion of all four wheels:

$$\begin{pmatrix} \mathbf{I} \\ \mathbf{I} \\ \mathbf{I} \\ \mathbf{I} \end{pmatrix} {}^R\dot{\mathbf{p}} = \begin{pmatrix} \mathbf{J}_1 & 0 & \cdots & 0 \\ 0 & \mathbf{J}_2 & \ddots & \vdots \\ \vdots & \ddots & \mathbf{J}_3 & 0 \\ 0 & \cdots & 0 & \mathbf{J}_4 \end{pmatrix} \begin{pmatrix} \dot{\mathbf{q}}_1 \\ \dot{\mathbf{q}}_2 \\ \dot{\mathbf{q}}_3 \\ \dot{\mathbf{q}}_4 \end{pmatrix}$$

with $\mathbf{I}$ as a (3×3) identity matrix.

Kinematic solutions of an omnidirectional mobile robot

- *Sensed forward solution*
  First, the platform velocity is determined in dependence of the measured wheel velocities $\dot{\mathbf{q}}_i$ by applying the sensed forward velocity solution:

$$\begin{pmatrix} {}^{\overline{R}}v_x \\ {}^{\overline{R}}v_y \\ {}^{\overline{R}}v_\omega \end{pmatrix} = \frac{R}{4(a+b)} \begin{pmatrix} -(a+b) & (a+b) & -(a+b) & (a+b) \\ (a+b) & (a+b= & (a+b) & (a+b) \\ 1 & -1 & -1 & 1 \end{pmatrix} \begin{pmatrix} \omega_{1x} \\ \omega_{2x} \\ \omega_{3x} \\ \omega_{4x} \end{pmatrix}$$

where ω_{ix} are those elements of wheel velocities $\dot{\mathbf{q}}_i$ describing the rotation of the wheel around the hub. If the platform is controlled in floor coordinates, ${}^W\dot{\mathbf{p}}$ can be obtained by a coordinate transformation of ${}^{\overline{R}}\dot{\mathbf{p}}$.

- *Actuated inverse solution*

  In a second step the platform velocity is integrated over each sample period to get the actual position ${}^{\bar{R}}\mathbf{p}$ or ${}^{W}\mathbf{p}$ respectively. After applying the control algorithm to the position error, the desired wheel velocities $\omega_{ix}(i=1,2,3,4)$ can be calculated using the actuated inverse solution:

$$\begin{pmatrix}\omega_{1x}\\ \omega_{2x}\\ \omega_{3x}\\ \omega_{4x}\end{pmatrix}=\frac{1}{R}\begin{pmatrix}-1 & 1 & (a+b)\\ 1 & 1 & -(a+b)\\ -1 & 1 & -(a+b)\\ 1 & 1 & (a+b)\end{pmatrix}\begin{pmatrix}{}^{\bar{R}}v_x\\ {}^{\bar{R}}v_y\\ {}^{\bar{R}}v_\omega\end{pmatrix}$$

Feedback control of an omnidirectional mobile robot

If for any reason no dynamic model of the robot is available, a kinematics based control system can be applied [13]. Nevertheless, better results will be achieved by using the dynamic model of the mobile robot (figure 5) [5]. As usual, a reference trajectory for the robot is provided by a trajectory planner (see chapter 7). The trajectory (e.g. a spline curve) is split into a sequence of points. These points are given to the control system, whose task it is to produce signals for the motors. The position of the robot is estimated by odometric means. The structure of the feedback control can be divided in three main parts: wheel velocity control, path control, and wheel coupling (see section 5.2). With this, the structure is set up by a path control loop with underlying single wheel control loop. The latter is supplemented by a coupling, acting directly on the wheel control loop.

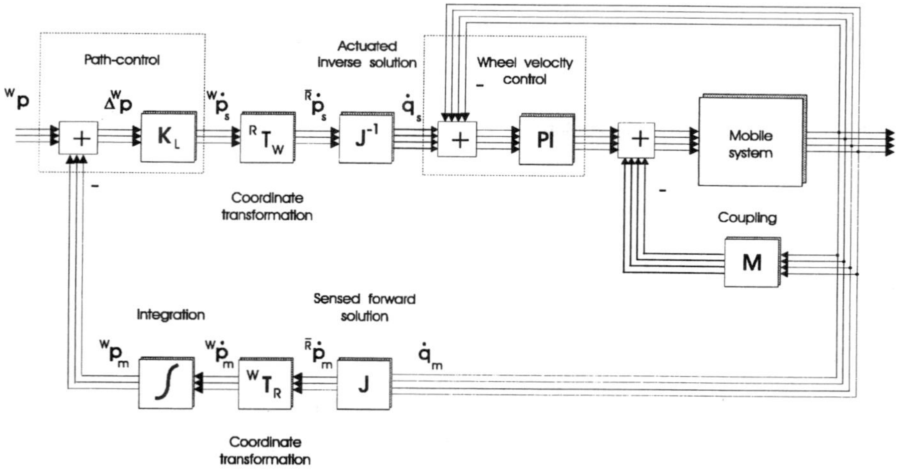

Figure 5. Feedback control of Mecanum-platform

5.2 System Coupling - Methods for Reducing Wheel Slip in Over-Determined Systems

The driving structure of a four-wheeled omnidirectional mobile robot is over-determined (just three wheels are necessary to achieve omnidirectional behaviour). This means, that it is not robust and an actuator conflict may occur. Solving the kinematic velocity equations, it follows that all four wheels need to be synchronised to avoid translational wheel slip. With appropriate measures of system coupling, it is possible to control omnidirectional vehicles in a way that translational wheel slip resulting from possible actuator conflicts is minimised and the overall dynamic behaviour of the vehicle is influenced systematically [6].

Using the vehicle from figure 4, two conditions must always be met:

$$\omega_{1r} = -\omega_{2r} \qquad \omega_{3r} = -\omega_{4r}\text{, and}$$
$$\omega_{1x} + \omega_{2x} - \omega_{3x} - \omega_{4x} = 0$$

To avoid wheel slippage, these *rolling conditions* must be observed. In figure 5, the coupling part is set up as described in [6]. The behaviour of the system is improved in two ways: The accuracy of the path is higher; and abrasion of the rollers as well as of the floor is reduced.

The same holds for non-holonomic devices with more than two independent driving/steering devices. Examples are tricycles with two independently driven back wheels plus one steered front wheel.

6. Case Studies

At present, there is a number of mobile devices designed for application in health care services in a broad sense. Many of them are laboratory devices, but there are also some commercial ones. All examples listed are randomly chosen, they are neither complete nor any indication for quality [16][17].

- *Automated Guided Vehicles (AGVs)*. These devices are intended for transportation of materials in different environments, like industry or hospitals. They are commercially available in a great variety, according to the applications demands.
  Examples are Omnidrive from MIAG in Germany and HelpMate from Pyxis in the USA.
- *Service-Robots.* There is an increasing number of application areas where service-robots are available or under development. Examples are:
  - Floor-cleaning (subway stations, supermarkets),
    e.g. BR 600, Kärcher, Germany; AUROR, Cybernetix, France; ST-81, Siemens, Germany,
  - Information and guide systems (museums),
    e.g. Rhino, Bonn University, Germany.
- *Rehabilitation (e.g. wheelchairs)*. This field of application is somewhat different from the other ones. Unlike other ranges of application, there is *always* a person on the system. In principle, this user is able to control it, though he/she might need some assistance in

doing so. In any way, the user must be able to assert himself. Furthermore, there are other persons in the environment of the device. Therefore, both security and intentions of all persons concerned must be observed. Examples of current developments are Maid from FAW Ulm in Germany, OMNI from Hagen University in Germany, and SENARIO from Zenon in Greece.

- *Planet exploration.* Though remote-control in principle is possible, autonomy is desired due to communication delays or temporary loss of communication.
  The best known example is the Sojourner from JPL in the USA.
- There is a lot of *other application areas*. To mention only a few of them: tube inspection (KURT/LAOKOON, GMD, Germany), wall/window cleaning (Comatec, France), wall construction (Akatsuki 21, Fujita, Japan).

7. Safety

The application of mobile robots in health care services is much more critical than in industrial applications. The first reason is that persons using the robots or that might get in contact with them are not accustomed to robots. The second one is that especially in this context robot motions are not cyclic and often unpredictable. This is due to the partially unstructured environments, changing tasks of the robots, and sensor-driven online collision avoidance. This induces the necessity of inherent security measurements:

- Reliable, redundant sensor systems,
- Reliable software,
- Smooth surfaces,
- Low speed.

Designing robots for health care applications, a number of topics particular to this scope need to be considered:

- Users and other persons are in the range of the system,
- Conflicts between functionality and safety have to be solved,
- Safety facilities require redundancy,
- Active or passive collision avoidance must be implemented (i.e. searching for a collision free path or slowing down),
- Use of standard hardware and software, interfaces, and components (as far as possible),
- Uniform look and feel of the human-robot interface (icons etc.) to avoid confusion in critical situations,
- Training of users to familiarise them with potential dangers and possibilities of the devices.

In general, three levels of safety should be implemented to avoid any risk both for the user and persons in the environment of the robotic device:

- First of all, *passive safety* (mechanical safety).
  Under worst-case conditions, passive safety largely depends on electro-mechanical design:
  - Low inertia of moving elements,
  - Limited motor velocities at maximum voltage,
  - Limited static motor torques at stall,
  - Possibility of passive movements,
  - Design avoiding sharp edges and protrusions, scissors effects, exposed gears etc.,
  - Fire resistance.
- Second, *supervised safety*:
  - Watch dog, safety monitor,
  - Forbidden zones,
  - Velocity limits,
  - Force and torque limits,
  - Strategies for safe homing and (pre)programmed motions.
- Third, *interactive safety*:
  - The user must always be able to switch off the system,
  - Independent alarm system,
  - Avoiding of 'control-blocking conditions' with the user loosing access to the control transducers (transducers get out of reach).

The most important means of safety for mobile systems is braking. It must always be possible to stop the motion of the device by one of the following conditions:

- *Emergency stop*:
  - System shutdown due to an unrecoverable hazard condition,
  - Initiated by the user or a hardware/software watchdog.
- *Intrusion pause*:
  - System pause due to an external hazard,
  - Initiated by a sensor,
  - The user may restart when the hazard has removed.
- *User pause*:
  - System pause due to a potential problem recognised by the user,
  - Initiated by the user,
  - The user may restart or cancel the operation when the problem has been rectified.

Besides these basic safety rules for mobile robots in health care applications, it is self-evident that all other applicable standards and safety regulations both for mobile systems and for robots need to be applied.

8. Design Principles for Mobile Robots in Healthcare

The principal properties of the workspace where a mobile robot in the healthcare sector will perform in are:

- Indoors,
- Crowded with people - limited space,
- Structured environment (partially),
- Several levels.

The indoors property implies that the floor will be levelled in the typical case and there will be available ramps or elevators (those to be used by wheelchair users). This excludes the need to employ very complicated mobility designs like legged robots (stair climbers). The environment may be assumed structured therefore special designs may be avoided because the organisation that would host the application would be willing to adapt the environment to the mobility need of the robot and subsequently the people it is servicing. The presence of obstacles of any kind (stair cases, overhanging obstacles, forgotten objects) will be detected by the on-board obstacle avoidance facilities, thus the mobile platform will implement a by-passing or another avoidance strategy instead of stepping over the potential obstacle or climbing the stair case.

Presence of people implies that the robot has to implement smooth motion and tries to use the minimum space in order to leave corridors', bedsides', and elevators' room free for people that are using the very same space. It is evident that high manoeuvrability is the strongest demand. The ultimate solution in achieving the maximum in manoeuvring capabilities is to select an omnidirectional kinematic configuration. Omnidirectional robots present features that enable them to move instantaneously to any desired direction as well as rotate by any point the control system may select. Given that the control algorithms are optimal, omnidirectional configuration enables the robot to use the minimum space required for a manoeuvre compared to any other kinematics configuration. In addition, omnidirectional configuration may implement the tracks that would be followed by any other kinematic configuration. For example, this could be a car-like one if this is an application demand, i.e. if the user driving the robot is used to this type of vehicle behaviour.

The main drawbacks in omnidirectional configuration are the limitation to indoor applications (the floor has to be smooth, flat, and preferably clean), small ability to overcome common obstacles (very heavy carpet e.g. 4cm thick would be a problem), the increased complexity in the hardware (at least three motors instead of two in the typical case), the increased cost of the omnidirectional wheels in comparison to the conventional ones.

9. References

[1] Angeles J., *Fundamentals of Robotic Mechanical Systems*. Springer, Berlin 1997.

[2] Borenstein J., Everett H. R., Feng L., *Navigating Mobile Robots - Systems and Techniques*. A K Peters Ltd, Wellesley 1996.

[3] Guldner J., *Intelligentes hierarchisches Regelungskonzept für autonome mobile Robotersysteme*. VDI Verlag, Düsseldorf 1995.

[4] Hinkel R., *Konzeption eines echtzeitfähigen, autonomen, mobilen Systems*. Kaiserslautern 1989.

[5] Hölper R., Intelligentes, flexibel konfigurierbares Steuerungssystem für mobile Serviceroboter. VDI Verlag, Düsseldorf 1997.

[6] Jochheim A., Reglerentwurf für Mehrgrößensysteme unter der Nebenbedingung vorgegebener Ausgangsgrößenverkopplungen. VDI Verlag, Düsseldorf 1995.

[7] Katevas N., "Intelligent Autonomous Mobile Robots - Contribution to System Architecture and Path Planning"., *Ph.D. dissertation*, National Technical University of Athens, Athens 1997.

[8]Katevas N., Tzafestas S. G., "The Active Kinematic Histogram Method for Path Planning of Non-Point, Non-Holonomically Constrainted Mobile Robots". In: *Advanced Robotics, the International Journal of the Robotics Society of Japan, Special Issue on Intelligent Mobile Robots*, 1998, Vol. 12, No. 4, pp. 373-395.

[9] Latombe J.-P., *Robot Motion Planning*. Kluwer Academic, Boston, MA 1990.

[10] McCloy D., Harris M., *Robotics - An Introduction*. Open University Press, Milton Keynes 1986.

[11] McKerrow P. J., *Introduction to Robotics*. Addison-Wesley, Sydney 1991.

[12] Meystel A., "Autonomous Mobile Robots". *World Scientific*, Singapore 1991.

[13] Muir P. F., Neuman C. P., "Kinematic Modelling for Feedback Control of an Omnidirectional Wheeled Mobile Robot". In: Cox I.J., Wilfong G.T. (editors): *Autonomous Robot Vehicles*. Springer, New York 1990.

[14] Muir P. F., Neuman C. P., "Kinematic Modelling of Wheeled Mobile Robots". *CMU-RI-TR-86-12*, Pittsburgh 1986.

[15] Paul R. P., *Robot Manipulators: Mathematics, Programming, and Control*. MIT Press, Cambridge 1981.

[16] Prassler E., Dillmann R., Kuntze H.-B., *Robotic in Deutschland*. Shaker, Aachen 1998.

[17] Schraft R. D., Schmierer G., *Serviceroboter*. Springer, Berlin 1998.

[18] Song S.-M., Waldron K. J., *Machines that walk*. MIT press, Cambridge 1989.

[19] Vukobratovi M. et al., *Biped Locomotion*. Springer, Berlin 1990.

Chapter 8

Global and Local Strategies for Mobile Robot Navigation

by Nikos I. KATEVAS, Spyros G. TZAFESTAS, Fernando MATÍA

Mobile Robotics in Healthcare
N. Katevas (Ed.)
IOS Press, 2001

Chapter 8

Global and Local Strategies for Mobile Robot Navigation

Nikos I. KATEVAS, Spyros G. TZAFESTAS, Fernando MATÍA

1. Introduction

Path planning or trajectory planning has been extensively studied by the scientific community and methods tackling the problem from various perspectives have been proposed. Initially the efforts were focused on the development of reliable off-line programming tools that would utilise exact geometric features of the environment, assumed to be available. However, navigation mobile robots introduced the need to heavily incorporate perception into the control loop and dropped the assumption of accurate and reliable environment representation. The first demand was to implement obstacle avoidance behaviour. Over the years, several control strategies for collision avoidance targeting mobile robots have been developed. These were based on information provided by environment perception devices such as ultrasonic sensors, infrared or visible light sensor, laser range sensors, cameras, tactile sensors etc. A great amount of effort has been given to develop systems that employ perception based on machine vision but the later was rapidly exchanged by the use of simpler sensing principles targeting specific applications. Only the last years seems that all together the related technologies are reaching the maturity required to realize navigation strategies based on machine vision meeting the efficiency demanded by real-time, real-life applications.

The chapter begins with the presentation of representative families of global and local strategies for mobile robot navigation. The overview of the families is not exhaustive, nor complete. The aim is to present the methods and trigger the reader to select/combine one or more of those for the mobile robot he/she is designing. The chapter concludes, presenting case studies of the navigations control methods used in mobile robots for healthcare services.

The main assumption in the chapter is that the robot knows with the required accuracy its position in the space.

2. Global Strategies: Path Planning Based on Geometric Features

2.1 Definitions

The first approaches tackled the mobile robot path planning problem by following a strategy that attempted to extract the path from an initial point to the goal, based on the geometric features of the space. The most considered point-sized robots and fitted polygonal lines in the space between the 2D representations of the robots' environment. When applications demanded to consider the actual size of the robot the very same methods applied using the approximation of: i) obstacles expansion ii) reduction of obstacles list.

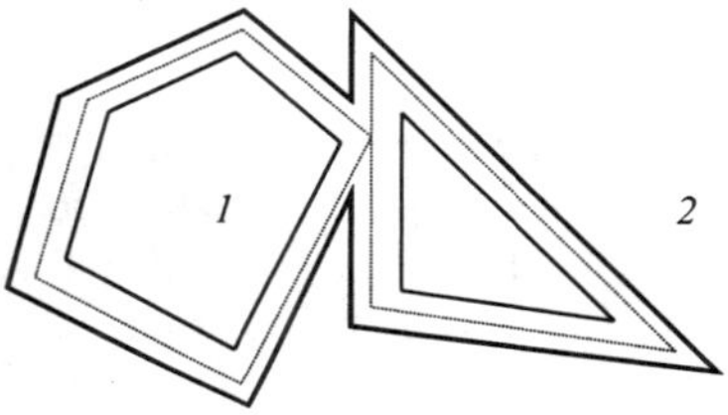

Figure 1. Obstacles expansion and list reduction

The term obstacles expansion or obstacle growing is used to declare the enlargement of the obstacle space by the robot dimensions [1]. This activity enables the safe assumption and representation of the robot body as a point. Reduction of obstacles list is the activity that merges the obstacles that are overlapping or touching each other after the obstacles expansion task.

A proposed representation for the robot sequential movements on the plane is consisting of the *robot configuration* vector (x, y, z), defined as the location x, y and heading z of the robot with reference to the origin and X axis respectively, of the world two dimensional space coordinate frame. It is assumed that the robot is able to perform turns on the spot. By this assumption the problem is reduced to the search of the sequential robot locations x, y rather than robot configuration vectors.

By the definition of the *free configuration space*, the robot configurations (locations) are not internal to an obstacle. It is obvious that the shortest path between start configuration and goal configuration is the line segment connecting the start point $\boldsymbol{s}$ and goal point $\boldsymbol{g}$ while the robot is having constant heading from $\boldsymbol{s}$ to $\boldsymbol{g}$. By definition the configurations $\boldsymbol{s}$ and $\boldsymbol{g}$ are belonging to the free configuration space. The line segment (s, g) is defined as the *optimum path*. Because of the use of recursive algorithms there is the need to define also the use of the terms *current optimum path*, *current start* and *current goal*, which are respectively the optimum path, start and goal points of each step of the recursion. It is obvious that in the first step of the recursion the optimum path and the current optimum path are identical. As *successful path* is defined the set of sequential robot's configurations that are giving a collision free path from start to goal. The configurations ***s*** and ***g*** are included as head and tail in each successful path.

The initial idea is based on the principle that the best path between start and goal is the straight line that is connecting start to goal. All approaches presented here are based on the *straight line principle* for solving the critical problem of successful path construction. In the following paragraphs the four approaches are presented from the simplest to the most sophisticated one as presented in [2].

2.2 Vertical Turns Algorithm (VTA)

According to the simplified navigation strategy of the *Vertical Turns Algorithm (VTA),* the robot is moving on straight lines, beginning with the optimum path. Each time the robot intersects or overcomes an obstacle edge or the initial optimum path, it turns by a 90^0 angle. In the case of intersection or overcome of an obstacle edge there are three alternatives: i) to follow the right direction ii) to follow the left direction iii) to go backwards. The direction towards the target is characterized as *friendly direction* and is selected first, but does not imply that this direction will lead to a successful path. The selection is made among the free directions and is based on the criterion of the *most friendly direction.* The most friendly direction has the smaller anti-clockwise positive angle with the current optimum path (the vector from current position to goal).

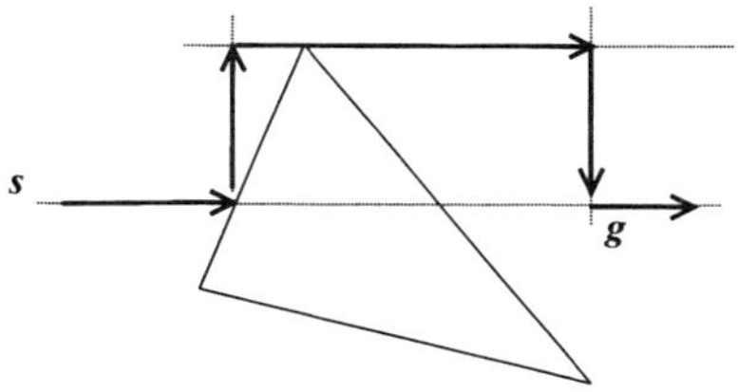

Figure 2. Vertical Turns Algorithm (VTA)

2.3 Edges Following Algorithm (EFA)

This approach is an extension of the Vertical Turns Algorithm and it the next progressive step towards the Convex Hull Method algorithm described later in this chapter. Initially the robot moves on the optimum path. Each time the robot intersects or overcomes an obstacle edge, turns by the angle enabling it to follow the intersected edge. The current optimum path has always the highest priority in direction selection and the edge following rule is violated only in this case.

In both VTA and EFA algorithms, when the robot changes direction, there is a possibility of the existence of another possibly successful path. This alternative path is that of the opposite direction of the chosen one. The points where a turning decision was performed are stored in the *Return Points List (RPL)* and they are indicators of alternatives paths. The results need to be further processed with reduction of path length procedures. These procedures lead to increased algorithms complexity.

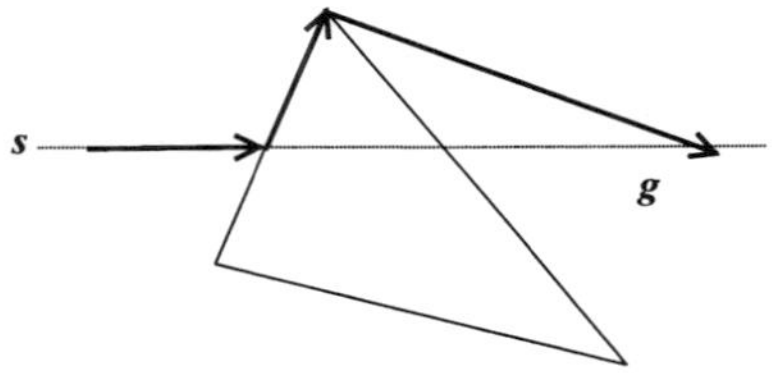

Figure 3. Edge Following Algorithm (EFA)

2.4 Perimeter Following Algorithm (PFA)

The *Perimeter Following Algorithm (PFA)* is the last progressive step towards the Convex Hull Method Algorithm. The algorithm is using the optimum path principle to begin. When an intersection with an obstacle edge occurs then the path is following the perimeter of the intersected obstacle until the point of the second intersection of the same obstacle and the current optimum path. According to the PFA, the deviations from the optimum path are on the obstacle perimeter. The algorithm is giving successful paths that are not optimised.

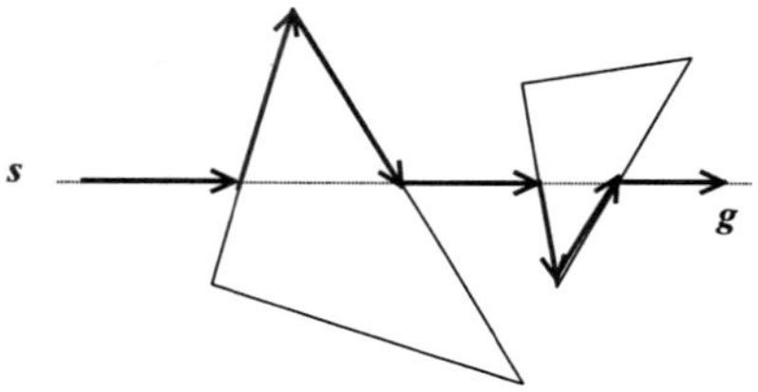

Figure 4. Perimeter Following Algorithm

2.5 Convex Hull Method Algorithm (CHMA)

According to the *Convex Hull Method Algorithm (CHMA)* the robot tries to move on the optimum path or by the obstacles edges. On intersection with an obstacle edge the robot follows the convex hull of the intersected obstacle, while checking the possibility to follow the current optimum path which is preferred if feasible.

Convex Hull Method Algorithm receives two arguments: Start point (s) and Goal point (g). Initially s is pushed into the *Successful Path List (SPL)*. Then the Convex Hull Path Planning algorithm is called with s and g. The algorithm checks if there is an intersection between current optimum path (s, g) and the list of obstacle edges. In other words, checks if the current optimum path does not belong to the free configuration space. If this is not the case and there is an intersection with an obstacle edge then the algorithm checks whether the intersection comes from (internal or an external direction of the obstacle).

If the intersection was caused from an external direction then there are two recursive calls of the algorithm that are dividing the successful path finding problem into to sub problems. i) Convex Hull Path Planning from 'Start' to 'one vertice of the intersected obstacle edge' and ii) Convex Hull Path Planning from 'the same vertice as above of the intersected obstacle edge' to 'Goal'.

The algorithm is continuing, solving recursively the path finding problem from 'Start' to 'one vertice of the intersected obstacle edge'. It is necessary to find a solution for this sub problem in order to continue with the second part of the problem. If any of the recursive call returns without success then a second pair of recursive calls is made for the 'other vertice of the intersected obstacle edge'. These recursive calls are having also the from: i) Convex Hull Path Planning from 'Start' to 'the other vertice of the intersected obstacle edge' and ii) Convex Hull Path Planning from 'the same vertice as above of the intersected obstacle edge' to 'Goal'. In parallel with the path finding the algorithm keeps track of the steps it is making in order to find the return point in a case of an unsuccessful path. The structure that hosts the points of return in the case of algorithm failure is named *Return Points List (RPL)* (as for EFA). The RPL is holding points elements and it is growing each time an intersection happens, because in this case there is a possibility of an alternative path that could be prove successful. So in the case of an algorithm failure during a recursive iteration, points are popped from the RPL and feed the recursive steps.

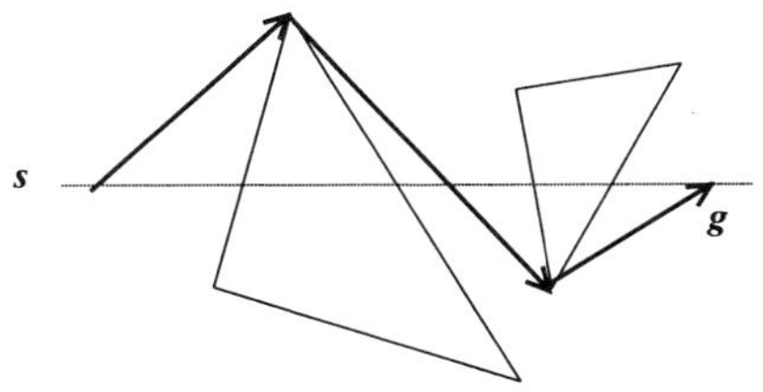

Figure 5. Convex Hull Method Algorithm

In the case that the intersection is caused from an internal direction of the obstacle then the algorithm continues with the next edge point of the current obstacle vertice (at the current algorithm step the current start should be an obstacle vertice, otherwise the intersection would be external).

Successful current optimum path implies no intersection with the obstacles configuration space. This is the only case that the algorithm pushes a point into the Successful Path List (SPL). This point is the current goal point. There is also a mechanism that pops points from the SPL in the case of algorithms failures. This mechanism is strongly related with the RPL manipulation mechanism.

The algorithm finishes when current start and current goal are identical, if the current optimum path is unsuccessful and there are no other points in the RPL to continue the algorithm's execution. The algorithm's output is the SPL, where all the successful paths are stored.

The proposed selection procedure of the points belonging in successful paths, results to minimized length paths. The algorithm outcome the set of length optimized, successful paths, thus the best path extraction is straight forward (if by definition the best path is the shortest distance from start to goal).

3. Local Strategies: Potential Field based Methods

The extraction of a feasible path using the potential field produced by the features of the environment space was and is still exploited by several researchers with quite impressive results. The family of methods is based on the principle that the obstacles space and the target itself produce potentials.

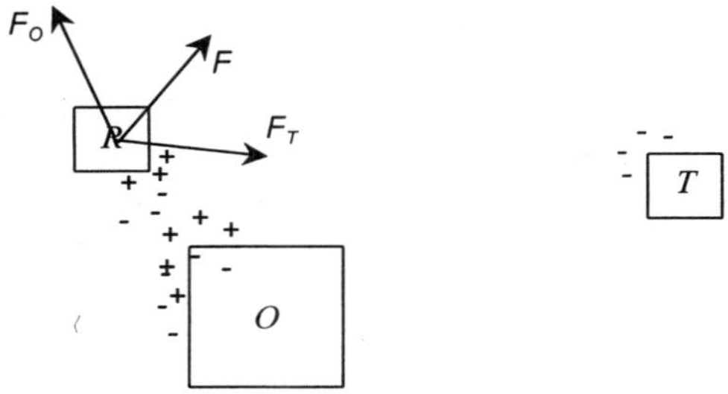

Figure 6. Attractive and Repulive Forces

The electric analogue is the most descriptive (Figure 6). One may assume: i) a positively charged object *R* (the robot - at the starting configuration) able to freely move into the configuration space, ii) a negatively charged fixed object *T* (the target - the goal robot configuration) and, iii) a positively charged fixed object or set of objects O (the obstacles - the obstacles space). According to the electric analogue object R will move towards the goal governed by the sum $\vec{F}$ of two forces: i) one attractive to the goal force, $\vec{F}_T$ produced by potential applied by the negatively charged object *T* to the positively charged object *R*, and ii) one repulsive from the obstacles force, $\vec{F}_O$ produced by potential applied by the positively charged object(s) *O* to the positively charged object *R*.

The principle is simple and effective. In the following sections several approaches based on the potential field method are presented. The main differences of the methods are on the approach they use to calculate the amplitude and direction of force applied to the robot by the obstacles and/or the goal. The most associate the amplitude of the force conversely to the distance between the robot, and the obstacle and the goal respectively, thus applying higher force values for a "charge" close to the robot and lower for a "charge" away from the robot. In order to measure distances the methods use environment information coming from the robot perception and correlate sensor values to charges, forces, potentials etc. Differences appear on the forms used to represent this information (certainty grids, direct sensor readings, histograms, histogramic grids, quad trees, etc.). In the various forms of environment representations the efforts is given to include the most of the principle elements into the calculation. Thus, distance from the obstacle might not be enough or accurate, so the estimation of the possibility being in the place reported maybe also incorporated into the value. The same might happen for other constants or factors that influence into a particular way the overall navigation strategy behaviour originating from the lowest levels of path planning calculations.

Differences are also presented in the methodology they use to select the final direction that would be traced by the robot. In the common case the notions of *peaks* and *valleys* on *histograms* are used to identify the candidate direction. Histograms are representing the angular two dimensional space of the obstacles around the robot. Valleys are representing angular sectors or directions, which hold high probability of obstacle presence or where obstacles are close to the robot. Peaks represent the opposite, although depending on the implementation the named might appear vise-versa and the values on the histogram might be interpreted neither as distance or a kind of confidence value.

The results of the application of the method are impressive, especially when the high priority is on the provision of a fast reactive behaviour.

However there is an inherent drawback in the method, well known as the *local minima* problem. Local minima problem is caused by the local minima might be produced in the potential field. When the robot falls into an area of a local minima is trapped. Thus, the robot may be stuck in a local minima situation even a few inches away from the target. The robot will remain trapped on spot corresponding to the lowest potential of the filed, unless either:

(i) the sources producing the trapping field change: a) the obstacles and/or the goal changes position - the robot is assumed immobilised when in the trapped situation or moving in a course that will conclude to the trapped situation, or

(ii) the "charges" of the obstacles, the goal and the robot itself, change.

To avoid the phenomenon several methods have been proposed. A discussion on those is included in the conclusions of the this chapter.

3.1 Virtual Force Field (VFF) Method

The Virtual force field's (VFF) principle of operation has originally been presented by O. Khatib in [3], based on which, J. Borenstein [4] produced the VFF method. In order to extract from the environment the data that would produce the desired filed, features of the environment where associated to the angular values of a histogram. The histogram represents the confidence of the system in the presence (or absence) of an obstacle at a particular direction from the robot heading. In order to rapidly construct the histogram the histogramic in-motion mapping (HIMM) method [5] was proposed. This, along with other methods, is based on the basic principle of the electric analogue, incorporating various factors & calculation methods.

By applying the potential field the probabilistic sensor information captured on the histogram can be used efficiently to control the robot as presented in [6]. The navigation strategy is analyzed as follows. The region around the mobile robot (also called active window) covers cells/grids in a grid environment representation, each one applying a repulsive force $\underline{F}_r$ (virtual) against it. The sum of these forces is computed. A constant in magnitude attractive force $\underline{F}_t$ (also virtual) is applied to the vehicle by the target. The final resulting force vector applied to the vehicle, is computed as $\underline{R} = \underline{F}_r + \underline{F}_t$ as the electric analogue.

3.2 Vector Field Histogram (VFH) Method

The VFH method is based VFF method representing better behaviour compared to the later in environments with high obstacle density. A two-dimensional map (a kind of occupancy grid) is generated and updated to hold the environment representation information. A one-dimensional structure, called *Polar Histogram* [7] (a histogram) is computed around the mobile robot's momentary location. Each sector in the histogram holds the polar obstacle density in that direction. The robot direction is aligned with the direction of the fittest sector. A function using peaks and valleys information is used to calculate the candidate direction.

3.3 VFH+ Method

This algorithm is based on the VFH method. Its advantages are that it reduces some of the parameter tuning of the original algorithm and the robot trajectory is better estimated.

The input to the algorithm [8] is the two dimensional map of the environmental data as mentioned in the two previous methods. There is a dimension reduction performed on the map and brought to a one-dimensional polar histogram, again constructed around the robot's momentary location. Based on further computations, which take in account robot dynamics the histogram provides the directions that are possible. From the set of possibilities, a set of candidate directions is selected. An optimisation follows based on a special cost function.

3.4 Active Kinematic Histogram (AKH) Method

This potential field path planning method applies to non-point, non-holonomically constrained mobile robots. It is based on features extraction by the one dimensional representation of the vehicle and obstacle space as they are derived by the available information on the robot's exact dimensions, kinematic configuration and sensor information. It is capable of providing the information for potentially collision free path. In previous methods robots were assumed to be point wise, and in the best case algorithms were applied several points on the robot catering for its geometry partially, hence inheriting the deficiencies of the method, and still not completely compensating for the entire geometry of the robot. With this method an 'exact' map of the obstacles as well as the robot is generated, hence having a very clear picture as to were the robot may navigate safely avoiding collisions to the best possible degree.

The AKH method [9] is using the histogramic environment representation of the VFH method (a histogram). The major difference in the way the environment is represented in AKH is that the method utilises two histograms instead of one. Figure 4 depicts the *obstacles active kinematic histogram*, AKH(o) and *the robot's active kinematic histogram*, AKH(r). The light grey area represents free space. AKH(o) is represented in dark grey colour, AKH(r) is represented in white.

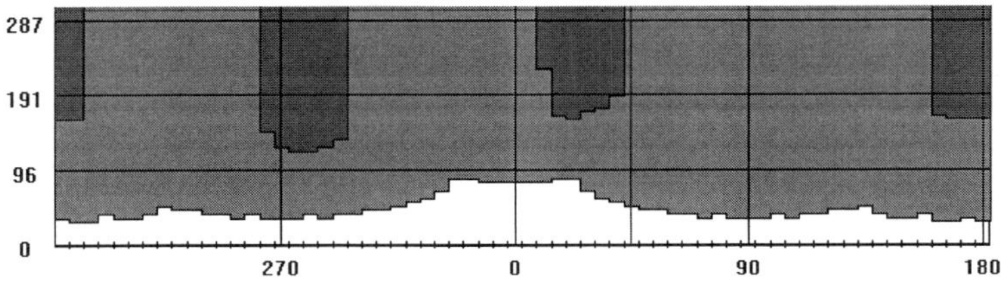

Figure 7. The Active Kinematic Histogram - obstacles (drark grey), - robot's (white)

Initially, according to the AKH method, the collision free rotational limits of the mobile robot are determined. Adaptive thresholding is employed in order to reduce collisions. The path around the obstacle is being planned. Sectors are classified as free or blocked. Candidate valleys are defined as the sets of sequential free sectors. The minimum angle necessary for the mobile robot to pass through a gap in the polar space is estimated. The shape and dimensions of the robot are included in the process of the method.

4. Case Studies and Examples

The section presents examples of local versus global navigation strategies. The case studies presented use the *Adaptive Fusion of Reactive Behaviours* (AFREB) architecture discussed in the next paragraph to implement the different cases of the examples. On one hand, AFREB is a hybrid scheme that needs an off-line path planner that, using a static map of the environment, sets the controller path reference, while, under it, a reactive control system performs the task, processing a high amount of on-line sensor information for on-line obstacle avoidance. On the other hand, and at the same time, it is a good example of the use of intelligent control algorithms for reactive navigation

4.1 The Extended AFREB Architecture

The architecture is composed of three control layers. At the bottom, several *low-level controllers* are able to implement behaviours, such as *turn*, *go back*, *follow a path*, *follow the contour of an obstacle*, and *follow a corridor*. Each of those uses direct sensor information as data source. PID or fuzzy controllers are adequate to implement these basic behaviours.

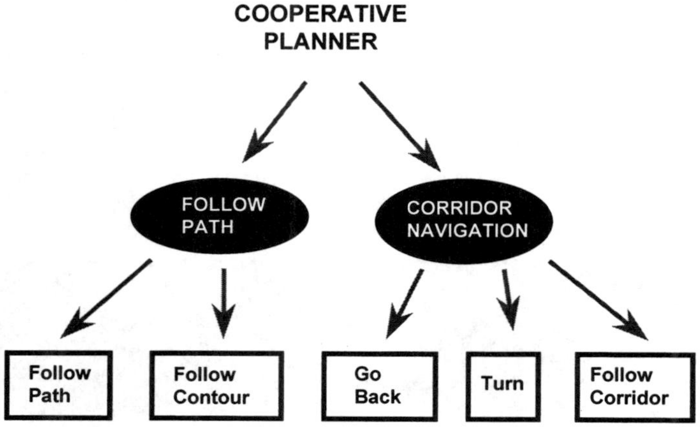

Figure 8. The Extended AFREB architecture

Over it, an intelligent decision system (control supervisor) is used to reach the target: *follow a path*, or *follow a corridor*, by using in both cases collision avoidance algorithms. The name of the architecture, *Adaptive Fusion of Reactive Behaviours* (AFREB), comes from the fact that the previous primitive behaviours are fused to complete the desired task, originating an emergent behaviour. The supervisor must determine the most adequate values for the behaviour weights used to fuse them. In such a way, the fusion process consists of determining the contribution of each primitive to produce the final movement or emergent behaviour. A static path planner for trajectory generation is only used off-line to set the reference for the supervisor. As stated above, two tasks were implemented: follow path (both by means of fuzzy logic and neural networks) and follow corridor (by means of heuristic rules). A modified version of the follow path supervisor using fuzzy logic, was also implemented for mobile robot avoidance, taking also into account the location of the closer robot to itself.

The higher level is the *co-operative planner*. In fact it is an extension of the AFREB architecture to allow the combination of different supervision modules as well as to co-ordinate multiple robot movements in a shared environment. The planner checks continuously the location of the robot to determine if it is entering a narrow corridor (a door or in between two obstacles). In such a case, first it checks if other robot is already inside the corridor. If so, it starts until the situation finishes. If not, it replaces the follow path supervisor with the corridor navigation supervisor and enters the corridor.

4.2 The Behaviours

The *follow path* behaviour was designed by using a simple nine rule fuzzy controller. It attempts to reach the next point of the path, by reducing the distance to it. It acts as a PD controller (proportional and derivative actions). No proximity sensors are checked, so the behaviour just drives the robot with odometry sensors, and without obstacle avoidance. Figure 9 depicts the laboratory room in which the mobile robot is following a path. Some fixed furniture and obstacles are represented. A risk management system cancels the behaviour action when an obstacle is too close to it.

The *follow contour behaviour* (right or left) keeps the robot parallel to the detected contour (right or left), by using two ultrasound sensors. No reference distance exists, although the minimum one is 30 cm. The velocity is lowered when this distance is low. The controller input is the deviation angle, while the output is the robot curvature. A PD controller is utilized. If the distance from the front corner to the wall is closer then the distance from the side, then the curvature (that will be stronger) is calculated as proportional to the difference between the distance and a reference value. Figure 10 shows the robot behaviour following the left wall. The contour of both, the small obstacle and the closed door are perfectly followed. The initial obstacle is also followed from the beginning of the movement.

The *go back behaviour* (as well as the turn behaviour) is designed for cases that cannot be solved by the other methods. It tries to follow a straight line except in the case an obstacle is obstructing the line. In such a case it turns to avoid the collision. In the trivial case, the linear velocity is constant and the angular velocity is zero. It is based on the idea of the follow corridor behaviour, although it is much simpler. Special attention is paid to the fact that in mobile robots with differential steering kinematics configuration the backward turn differs to the forward turn.

The *turn behaviour* is used to turn without linear velocity, constant angular velocity and with obstacle avoidance. It is possible to assign a turn direction, or the behaviour will select one depending on the surrounding space. The robot requires at least half a meter to turn, and this condition is checked. While the robot is turning, if an obstacle appears in the area, the behaviour stops and changes the turn sense trying to reach the goal through the free space sector.

Finally, the *follow corridor behaviour* tries to follow two walls (obstacles) at the same time. It is useful for navigation in narrow corridors, forgetting the path and solving the immediate problem. The simple case shown in figure 13 is solved in a similar way than the follow contour behaviour. The deviation from the straight line in the robot movement is due to the derivative action of the PD controller. The path to follow is not taken into account inside the corridor. But when the walls disappear, the robot returns to the path to follow.

4.3 Special Cases

Some special cases are directly called from the behaviours servicing safety purposes. These cases are triggered in the case where the robot approaches too close to an obstacle. These three cases are *frontal obstacle*, *side obstacle* and *back side obstacle*. In the case of the go back behaviour, the frontal corresponds to the back part of the robot. The first action performed is the reduction of the speed. Then are two possible speeds that may use for safety purposes: low speed and null speed.

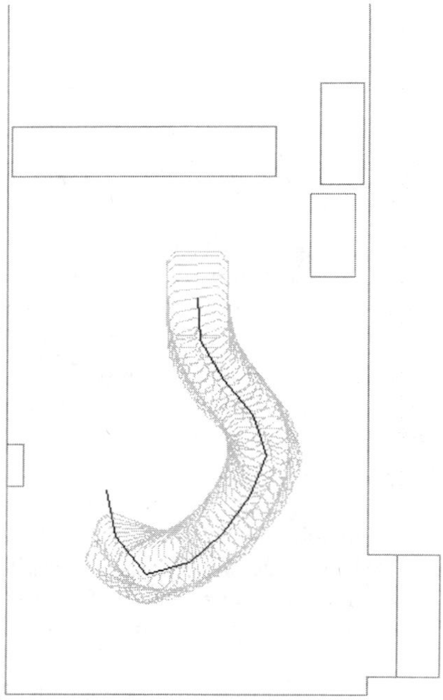

Figure 9. Follow path behaviour

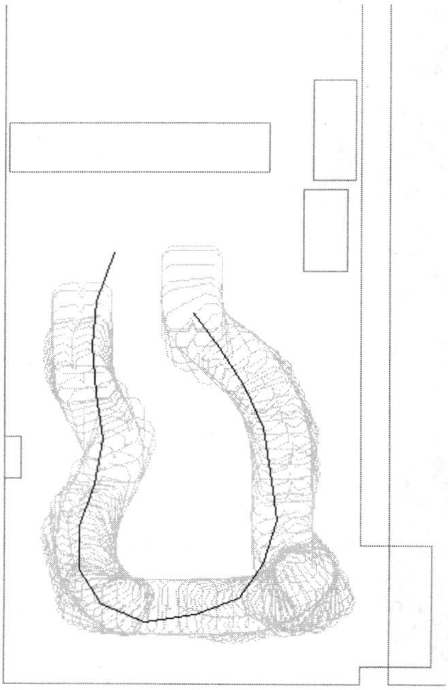

Figure 10. Follow contour behaviour

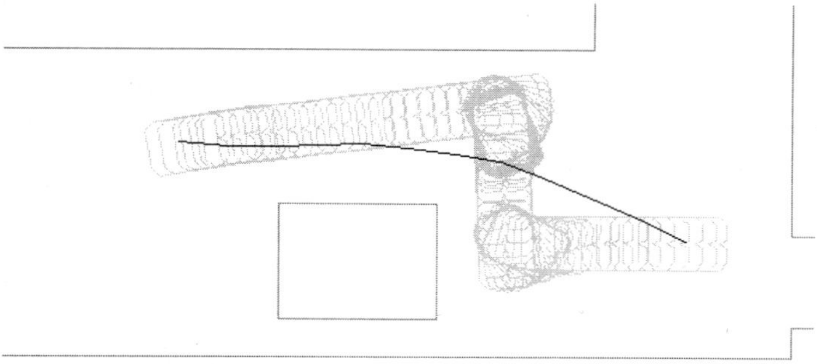

Figure 11. Go back behaviour

The *frontal obstacle* case directs the robot to the direction where wider free space is found. The turn maybe performed in low or null velocity, depending on density of the surrounding obstacles. If there is no free space to make the turn feasible, the robot will stop.

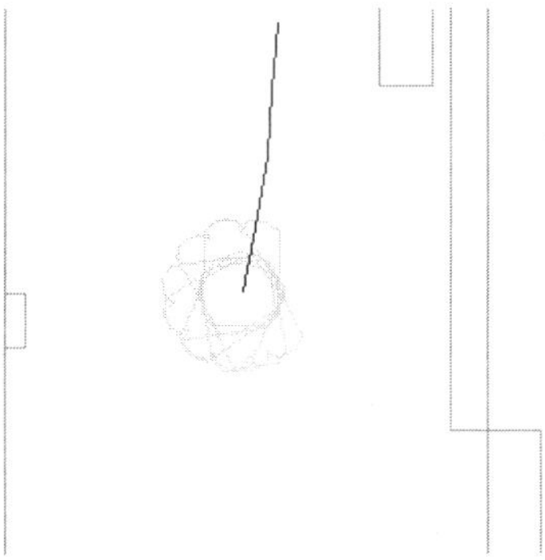

Figure 12. Turn behaviour

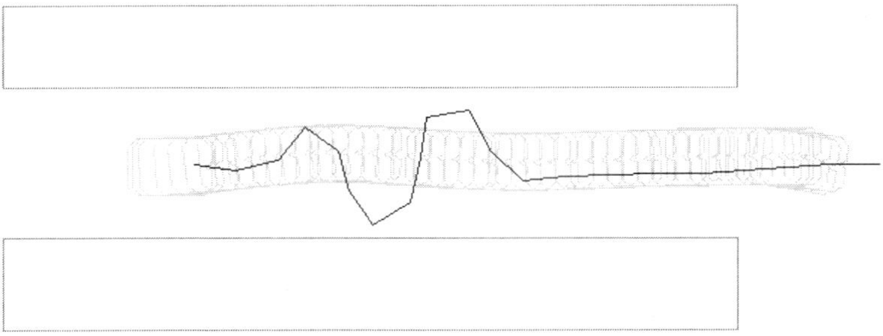

Figure 13. Follow corridor behaviour

The *side obstacle* case directs the robot in the opposite direction of the side that caused the minimum distance alert. There is also the necessity also to implement the *back side obstacle* case. This is because the robot kinematics will produce a different behaviour when turning backwards.

4.4 The Supervisors

Artificial Intelligence techniques (expert systems, fuzzy logic and neural networks) are used to implement the supervisory decision system. For instance, a fuzzy decision system may be implemented with rules like:

"if the distance to an obstacle is large, then follow path behaviour is very strong"

"if the distance to an obstacle is small and the obstacle is on the right hand, then follow path behaviour is weak and right contour following behaviour is strong"

4.5 Case Studies

The cases studies will be devoted to the follow path and follow corridor supervisors. The follow path supervisor was designed to follow a path with obstacle avoidance and is intended to be used and work fine in wide areas. It uses two behaviours: follow path, when no obstacle is present, and follow right/left contour when an obstacle appears at the right/left side. It is based on a fuzzy rule based system with about 30 rules. It takes into account the sonars distances (grouped in five sectors: left, left front, front, right front and right), the deviation angle in respect with the next point of the path, and a history of the previous behaviours used. An example is shown in figure 14.

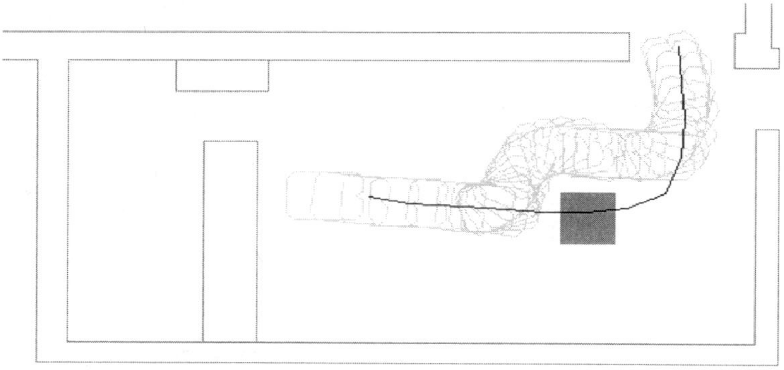

Figure 14. Follow path supervisor

The corridor supervisor is much complicated. It is designed for narrow corridors, door passages or areas cluttered with obstacles. The supervisor utilises three behaviours: follow corridor, turn and go back. Under normal conditions, the follow corridor behaviour is used.

In special cases such as a bifurcation or a dead end corridor, it activates the others. If the minimum distance alert comes from the sensors on the right or the left side, the supervisor calls the follow corridor behaviour. If the minimum distance corresponds to the frontal left or right sides, there are two possibilities:

- If the distance is too short or if the frontal distance is short, the supervisor calls the go back behaviour.
- If the distance is not too short, the follow corridor behaviour is used.

Finally, if the minimum distance comes from the front of the robot, the turn behaviour is called, selecting the turn direction depending on the angle between the robot and the next point in the path. In such a way, a frontal bifurcation is solved choosing as destination the path (see Figure 15).

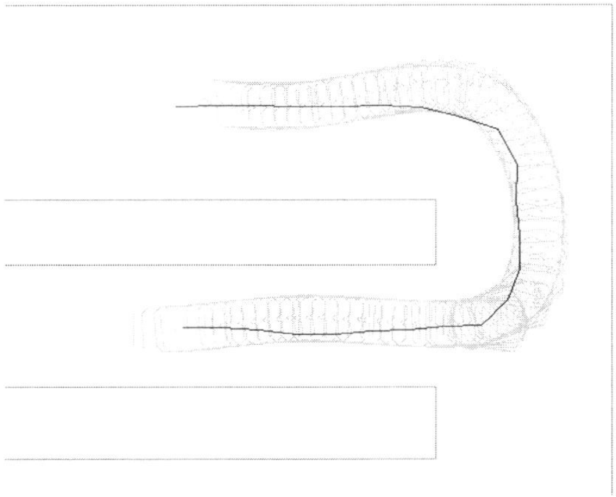

Figure 15. Frontal bifurcation

A more difficult case is shown in figure 16. The robot approaches the bifurcation, turns adequately, leaves the corridor and reaches a wider area. The sonars have problems to find the sharp corner, but the robot avoids it without problems. After leaving the corridor, the robot turns to return to the trajectory.

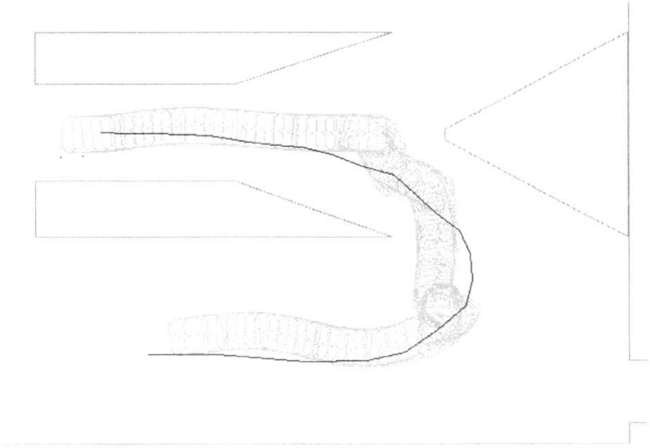

Figure 16. Frontal bifurcation with sharp corner

Another possible case is a dead end corridor. The robot will try to turn, using the turn behaviour, until the robot sees open space to continue. If there is not space enough to turn, the supervisor will call the go back behaviour, until the robot finds a wide area to continue with a forward movement.

The behaviours used in the past are also taken into account and are influencing the decision of the next behaviour selection. For example, if the last behaviour was the turn behaviour, the supervisor will continue calling it until the front distance is 1 meter at least; then it will change it to the follow corridor behaviour. In the case where the last behaviour was the go back behaviour, the supervisor will maintain it active while the right or left side there is 1 meter free at least and will replace it with the turn behaviour in the opposite case, so the robot can find a new corridor, by searching for the wider area.

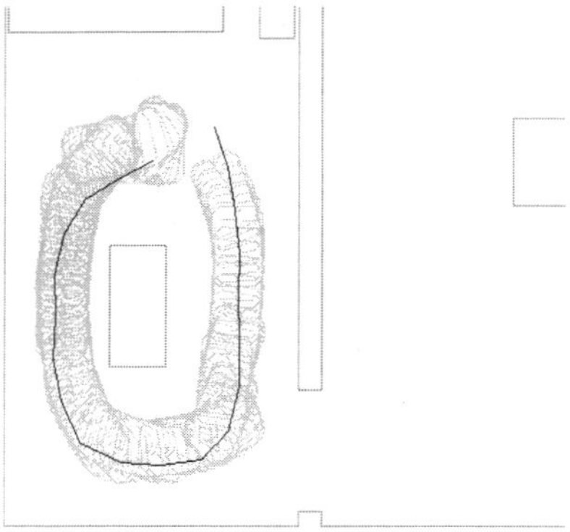

Figure 17. Surounding an obstacle

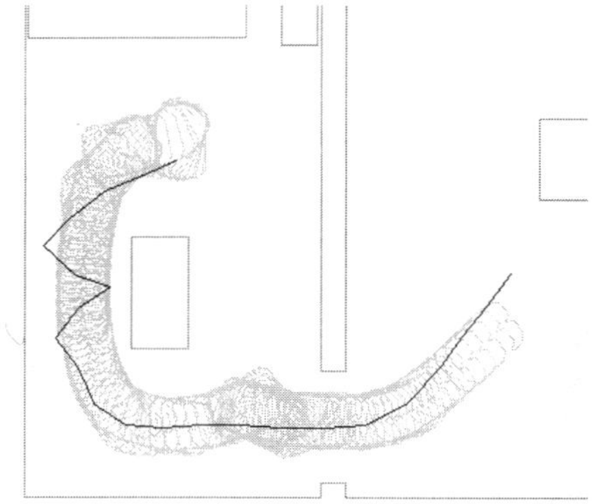

Figure 18. Passing through a door

Employing the corridor supervisor the robot presents a behaviour as follows. Figure 17 shows a simple case of the robot moving around an obstacle in the centre of the room. At the initial position, the obstacle is too close, so the turn behaviour is used turning towards the path. Then it moves around the obstacle until it reaches the open door. The bifurcation is solved by turning again towards the path. The second case is similar, but now the path drives the robot out of the room (figure 18).

A more complicated test is to navigate through an amorphous set of corridors. The robot always has its goal in the path to follow (see figure 19). The robot starts close to a wall, so the initial turn is big. A small oscillation appears and then the path is followed.

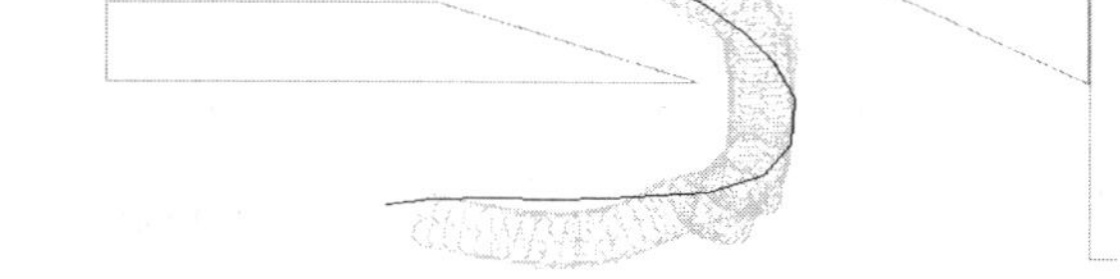

Figure 19. Passing several bifurcations

The final case shows what would happen using only the follow corridor behaviour. A lateral bifurcation is more complicated. Under such a bifurcation, this behaviour uses to follow the wider corridor. This is what initially happens in figure 20.

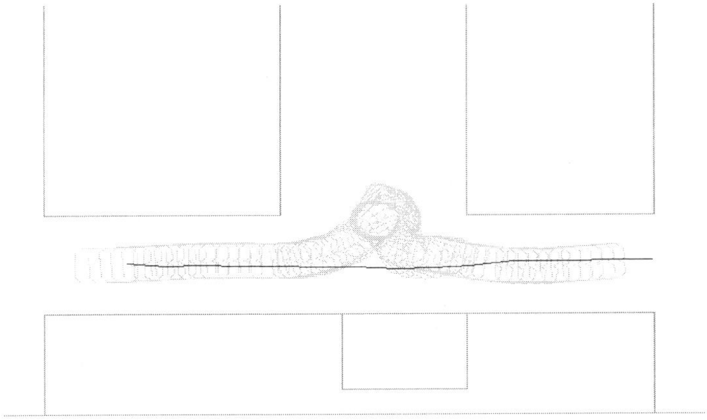

Figure 20. Lateral bifurcation

Initially, the wide corridor is followed, until the supervisor detects this situation. Then it changes to the turn behaviour to recover the correct path, entering into the narrow corridor.

5. Discussions

The chapter presented a family of methods for mobile robot navigation based on workspace geometric features or geometric representations of the features extracted from the robot's environment. The methods are presenting impressive results when planning the long paths.

However, the produced paths are not smooth and they present high oscillating behaviour or very sharp turns. Dealing with robots in healthcare care, there would be several instances where the robot would be instructed to carry sensitive material or even persons. We call *path smoothness* the value of the max curvature of the path measured at each segments of 7 cm and over the full path length. Smoothness is a measure of how comfortable the journey for the potential rider of the robot. The notion of smoothness was developed during tests in real healthcare environment and was designed to be one of the comparison criteria for robot navigation algorithms.

Comparing global and local navigation strategies one may comment that in the common case the local navigation strategies produce smooth paths. On the other hand as already discussed in section 3 of this chapter, local navigation strategies suffer from the local minima problem. In fact what characterises and labels a navigation strategy as global or local is its ability to overcome the local minima problem or the path smoothness problem respectively.

Figure 21 gives an example of the advantages and drawbacks of both a typical global and local path planning method.

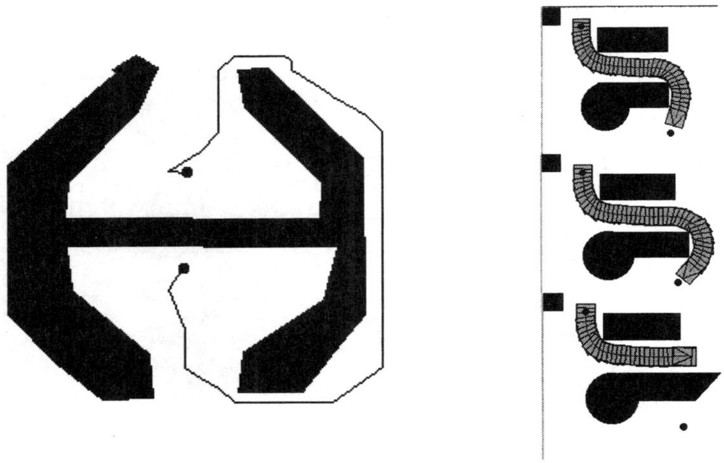

(a) *(b)*

Figure 21. (a) Global path planning, (b) Local path planning

Figure 21 (a) depicts the path planned by the approximate cell decomposition method with local node refinement [7]. It is important to notice that even if the method introduces local features of the workspace in order to smooth the path produced by the cell decomposition method, the path produced includes segments with high curvature values. For example there is a sharp turn in the initial steps of the path (in the upper half part of the figure). This is a result of the nature of the method and is caused by the digitisation of the space in cells. Incrementing the cell decomposition depth might eliminate the phenomenon in that particular area but may arbitrarily present it somewhere else in the workspace. The enhancement of the method by the local node refinement proves inadequate to improve the method in this specific case, because the enhancement targets the smoothness of the path in the vicinity of obstacles. At relatively free areas, the local node refinement is not influencing the path at all or its influence is minimal.

On the other hand one should mention that the method presents impressive behaviour driving the robot out of the H-shaped obstacle of Figure 21 (a) which is considered as one of the most difficult cases. A direct application of the optimum path principle of section 2.1 would drive the robot directly toward the separating - of the H-shaped obstacle. However, as described in section 2 the algorithm finds an escape from this situation, which is in fact a local minima trap.

In Figure 21 (b) the navigation strategy, which is in this case a local path planner namely the AKH, is given a series of simpler problems. The method manages to reach the goal in the first two cases, but in the last case when the obstacle fully obstructs the way to the goal, the method fails to find a path to it although one exists and stays trapped in the local minima in front of the obstacle. On the other hand, one should notice that the all the paths produced are smooth and the robot is travelling even adapting its speed according the obstacle configuration.

The benefits and drawbacks of each of the local and global strategies do not allow the researcher to be based on of those in order to resolve the navigation problem in healthcare environments. The application sector needs the features of both. The typical approach would be to incorporate in two loops a global and a local path planner. The structure could be as follows:

> Go to Goal (*initial position, final goal*)
> While not at *final goal*
>   *next sub goal* = Global Path Planner (*final goal*)
>   Local Path Planner (*next sub goal*)
>   while not at *next sub goal* and not *blocked in local minima*
>   Drive the robot toward *next sub goal*
>   If *blocked in local minima*
>   Call recursively the Go to Goal algorithm with *start* operant the *current position* and *goal* operant the *final goal*

The global path planner warranties that if there would be a path from the initial position to the final goal this would be found. In order to achieve smooth motion the local planner gets the sub goals produced by the global planner and drives the robot towards them avoiding obstacles in the robot's vicinity. Each time the local planner reaches a sub goal the control returns back to the global path planner which calls again the local planner with the next sub goal.

It is evident that the efficiency and reliability of the local minima detection highly affects the performance of the method. Several techniques have been proposed for that. Some are calculating the distance travelled within the same area, some other calculate the time within a circle of a predefined radius, etc. However, if the local minima situation is detected there the global path planner is called to escape from the situation. An approach is to call the global path planner to plan a new path from the current position to the final goal. Another alternative could be to plan the new path from current position to the sub goal that was not achieved or the next to that sub goal. By this the global path planner is activated in the local problem subdividing it into several sub problems and calling the local path planner to resolve each of those. Given the features of local and global planner it is highly probable that in one hand the local minima will be avoided and the path will be smooth.

There is also another point that needs the attention of the researchers intending to follow this approach. This is the behaviour that the robot may present during the transition between the old goal (reached) and the new goal (to be reached). When a sub goal is reached, the local planner gets the next sub goal to drive the robot to. The robot may tend to oscillate or make sharp turns due to the high or weak potentials produced by nearby obstacles or the far goal respectively. This phenomenon may be avoided by the employment of an adaptive mechanism of the weights used the repulsive and attractive elements of the virtual potentials.

Beyond this approach the researchers employed other schemes like those reported to implement the behaviours described in section 4. Fuzzy logic based navigation algorithms gained the interest of the researchers because of the mimics they use in the way the humans or animals take decisions. In [13] an exhaustive discussion takes place on the use of fuzzy logic for autonomous mobile robots navigation and control and the reader is recommended to address the reference for more details.

The main assumption used in the chapter is that the robot has the knowledge within a degree of accuracy of the actual position (configuration in the workspace) it is in at any given instance. The reader is encouraged to address Chapter 14 dealing with those matters.

6. References

[1] Borenstein J. and Koren Y., “Real-Time Obstacle Avoidance for Fast Mobile Robots”, *IEEE Transactions on Systems, Man and Cybernetics*, Vol. 19, No. 5, pp. 1179-1187, 1989.

[2] Borenstein J., and Koren Y., “Histogramic In-Motion Mapping for Mobile Robot Obstacle Avoidance”, *IEEE Journal of Robotics and Automation*, Vol. 7, No. 4, pp. 535-539, 1991.

[3] Borenstein J., and Raschke U., “Real-Time Obstacle Avoidance for Non-Point Mobile Robots”, *Fourth World Conference on Robotics Research, Society of Manufacturing Engineers*, 1994.

[4] Borenstein J., et al., "VFH+: Reliable Obstacle Avoidance for Fast Vehicles", *Proceeding of IEEE Robotics and Automation Conf.*, 1998, pp. 1572-1577

[5] Borenstein, J. and Koren Y., “The Vector Field Histogram - Fast Obstacle Avoidance for Mobile Robots”, *IEEE Transactions on Robotics and Automation*, Vol. 7, No. 3, pp. 278-288, 1991.

[6] Katevas N., and Tzafestas S. G. “The Active Kinematic Histogram Method for Path Planning of Non-Point, Non-Holonomically Constrainted Mobile Robots”, In *Advanced Robotics, the International Journal of the Robotics Society of Japan*, Special Issue on Intelligent Mobile Robots, 1998, Vol. 12, No. 4, pp. 373-395

[7] Katevas N., Tzafestas S. G., and Pnevmatikatos C. G., “The Approximate Cell Decomposition with Local Node Refinement Global Path Planning Method: Path Nodes Refinement and Path Parametric Interpolation”, In *Journal of Intelligent and Robotic Systems, Special Issue on Autonomous Mobile Robots in Health Care Services*, Kluwer Academic Publishers, 1998, Vol. 22, No. 3-4, pp. 289-314.

[8] Katevas N.I., and Tzafestas S.G., “Path Planning Algorithms for Mobile Robots among Polygonal Obstacles”, *3rd IFAC/IFIP Workshop on Algorithms and Architectures for Real-Time Control (AARTC ’95)*, 31 May -2 June 95, Ostend, Belgium, pp. 95-100.

[9] Khatib O., "Real Time Obstacle Avoidance for Manipulators and Vehicles", *IEEE International Conference on Robotics and Automation*, March 25-28, 1985, St. Louis, pp. 500-505.

[10] Matia F., Jimenez A., "Multisensor Fusion: An Autonomous Mobile Robot". *Journal of Intelligent & Robotic Systems* (1998).

[11] Matia F., Moraleda E., Mena R., Puente E.A, "Fuzzy Systems for Reactive Planning and the Cooperation of Autonomous Robots" *EFDAN'96*, Dortmund (Germany), 20-22 May 1996.

[12] Moraleda E., Matia F., E. Puente A., "ARCO: Architecture for Autonomous Mobile Platforms Co-Operation in Industrial Environments" *3rd IFAC Symposium IAV'98*, Madrid (Spain), 25-27 March 1998.

[13] Saffiotti A., "The Uses of Fuzzy Logic in Autonomous Robot Navigation", *Soft Computing*, 1997, Vol. 4, No. 1, pp. 180-197.

[14] Tzafestas S.G., and Hatzivasiliou F.V., "A Path Planning Method for Mobile Robots in a Structured Environment" in *Robotic Systems-European Robotics and Intelligent Systems Conference (Ed. S.Tzafestas)*, 1991, pp. 261-270. Kluwer Academic.

Chapter 9

Communicating Robots in a Healthcare Environment

by Fergal J O'HART, Richard J GREENANE, Gerard LACEY, Darren WENN

Mobile Robotics in Healthcare
N. Katevas (Ed.)
IOS Press, 2001

Chapter 9

Communicating Robots in a Healthcare Environment

Fergal J O'HART, Richard J GREENANE, Gerard LACEY, Darren WENN

1. Introduction

Many new network technologies[1] are now concerned with dynamically connecting devices to networks that may ultimately allow access to the Internet. The wide availability of the Internet has led most businesses going online into the dynamic world of e-Commerce. Manufacturing systems have large dedicated control networks to allow machinery to be controlled and audited by many different systems. In some cases these two technologies have merged to create a single virtual network populated by physical machines, people and agents that interact to perform complex tasks.

A good example of the collaboration between computer systems is the SETI@HOME project. This project strives to achieve the performance of a super-computer through the collaboration of PC users around the Internet. Home internet users run a background task, which takes small pieces of radio telescope data and searches it for anomalies. Each user processes different data, thus allowing large amounts of data to be processed in parallel with only a small overhead. Similarly an *Intelligent Building* can be made up of several thousand devices each of which has the capability to process small amounts of data. Communication between these devices can enable large amounts of data to be processed while distributing the resources across a large area.

Research within the MobiNet project has focused on healthcare robotics; these are primarily indoor robots that work within highly structured but dynamic environments. Our research has focused on the development of robots that are elements within a larger

[1] At the time of writing WAP, Jini and Bluetooth show some potential to achieve a measure of success in creating dynamic ad-hoc networks.

Healthcare Intranet. This approach is similar to the *Domotic approach*[2], however we focus on the institutional and inter-institutional network and systems rather than those in the home. Within a healthcare context the use of wireless networks and the integration of heterogeneous networks to create a single virtual network facilitate the integration of Medical Informatics, online Health Monitoring using smart bio-sensors, tele-medicine and other IT supports to healthcare service delivery. Mobile robotics is facilitated in this context when sensors are distributed around the building and actuators are fitted to doors, windows, etc. We also advocate the redistribution of large elements of robot control from the mobile robot to the building. The implications of this approach are best captured by the phrase "smart building – dumb robot".

This approach has several important consequences:

- The infra-structural costs of refitting the building are balanced by benefits in many different applications.
- The cost factor, so long an impediment to the fielding of mobile robots, is significantly addressed.
- The capabilities and response times of robots will significantly be improved because of access to off-robot computation and communications.

2. The Building Control Network

With the increasing popularity of the Intelligent Building for the home user and offices in the industrial sector, the convergence between home and office is likely to be achieved with greater efficiency. Research has been undertaken to increase the possibilities of controlling the home and the office from one small device. These devices can take the form of PDAs (Personal Digital Assistants), where new software is written so that the PDA device acts as a buildings' remote control, in the same way as a TV remote control. They can also be made up of small mobile robots who can control the building depending on the route they take on the move.

Many networked structures already exist in the office environment. These not only include standard Ethernet cabling, but also PCM telephone connections and small amounts of video cabling. The existing cable structure within buildings can be used to connect a series of small devices allowing the control and monitoring of building services. These devices can communicate with one another, so that an event which occurs while monitoring, can cause a control event to activate a remote actuator. For example, Figure 1 shows a network of two devices. A light sensor monitors the light levels within a room. The lights are controlled by an actuator that can adjust the levels of the lights. When the light levels drop in the room, the sensor records this and triggers an event that propagates itself on the network and causes the actuator to adjust the lights so that the levels are the same. Figure 1 only shows two devices in a network, however, it is possible to control several thousand devices in a network using

[2] The Domotics project at the ARTS Lab, Scuola Superiore Sant'Anna, Pisa. For more information see http://www-arts.sssup.it/

the same ideas. Furthermore it is possible to control elevators and doors and by using a large number of devices it is possible to achieve a "smart" environment.

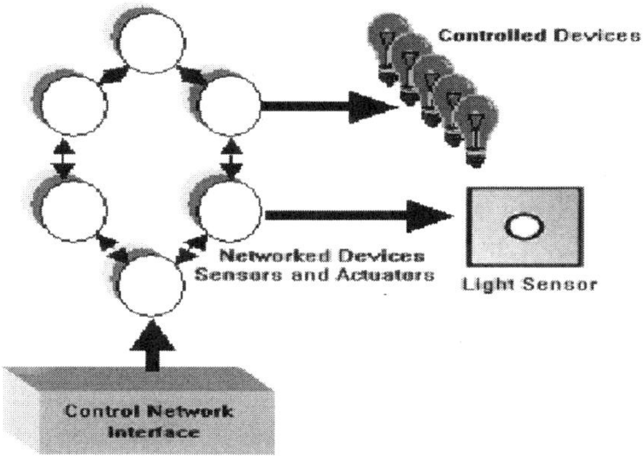

Figure 1. Network of two devices

Control networks are designed to contain small devices each with their own schedule and operational parameters. Movement of data is achieved through packets which are highly optimised to make them faster as the bit rate for the networks is usually quite slow.

For some applications a high bit rate is needed. This would almost certainly be the case if one was trying to stream audio or video data between devices. Ethernet is an ideal network structure to use in this situation. Ideally, a direct link between the control network and the Ethernet network is needed to allow a seamless interaction between high bit rate and low bit rate work.

This has been achieved with the use of CORBA (Common Object Request Broker Architecture). CORBA is an OMG (Object Management Group) designed architecture that can transfer data objects to and from multiple computers. In other words, it allows software to be executed on many different machines throughout the world while still interacting in an efficient manner. This architecture lends itself to be used as a bridging tool between a control network and a standard Ethernet network. As part of the MobiNet project, interest in intelligent environments and the fields use in robot navigation has lead to the development of a bridge between a control network and an Ethernet network, using CORBA technology [10].

The control network is supplied with an API (Applications Programming Interface) that allows the programmer to monitor and control events and devices. The bridge that has been developed, uses this interface to broker events and control instructions between a server and the control network devices via an interface card that is connected to both the control network and the server. As the server uses CORBA, clients can be written for the server with operating systems that were previously unavailable to the control network developer. This means that a greater number of people can benefit from the control network, for not only research and development purposes, but also for the monitoring capabilities within the building structure. Figure 2 shows the complete network structure with the newly developed

CORBA bridge in place. The bridge is layered with the other components which allows additions and revisions to be made with relative ease.

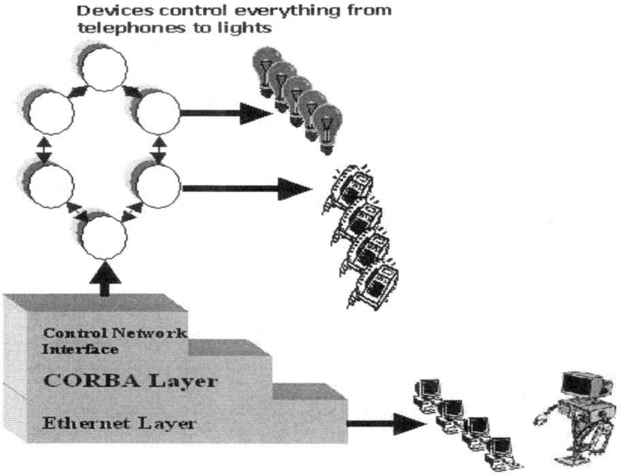

Figure 2. Network structure incorporating CORBA bridge

2.1 CORBA Services & Access to Control Network

The robot responds to events received from a CORBA Service client to a LonWorks network. The LonWorks fieldbus is a control network devised by Echelon Corporation. This network interconnects nodes distributed around the building. Nodes consist of a Neuron microcontroller and some sensor or actuator. The Neuron consists of three 8-bit microcontrollers. One microcontroller is used for processing the application code, the other two manage the network interface. These nodes communicate via twisted-pair using a *free-topology tranceiver* (FTT). An FTT allows the designer of the control network to choose any topology that suits the infrastructure. The network is installed using a structured cabling approach. The structured cabling approach uses unshielded CAT5 cabling. It allows for an extendable network to be installed. Prior to the adoption of this approach, control networks tended to be daisy-chained. This meant that any time network modification was required, the network was brought offline and rewired to incorporate new nodes.

3. The Robot Architecture

The robot is built on top of a Transitions Research Corporation (TRC) Labmate chassis. The Labmate is a servo-controlled mobile robot platform which can carry heavy loads (100kg) at velocities up to 1m/s. The base is approximately 70cm^2. Linear and angular velocities, accelerations, goal distances, and point-to-point motions are available. Trajectory and servo control is managed by an on-board microprocessor. The robot has a ring of 24 Polaroid ultrasonic sensors and a pan-tilt camera. The robot software is implemented in C/C++ on a Debian Linux OS.

The robot's software is partitioned as a three-layer architecture. Three-layer architectures generally consist of: [9]

- A reactive feedback control mechanism, known as either the *controller* or *skill layer*
- A reactive plan-execution mechanism, known as either the *sequence* or the *sequencing layer*, and
- Some mechanism for performing deliberative computation, known as either the *deliberator* or the *planning layer*.

All robot software components in this implementation communicate using the Task Control Architecture (TCA) [24]. TCA provides a general-purpose framework for building robot systems that need to combine deliberative as well as reactive components. High-level support for distributed communications, hierarchial task decomposition and task sequencing is provided for. It also provides resource management, error recovery and monitoring of execution.

3.1 Layer 0

The lowest layer in our implementation employs several well known techniques for obstacle detection and avoidance.

The VFH+ algorithm [26] is used for obstacle detection and metric map making. For further information on VFH+ please refer to Chapter 8, Section 3.3

3.2 Layer 1

In this implementation, layer 1 is responsible for place recognition. Place recognition consists of matching current perceptions with those previously learned to determine the robot's current location.

Topological Mapping

In grid-based approaches to map generation, each grid cell contains a value that indicates the presence or absence of an obstacle in the corresponding region of the environment. Topological approaches on the other hand represent robot environments by graphs. Nodes in such graphs correspond to distinct places, e.g. corridor junctions, doors, etc. If there exists' a direct path between two such distinctive places then a corresponding arc between them in the graph indicates this.

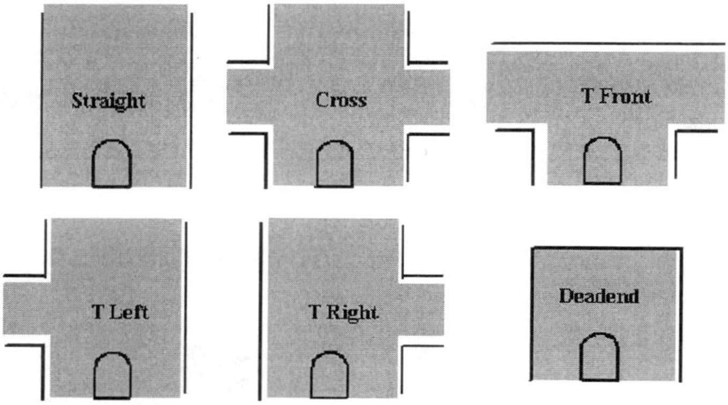

Figure 3. Typical cooridor junction cases

Horswill's Carpet Blob Detector

A vision system, as developed by Ian Horswill in his thesis [14] and implemented on Polly [12][13] and more recently in HERMES [4] is used to give a direction of motion for the robot. The algorithm treats the lack of texture on the floor as a positive feature of the environment. The algorithm executes the following steps:

1. Smoothes the input image with a 3 x 3 filter to remove camera noise.
2. Finds the textured pixels in the image. Image pixels are categorized into either black or white. White pixels differ from their neighbours above and to the right by a total of at least 15 grey levels. Black pixels differ by less than 15 grey levels.
3. Extracts the *carpet blob*. Because the camera is mounted facing downward towards the floor, that part of the image corresponding to the floor is at the bottom of the image. Starting from the bottom of the image, the *carpet blob* is computed by tracing up each image column until a textured pixel is found. The set of pixels skipped over is the *carpet blob*. In other words, a one-dimensional simple gradient filter has been applied, scanning the image from bottom to top and left to right for contour points that mark the transition between obstacle free areas and obstacles.
4. Turns in the direction in which the *carpet blob* is tallest.

This algorithm is essentially a first-order approximation of the direction of motion to pursue. If this set of resultant values is appropriately thresholded, that subset above the threshold may indicate that the robot is observing a distinct place within the building. A distinct place correpsonds to a node in a topological graph. However, certain places in the environment are more distinctive than others, corridor junctions are an example. Using knowledge of the types of junctions present in the building and their relative locations to one another from the topological map, similiar places can be distinguished from one another. Place recognition is important as it effectively means that the robot has been able to localize itself within some global coordinate system. Localization is particularly important for map-based approaches that learn their maps, since the accuracy of a metric map depends crucially on the alignment of the robot with its map. Place recognition allows the robot to invoke a reset of its path-following algorithm and allows the path-planning and scheduling techniques in Layer 2 of the architecture to proceed.

3.3 Layer 2

For a robot to perform effective path planning requires detailed knowledge of the environment. The robot requires a plan to be given to it so that it can navigate its required route. There are several important constraints that need to be satisified when producing a suitable plan. These include:

- Robot constraints
- Task constraints – governed by the scenario in which the robot is "embedded".
- Topological constraints
- Human constraints
- Temporal constraints – the delivery of a quality of service dictated by inter-task relationships.

In this implementation planning focuses on the use of *Discrete Event Systems*, in particular the use of *Coloured Petri Nets* for the specification and supervised satisfaction of these constraints. Discrete Event Systems are useful for describing the relationships and the ordering that should take place between events in the evolution of a task. Petri Nets, for example, have been widely used in the control of *Automatic Guided Vehicles* (AGV) [3] [19].

Discrete Event Systems (DES)

A DES is a dynamical system whose state space is an unordered collection of events or symbols. A DES is a discrete-state, event-driven system, that is, its state evolution depends entirely on the occurence of asynchronous discrete events over time. DESs are used to provide organisational descriptions of communication networks and process-oriented tasks including delivery and industrial automation. These systems are discontinuous in that their behaviour is affected by sudden changes in operational flow. These systems are by their nature non-deterministic. In DES, observations and actions are treated as events. Events correspond to the transitions between states and model abrupt discrete changes in the system's behaviour. The event-space is partitioned into what is controllable and what is uncontrollable. Controllable events are enabled or disabled in order to ensure the correct behaviour of the system. Uncontrollable events are observable events over which the system has no control. These may include sensory observations of the environment, or the effects of actions performed by the subject of control.

There has been little adoption of DES to the control of mobile robots. In [16] Kosecka models elementary sensing and control strategies through appropriate finite state machine abstractions, capturing the discrete event aspects of continuous models. A task specification language is employed to compose elementary strategies to form complex missions. *Supervisory Control Theory* (SCT) is used to synthesise a supervisor for a run-time scheduler and task monitor. Kosecka employs an Input/Output semantics rather than the Generator semantics typically used in SCT. This allows the *plant* and *supervisor* to be fully synchronised. The role of the supervisor is to force controllable events on the plant while monitoring the plants responses. In [2] the mobile robot is modelled as a set of differential equations describing its motion. The discrete event controller, modelled as an automaton, describes task level decision making. The system also comprises of an interface layer which serves as the communication between the mobile robot and the decision module. Behaviours are implemented via constraint maintenance. The robot is seen to be constrained by the obstacles in its environment. It is also constrained by its own dynamics of motion. Discrete events in this system are the gain and loss of constraints due to obstacles.

In both of the above applications of DES to mobile robotics, only DESs' based on *Finite Automata* (FA) are considered. The only constraints tackled in these systems are partial environmental constraints, i.e. obstacle constraints, and the constraints due to the dynamics of motion of the physical robot. There is no evidence of tackling constraints imposed on a system by the task, the topology in which that task is centred, or the temporal constraints of the task as performed by the robot. The primary reason is in the synthesis of a supervisory controller. The state-space is in the general case very large. In any real world process, a computational explosion in the state-space is encountered when trying to synthesise a controller. In the supervisory control of discrete-event systems based on controllable languages, a standard way to handle state explosion in large systems is by modular supervision. The overall specification for system behaviour is decomposed into a set of modular specifications. These modular specifications are used to synthesise a set of modular supervisors, so that the state-space over which the supervisor synthesis procedure iterates is reduced. However, modular supervision implies concurrency. FA's are only capable of modelling conflict, not concurrency. Decentralised DES is usually studied under the framework of Petri Nets. In decentralised control, modular supervisors that are individually non-blocking for the plant may produce blocking, or even deadlock, when operating online concurrently. Petri Nets can therefore manage the concurrency but not conflict. Because control is distributed across multiple controllers, any individual controller can only partially observe the system state. An individual controller has only limited control over the system. The controllers must interact to ensure that the system will not reach a state satisfying a forbidden condition. In [23] the problem of shared events is considered. It is important that control in one subsystem does not cause blocking in another. This is achieved by ensuring that for a set of local specifications, local synthesis and control achieves the same behaviour as that of a global optimum design for the overall specification. When a problem cannot be solved using fully decentralised supervisors, reasoning about knowledge may provide guidelines for incorporating communication and pooled information into the model [21].

Coloured Petri Nets

A Petri Net (PN) is a directed bipartite graph consisting of places P and transitions T. Places are represented by circles, trasitions by bars. Places and transitions are connected by arcs. The difference between a PN and an FA is that a FA is a restricted class of PN. A PN is a FA or state machine if each transition $t \in T$ has exactly one input place and exactly one output place. The state of a Petri Net is in its marking. $M = [m(p_1), m(p_2), \cdots, m(p_n)]$ This marking can be finite or infinite. Petri Nets can model an infinite system with a finite number of *places*. A Coloured Petri Net (CPN) is an extension of a regular PN. In a CPN , a set of colours is associated with each place $p \in P$ and transition $t \in T$, and a transition can fire with respect to each of its colours. Coloured Petri Nets allow us to model conflict as well as concurency. A regular Petri Net is a free-choice PN, that is, a token in a place enables all the output transitions of that place, and any one of the output transitions can be chosen to fire. In a CPN, if a transition t_i is one of the output transitions of a place $p \in P$, then the tokens in place p that enable transition t_i must have the same colour b_i as the transition t_i. A token in place p may enable more than one tranisition simultaneously. Thus, the token has a colour set $\{ b_1, b_2, \cdots, b_k \}$ corresponding to a transition set $\{ t_1, t_2, \cdots, t_k \}$ with $k \geq 1$, implying that a token can fire any output transitions of place *p* with colour b_i, $i = 1, \cdots, k$.

The Planner

This research investigates path planning within an intelligent structured environment. Several scenarios for mobile robot use within health care environments have been considered within the context of the MobiNet project. These robots are generally categorised into delivery or assistive. Typical examples of delivery type robots for the health care industry are Helpmate [7] and FIRST [22]. An example of an assistive robot is PAM-AID [17][18] (See also Chapter 4). The PAM-AID project has constructed and field tested a prototype mobile robotic device which gives greater autonomy to elderly frail and blind patients.

In these scenarios the robot requires a plan of actions to be given to it so that it can perform its scheduled task. This plan may be a specification of the topological features that must be observed to satisfy a route. Within this specification, the constraints that must be satisfied are:

- Reach each way-point i.e. landmark, on the path, while
- Avoiding obstacles on that portion of the path, and
- Do so in the time allowable for that portion of the journey.

The planner responds to events that occur within the building. If, for example, another request for service of the robot is required, the planner will check if it can be accomodated within the context of the current plan by augmenting the Petri Net model of the process. In this sense, the robot is only ever dealing with partial plans; the constraints on the robot task can be altered dynamically. If the request cannot be serviced in the current context, then a time at which the request can be serviced is determined by look-ahead prediction of the PN model of current progress.

4. Robot Navigation and Intelligent Buildings

The navigation of a mobile base requires a large amount of peripheral equipment. This might include sonar, laser and optical sensors. This leads to a large and often cumbersome robot that can only move on one floor of a building and has difficulty in the navigation of doors. With the aid of a "smart" environment it is possible to aid the navigation of a mobile robot and reduce the number of sensors. Utilising wireless technology, e.g, IEEE 802.1, a mobile robot can access building services within the "smart" environment. Elevators can be requested by propagating the appropriate event on the control network. The device in the elevator receives the event and takes the robot to the correct floor. Office doors can also be easily controlled. If a robot needs to travel from one room to another then the robot needs only instruct the building to open the door that is blocking its path. Mobile robots often use maps to navigate through large areas, and local sensors to cope with dynamic situations. Provided that the starting point of the robot is known, the map is used as a method of localisation. These maps become very large as the building size increases. Devices that monitor and control a building can also contain a small map of their local area . A robot moving around a building can download one of these maps from the closest device, thus reducing the need for a large storage device situated on the robot. If the robot finds an error or omission in the local map then adjustments can be made and uploaded to the relevant device. This gives a dynamic method of map building, while reducing the cost of the robot and distributing expensive resources throughout the building architecture. Figure 4 shows the integration of the system, detailing the implementation of the robot architecture.

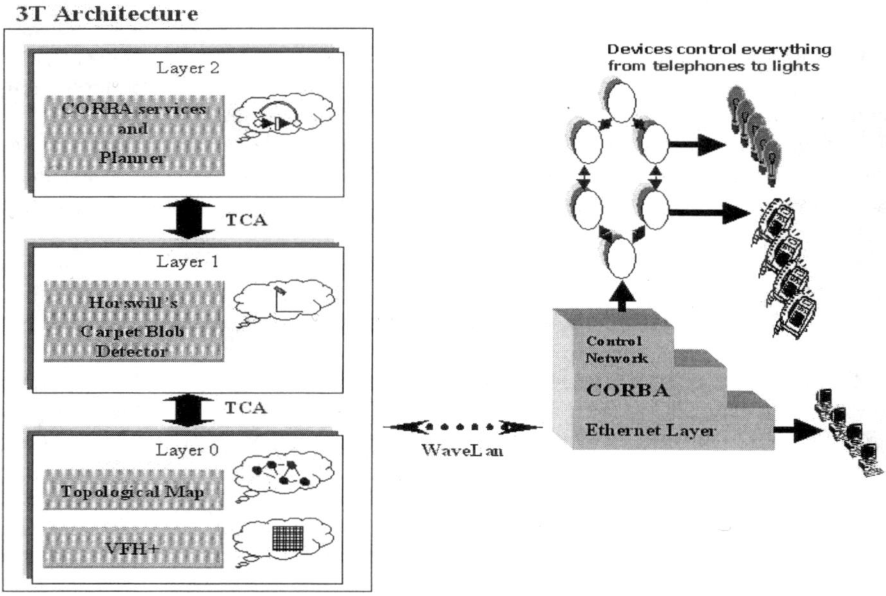

Figure 4. Integrated Robot-Building Architecture

4.1 Distributed Multi-Robot Communication.

Multi-robot communication is well studied, particularly in multi-agent research whereby many agents contribute to the solving of the task at hand by coordinating their efforts. Agents are modelled as having a defined set of beliefs about the environment in which they operate, but need to communicate to combine their beliefs to reach a global solution. The Contract Net protocol [25] has been recognized as an attractive way for task negotiation. However the main communication cost on Contract Net Protocol is caused by broadcasting task announcements. The LEMMING system [20] uses Case-Based Reasoning (CBR) to learn focused addressing to reduce the broadcasting overhead and message information discarded after each negotiation. Dealing with conflict locally among agents is required to maintain a global coherence of the system. In the MARTHA project [1] a Plan-Merging Paradigm is employed to achieve this coherence among a large number of robots. The robots incrementally determine the resources they require taking into account their execution context. MARTHA comprises of a central station and a fleet of autonomous robots. The robots have the ability to communicate with the central station and one another. They receive their missions from the central station, but communicate with one another to coordinate their actions, refine their plans, and update their trajectories. In AMADEUS [15], intelligent AGVs communicate with job-shop cells in an agent framework to allocate an AGV to a transportation task, and to coordinate multiple AGV actions so that their goals may be realised.

4.2 Multi-Robot Communication in Intelligent Buildings

The nodes of the control network are distributed throughout the building. Each node maintains a table of known "interesting" objects local to it. It also maintains an adjacency table of the nodes local to it.

The nodes in the control network are best viewed as agents. As in Actor[11], each agent is devoid of complex control structure. Actor systems are simple collaborative systems since a given series of computations are performed by several agents. These agents co-operate through a variation of the Contract Net Protocol [25], to select the nearest "idle" robot for a task, and use a signpost mechanism to guide the robot to its destination. The Contract Net Protocol provides dynamically opportunistic control, where agents help each other by sharing the computation involved in the subtasks for a problem. The protocol described here [8] provides optimal route selection through distributed search.

When searching for the location of a feature or device the node broadcasts a message to all other nodes on its subnet. The receiving nodes will then interrogate their local object model to see if the search feature is present. If it is then this fact will be relayed to the originator of the message in a confirm transaction. The node containing the feature then propagates a reply agent. If the reply agent has propagated back to the originator then the search is complete. Upon receiving an agent, the agent table is queried to see if this is a unique search. If so it is added to the table and propagated to adjacent nodes. The agent in the table contains a signpost to the next node. This signpost indicates the direction of travel for the most optimum route. If the search is not unique, that is, the agent has been propagated to this node by some other node, then a comparison is made between the two competing agents. The agent with the minimum cumulative cost is stored and the signpost adjusted accordingly. The previous agent is deleted. The network will eventually converge to a solution. This route can then be followed to find the desired feature. As the robot enters into an area controlled by a particular node, that node will indicate the direction of travel to complete the task.

Unlike other multi-robot systems, individual robots do not communicate directly with one another. They communicate through a distributed information space mediated by the intelligent building.

5. Conclusions

Demographic trends show that 25% of the European population will be aged over 60 by 2020 [6]. In the USA the percentage of over 65's in the population will increase from its current level of 12.5% to 20% by 2030 [27]. These projected trends have serious implications for the standard of care that will be available. There simply won't be enough carers. To alleviate this, it is suggested that robotic couriers should perform most of the non-essential tasks, e.g. fetch and carry. Robots for the visually impaired [17] will give patients more autonomy. In this way carers will be able to assist comfortably those with the most urgent needs.

So far there has been little market penetration by mobile robotic products due to the fact that fully autonomous systems are too expensive in both initial capital cost and also in maintenance. This chapter has proposed the use of a building managemnet system as a method of structuring the robot environment. The network, as part of the healthcare Intranet, acts as a management infrastructure for multiple robots so the robotic services can be coordinated across the building. This is good for the marketability of mobile robots as they can be integrated with the workflow of the institution. Reduced costs and a system that is readily inter-operable with existing hospital systems is much more marketable to hospital managers.

6. References

[1] Alami R., Fleury S,. Herrb M,. Ingrand F., and Robert F. "Multi-Robot Cooperation in the MARTHA Project". *IEEE Robotics & Automation Magazine*, Vol. 5, No.1, March 1998, pp. 36-47.

[2] Austin D.J., and McCarragher B.J., "Discrete Event Control for Mobile robots". *Proceedings of the International Conference on Field & Service Robotics (FSR'97)*, 1997.

[3] Barad M., and Sinriech D., "A Petri Net Model for the Operational Design and Analysis of Segmented Flow Topology (SFT) AGV Systems". *International Journal of Production Research*, Vol. 36, No. 5, pp. 1401-1415, 1998.

[4] Bischoff R., "Advances in the Development of the Humanoid Service Robot HERMES". *Proceedings of the International Conference on Field & Service Robotics*, August 29-31, 1999, Pittsburgh, Pennsylvania, pp. 156-161.

[5] Borenstein J., and Raschke U., "Real-time Obstacle Avoidance for Non-Point Mobile Robots". *SME Transactions on Robotics Research* Vol2, pp. 2.1-2.10, 1992.

[6] Eurostat: Regional population aging of the EU at different speeds up to 2025. *Statistics in Focus 4/99, Statistical Office of the European Communities*, 1999.

[7] Evans J., "HelpMate: A Robotic Materials Transport System". *International Journal of Robotics & Autonomous Systems*, 1989.
[8] Foster G., "Local Modelling Techniques for the Management of Distributed Control Systems". *Doctoral Thesis*, Dept of Cybernetics, University of Reading, UK, September 1998.
[9] Gat E., "Artificial Intelligence & Mobile Robots: Case study of Successful Robot Systems", *Chapter Three-Layer Architectures*, MIT Press, 1998.
[10] Greenane R., & Dobson S., "Integrating LonWorks into an Open Systems Control Environment". *LonWorld99*, October 13-15 1999, Amsterdam RAI, The Netherlands.
[11] Hewitt C., "Viewing Control Structures as Patterns of Passing Messages". *Artificial Intelligence*, No.8, 1977.
[12] Horswill I. Polly, "A Vision Based Artificial Agent". *Proceedings of the Eleventh National Conference on Artificial Intelligence* (AAAI93), 1993.
[13] Horswill I., "Analysis of Environment and Adaption". Artificial Intelligence – Special Issue on Computational Theories of Interaction & Agency, 1995.
[14] Horswill I., "Specification of Perceptual Processes". *PhD thesis*, Massachusetts Institute of Technology, 1993.
[15] Kamada T., & Oikawa K., "AMADEUS: A Mobile, Autonomous Decentralized Utility System for Indoor Transportation". *Proceedings of the 1998 International Conference on Robotics & Automation*, Leuven, Belgium, May 1998, pp2229-2236.
[16]Kosecka J., "A Framework for Modeling & Verifying Visually Guided Agents: Design, Analysis & Experiments". *Ph.D. thesis*, University of Pennslyvannia, 1996.
[17] Lacey G., & Dawson-Howe K., "Evaluation of a Robot Mobility Aid for the Elderly Blind". *Robotics & Autonomous Systems – Special Issue*, 1998.
[18] Lacey G., MacNamara S., & Dawson-Howe K., "Lecture Notes in AI: Assistive Technology & Artificial Intelligence", *Chapter Personal Adaptive Mobility Aid for the Frail & Elderly Blind.* Springer-Verlag, 1998.
[19] Lee C.C., & Lim J.T., "Deadlock Prediction and Avoidance based on Petri Nets for Zone-Control Automated Guided Vehicle Systems". *International Journal of Production Research*, Vol. 33, No. 12, pp3249-3265, 1995.
[20] Ohko T., Hiraki K., & Anzai Y., "Learning to Reduce Communication Cost on Task Negotiation among Multiple Autonomous Mobile Robots".
[21] Ricker S.L., & Rudie K., "Know Means No: Incorporating Knowledge into Decentralized Discrete Event Control". *Proceedings of the 1997 American Control Conference*, 1997.
[22] Sandt F., & Pampagnin L., "Distributed Planning and Hierarchical Control for a Service Mobile Robot". *Proceedings of the International Symposium on Intelligent Robotic Systems (SIRS94)*, 1994.
[23] Sang-Heon L., & Wong K.C., "Decentralized Control of Concurrent Discrete Event Systems with Non-Prefix Closed Local Specifications". *Proceedings of the 36th IEEE conference on Decision & Control*, 1997.
[24] Simmons R., Fernandez J., Goodwin R., Koenig S., & O'Sullivan J. Xavier, "An Autonomous Mobile Robot on the Web". *IEEE Robotics & Automation Magazine*, 1999.

[25] Smith R.G., & Davis A., "Distributed Problem Solving: The Contract Net Approach". Proceedings of the Second National Conference of Canada Society for Computational Studies of Intelligence, 1978.
[26] Ulrich I. & Borenstein J., "VFH+: Reliable Obstacle Avoidance for Fast Mobile Robots". *Proceedings of the 1998 IEEE International Conference on Robotics & Automation*, 1998.
[27] US Census Bureau. "Sixty-five plus in the United States". *Economics and Statistics Administration, US Department of Commerce*, May 1995.

Chapter 10

State of the Art on Manipulators

by Frithjof WEBER, Bart DRIESSEN, Gunnar BOLMSJÖ,
Stanislao LAURIA, William HARWIN

Chapter 10

State of the Art on Manipulators

Frithjof WEBER, Bart DRIESSEN, Gunnar BOLMSJÖ,
Stanislao LAURIA, William HARWIN

1. Introduction on Manipulators

Since the mechanical, electrical and computational structure of robots can vary considerably, it is difficult to make a clear distinction between the robot and manipulator concepts. Traditionally, the *manipulator* has been defined as a major component characterising a robot [8] although sometimes the term manipulator is used in a broader sense [4]. In our context, we understand the manipulator as a programmable element (*arm*) of a robot (in contrast to e.g. the understanding as a manually controlled manipulating device for pick and place operations). The manipulator may be thought to consist of a group of 'rigid bodies' called *links*, or linkages, connected by *joints*. The links are interconnected such that they are forced to move relative to one other in order to position the free end of the manipulator. In this way it is capable of movement in various directions and it is said to do the 'work' of the robot. This is the reason for which the terms 'robot' and 'manipulator' are often used interchangeably. PUMA, the Stanford arm, the Cincinnati Milacron and the RTX are some general-purpose manipulators.

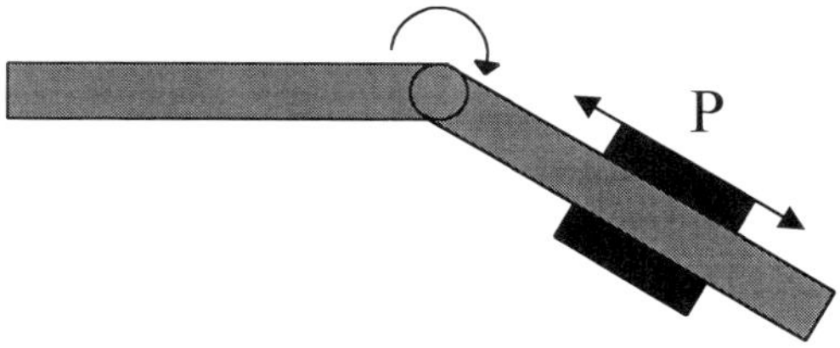

Figure 1. Translational and prismatic joints

Generally, joints of manipulator fall into two classes. The first one, *revolute*, produces pure rotary motion (Rotary joint or abbreviated as R). The second one, *prismatic*, produces pure linear or translational motion and as a result, it is often referred as linear joint (Prismatic joint or abbreviated as P).

Hence, a manipulator is considered to be a combination of links and joints with the first link connected to the world and the last link containing the 'hand', may be classified by the *type of joints* and their *order* (from the base to the hand). With this convention, the PUMA robot arm (Figure 2) can be classified as 6R, the Stanford arm as 2R-P-2R, the Cincinnati Milacron T3886 as 3P-3R and the SCARA (Figure 3) as P-5R. Other manipulator, or more in general robot, classification methods are possible [5].

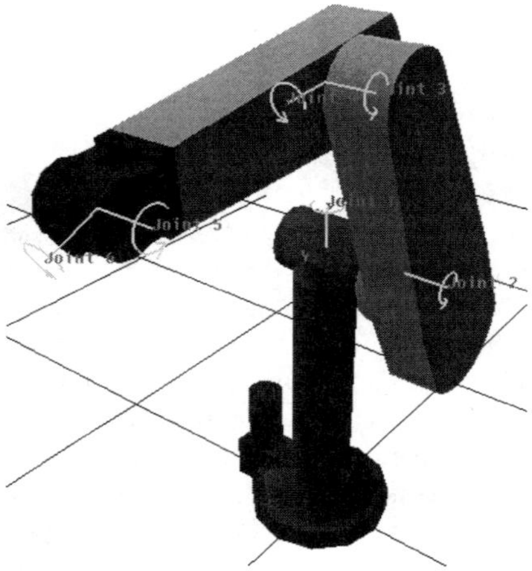

Figure 2. The PUMA robot arm.

1.1 Drive Mechanism

Various types of motors are used in robotics to drive the robot to its required position: stepper motors, DC motors, brushless DC motors and AC motors. There are also hybrid motors between these types. These motors all have varying characteristics with respect to price, size, weight, controllability etc.

Stepper motors are easy to control in position and velocity. Theoretically, no external sensors are necessary, since it can be assumed that the stepper motor follows exactly the number of steps that are sent by the motor driver. Unfortunately, sometimes the stepper motor misses steps, due to high external forces, or high friction in the mechanical construction. If this happens too frequently, extra sensors are still necessary, and the advantages of the stepper motors strongly reduces. A disadvantage of stepper motors is that they cannot be torque controlled: between two steps, the motor is in fact uncontrollable.

Another disadvantage is that stepper motors can not deliver much power. Not many robotic applications use stepper motors. An exception is the HANDY1 single task workstation [2].

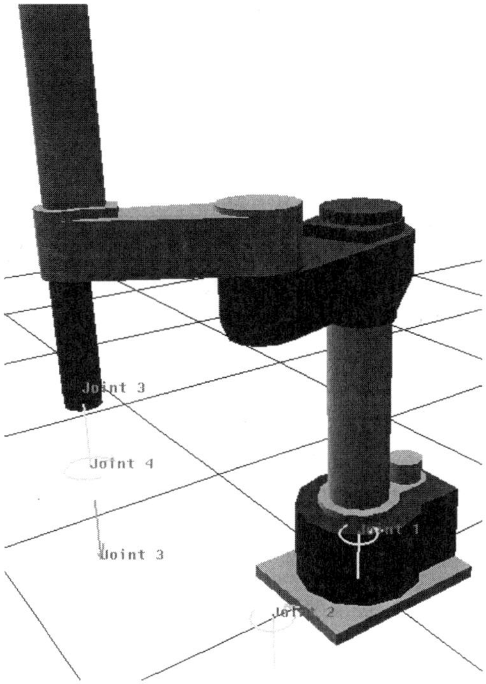

Figure 3. The SCARA robot arm

DC motors are more widely used in robotics. The stator of the motor typically contains permanent magnets, whilst the magnetic field in the rotor is controlled by the motor drives. Commutators make sure the direction of the magnetic field of the rotor is changed appropriately. The motor torque can be controlled by controlling the current through the rotor coils. Typically, the motor is driven using pulse width modulated drivers (PWM). For position or velocity control, extra sensors are required. Typically these are incremental or absolute encoders placed on the motor. DC motors are cheap, but cannot deliver high power. Due to the commutation between the rotor and the motor driver, the motor will suffer from wear. An example of a manipulator which uses DC motors is the MANUS manipulator.

Brushless DC motors do not have the commutators that normal DC motors have. The commutation is achieved by rotating the stator field, based on the position of the rotor. Typically Hall-effect sensors are used for measuring the position of the rotor, and based on this position, the field of the stator is rotated. In addition, an incremental pulse sensor is used for position control. Brushless DC motors have higher performance than normal DC motors, but are also more expensive. The (mechanical) impedance of brushless DC motors is very low, since no friction caused by the commutators exists. An example of a robot, which uses brushless DC motors, is the ASIMOV robot.

AC motors differ from brushless DC motors by the way the stator field is rotated. The direction of the stator field is rotated continuously for AC motors, using a resolver signal which measures the position of the rotor. AC motors are widely used by industrial robots, such as those from ABB and Motoman..

1.2 Internal Sensors

In the previous section various actuators for moving the manipulator links have been discussed. Nevertheless, without the ability to obtain information about the joint and/or end effector position, the manipulator control can be problematic. In particular position, velocity and acceleration must be measured to insure that the manipulator moves in a desired manner at the final position. For this, often potentiometers, resolvers or optical encoders are used.

The simplest device that can be used is to measure position is the *potentiometer*. Applied to manipulators, such devices can be made to monitor either angular position of a revolute joint or linear position of a prismatic joint. Linearity is the important feature for the potentiometer to be a useful position sensor. The inevitable presence of non-linearity in any potentiometer makes its use in systems where excellent accuracy measurement is required, difficult and often impractical, especially since the non-linearity will change, due to wear.

There are a variety of sensing devices and techniques that avoid this difficulty [9]. One of the earliest solution is the *resolver*. It consists of a rotatory transducer that converts angular displacement into an AC voltage or an AC voltage into an angular displacement. Based on these principles, several other devices have been developed to determine the position of a manipulator joint.

Another class of sensor, using optical hardware and techniques, which can quite frequently be used to perform the position determination task with relative ease and great accuracy is the *optical encoder*. This non-contact sensory device comes in two distinct classes: absolute and incremental. In the former case, the encoder is able to give the actual linear or rotational position whereas the latter only provides positional information relative to some reference point.

1.3 Programming and Control

The programming of a robot includes all activities with which the user instructs the robot about the activities to be performed. The actual performing of the activities (operation) is then matter of the robot control. Programming the robot is mainly about programming the manipulator and the gripper. Consequently we give an introduction into this subject in this section.

The major challenge in programming is the user's need to program the robot in an easy and fast way and without any ambiguity in order to avoid dangerous situations and harm for the environment or the robot. Within healthcare this is specifically demanding as the users are not necessarily experienced robot programmers but also 'normal' people, i.e. users with no specific training in programming. Following the approaches from industrial robots, two basic methods of programming can be distinguished:

On Line and Off Line Programming

With *on line programming*, the programming task is done by using the robot itself in a real environment. This is usually done by using a teach pendant to guide the robot to the desired positions, to store them and to define the logical instructions. In some cases these activities can also be separated and the positions are up-loaded to another computer where the instructions that define the motions, logistics and sequences, and using of the I/O of the robot are defined.

Off line programming on the other hand is a method that mainly uses other support than the actual robot that is programmed. The time spent at the robot station is much smaller than in the on line programming method. However, in practice, a teach up procedure is necessary to correct the positions. Due to its simplicity, on line programming is the most commonly used method. Some of the advantages of this method are:

- The programming is intuitive and direct and in most cases carried out directly by the operator that will operate the robot later during real operation.
- The programming is done under real conditions meaning that all equipment and objects around the robot are the same as under operation. This includes robot, gripper, objects to handle, etc. and provides immediate feedback which minimises geometrical and functional errors.
- Simple function checks during programming are supported as the program is developed more or less in an incremental way where parts of the program can be tested during this procedure.

There are of course some drawbacks with the method:

- The most obvious is that the robot itself must be used during programming, which means that it can not be used for other, more productive work. (However, this can be considered as more relevant for an industrial production line as a close down of a robot will affect the whole line and not the robot alone. Reprogramming robots at the same time in a line may need more programmers that the company has available for the task. In such cases on line programming is expensive.)
- Another drawback is that complicated programs with complex logistics, accurate motions and/or long cycle time are difficult to develop in the environment of e.g. a manufacturing plant or a hospital environment while maintaining a good structure. Even with a well prepared structure, there are numerous disturbances that may affect the programmer's concentration on the task. On the other hand, most work processes to be done by a robot need experience and knowledge of the operator so that the program generates the expected result.

It is therefore not always the case that off line programming creates "better" programs. On the other hand, the off line method encourages a more structured way of programming which, in many applications, leads to parameterised programmes that can be reused or adapted for similar applications. Thus, even if off line programming initially is more expensive, it is in general more effective in the long run. Due to this, off line programming is a method that is increasing and has the following advantages:

- Higher utilisation of the robot since the programming can be done while the robot is working in normal operation. In most cases, a final correction is needed for some of the programmed positions, but the downtime of the robot is considerably lower than the downtime during on line programming.
- Better documentation of programs and reuse of experience and knowledge. It is also in general easier to create programs with better structure applying a modular approach.
- Off line programming supports the use of simulation techniques. By this, programs can be analysed and tested from different aspects which is important if they contain complex logical statements. Other parts of the analysis include the generation of motions where collisions with other objects and singularities can be detected as well as the robustness of the program to get into such problems.

As mentioned above, off line programming requires in general knowledge within the field of computing that is not required or used otherwise and, at the same time, the programmer needs knowledge and experience about the process to be done by the robot. Based on the specific need, efficient programming of robots is a complex process that may involve people with different skills and expertise.

Finally, it has to be stated that on line programming receives specific attention in health care because the mechanism are the same as for controlling the robot directly. As both modes are relevant for a robot (i.e. automated control following the program or manual control following the user, e.g. for supporting the user in drinking a glass of water), the effort to implement and train the required functions is smaller.

Programming Languages

The way the robot operates is in general defined in a specific programming language. Most, if not all robot manufacturers, have defined their own language for their robots. In general terms, we may say that the robot specific languages are robot oriented languages. From an abstraction point of view, this is the lowest level and we may clearly see the following abstraction levels of programming languages: robot oriented languages and task oriented languages.

- In *robot oriented languages*, all instructions describe the task to be performed in direct relation to physical or logical operations in the robot system. All activities are described in great detail and they can also be referred to explicitly. This means that all data is stored as numerical data that specifies a direct action to be made, for example coordinate values for a target position or data to send out on a specific I/O port.
- In *task oriented languages*, sometimes referred to as objective or object oriented languages, the instructions refer to the task to be done by manipulation of objects, set of parameter data for a process to be controlled and so on. By this, the instructions describe the task to be done rather than the specific motions of the robot. Target

positions can be attached to specific objects if the objective is to manipulate the object. In such case, the robot will automatically adapt to changes and follow any new target position if the object position has changed. However, in operation, the robot must have access to world model data in order to adapt to changes. Otherwise, changes will not be known and the robot will operate in a static world which is based on the data defined when the executable program was generated.

Despite the different types of languages which are existing, most, if not all, are of the robot oriented type. This does not mean, however, that task oriented languages are of no interest. Instead, complex tasks can be described in a more structured way and an executable code can be generated using a translator for the specific target robot on demand. This technique is growing fast by combining off line programming, task oriented languages and simulation systems with graphical output capabilities.

Programming and Operation

If a program is generated on line, the instructions are generally defined "on the fly" by using a hand terminal that assists in defining the instructions, its arguments, etc. by using a menu system. Thus, the programmer does not need to remember the exact syntax of a specific instruction. In off line programming, the program instructions are generally defined in a text editor. The same type of assisting menus can be implemented in such systems, but free text gives the programmer more flexibility. Robot languages nowadays tend to resemble the structure of high level computer languages such as "C" or "Pascal". In addition, they also have the following basic functions:

- *Position and frame data types and corresponding mathematical operations:* Examples are the definition of reference frames and their use for defining positions for the robot motion. In an application this can be used for real time calibration by using sensors to measure the object frame and orient and translate it and all related positions. Another case is the manipulation of objects in a pattern. By applying mathematical operations on the positions, only a starting position is needed.
- *Motion description:* The motion can be of several types, where the most common ones are linear and circular motion in Cartesian space and a joint based motion in robot coordinates. In addition, a motion must be accompanied by a set of arguments that specifies how the motion is generated. This is strongly depending on the specific robot. In general, a velocity has to be defined, that specifies the velocity of a TCP, Tool Centre Point, located at a specific place from the last link on the robot. At the TCP, a frame is generally defined as well so that the motions are defined with both position and orientation. If the robot moves from position to position and we do not want it to stop during the motion, there must be arguments that specify how the motions should be generated.
- *Use of sensor information:* By using I/O signals, the robot can keep track of the world around and control the equipment. The most simple information relies on binary data, while more complex information can be provided through binary data ports with four or eight parallel data signals. Such signals are easy to implement and use in the application program. More advanced sensors, such as vision systems, force

sensors, optical seam trackers using laser triangulation, etc. are more complex and generate (or are able to generate) more complex data that, in an advanced application, may need careful programming. Problems that may arise if a sensor generates target positions for a robot are that the target position is out of reach, the robot switches configuration, the robot moves through a singular area, etc. Great care must be taken to secure any application that relies on sensors, especially if advanced sensors are used.

Besides the description of the robot task through a program, which can be seen as describing it from an external point of view, there is also an internal side of the operation of the robot which affects the way the robot executes a task. Depending on the configuration of the robot, the internal control and performance is in general highly non-linear. There is, for example, a high difference in torque needed depending on the position of the links of a typical arm robot. The performance is a compromise defined by the robot arm configuration, workspace, payload, general motions, etc. However, if the robot is to execute a specific trajectory with a specific payload under equal operating conditions (same temperature for example), an optimisation can take place that generates optimised control signals during the trajectory. Such adaptive control can normally be achieved by most advanced commercial robots and needs a learning trajectory to be run before the optimised control can take place.

2. Grippers

The gripper is the connector between the manipulator of the robot and the object. Its task is to pick up an object, to re-orientate it, to hold it in a stable position while the robot is moving or the object is being manipulated, and finally to put it down. The holding of the object can be based on different physical principles, as e.g. pneumatic, mechanical or magnetic forces. However, as it seems that within the healthcare sector there is no real application for these principles, this section will focus on mechanical grippers only[1]. The section provides an introduction into the theory of grasping, describes the major parameters characterising a gripper and outlines different types of grippers. Finally, it presents a variety of selected grippers from healthcare and beyond.

2.1 Gripper Theory and Characteristics

Gripping the object is only one activity within the overall grasping process: Mostly grippers are used with robots in order to transport objects and to assemble or manipulate them. Thus, a few types of motions can be distinguished for describing and programming the movements of the gripper:

---

1 However, the creation of the forces for these mechanical grippers or the control system are frequently based on pneumatic or hydraulic principles.

Grasping Process

Firstly, the gripper has to *approach* the object. Similar as for the movements of the overall robot in its environment, this approaching has to be in a safe way. A collision-free path has to be determined in order to avoid conflicts of the gripper with the object to be gripped and with the surroundings. For autonomous robots, this includes the decision whether the object can be accessed and gripped at all.

For the actual *grasping* of the object a stable grip has to be chosen. The gripper must have information about the characteristics of the object as e.g. shape, surface, allowed forces, or allowed positions, in order to decide on the parameters of the grip (gripping force, orientation, etc.). The different types of grip are described in more detail below in this section.

When *departing* and *moving* with the object, the same rules for collission-free movements as for the approaching apply. However, they are extended with additional rules about the object which now 'has become a part of the robot', i.e. which has to be considered as a moving element of the robot as well. Thus, the geometry of the robot has changed. Further, information about the allowed positions and movements of the object has to be considered (e.g. orientation limits and maximum acceleration for a glass with water).

After the target position has been approached and reached, the gripper *releases* the object. A sensor based release planning is necessary in order to identify unknown environments and assure a safe put-down. If the gripped object is to be *interlocked with other objects,* sensory supervised motions planning is required in order to achieve a successful mounting.

With these types of motions, a "*pick and place operation*" and a "*pick, manipulate, and place operation*" can be described completely. Further to the generic rules of path planning which apply to robots and manipulators in general, some additional elementary issues and conditions are to be considered for the grasp planning:

Grasping Constraints

For the feasibility of the grip, the gripper width has to be larger than the object width and the gripper must be able to reach the object without collision. Furthermore, the robot-arm must be able to reach the grasping point and with the gripped object to reach the final position. For this, the length of the gripper and manipulator must be long enough to reach the object. During the gripping, departing and transfer motion a stable grip of the object is necessary. This means especially that the object must not slip out of the gripper, but usually also that a rotary movement of the object has to be prevented.

If it is not possible to achieve a stable grip with the first grasping motion, *a regrasp operation* is necessary. This can be carried out by releasing the object and grasping it again, by the help of a second gripper, or by reorienting it in the gripper without releasing it. This latter process, however, imposes high requirements on the mechanical and control characteristics of the gripper.

Besides the stability of the object, the *stability of the environment* is required as well: If an object is taken away from the environment, it must leave the environment in a steady state. For example, if there are glasses on a tray, it is important that if one glass is grasped, the remaining glasses do not create a torque that will drop the tray to the ground. Unfortunately, these requirements increase the complexity of the grasping process significantly for autonomous robots, who must be able to detect and consider the environmental conditions [13].

2.2 Form and Force Closure Grip

As in any classical mechanical system, grippers can be distinguished by the physical principle of how they transfer force and torque to the object [11]. Two principles are distinguished:

- *The force closure grip:* The characteristic of the force closure grip is that the gripper keeps the object in a stable state by compensating all forces and torques created by the object. The sum of all forces and sum of all torques must equal zero ($\Sigma F = 0$; $\Sigma M = 0$).
- The force closure grip can be differentiated into a grip with friction and without friction. The force closure grip without friction is very idealised and not very common in daily use, therefore it is no further mentioned. The force closure grip with friction requires at least three contact points for gripping a planar object and at least 4 contact points for a three-dimensional object.
- *The form closure grip* is the second principle for gripping objects. This grip is feasible, because the gripper is a negative model of the object (or of a part of it) which limits the movement of the object within the gripper in any direction, also when changing the gripper orientation. The force is compensated on well specified contact surfaces. Tangential load, pressure load, and torque are not considered, but are instead reduced to the corresponding forces. The gripper must either make use of a special geometry (i.e. negative model of the object), or a significant number of fingers are required. Thus, a simple parallel jaw gripper can usually not be used for the form closure grip, except the jaws have the contour of the object. Some literature suggests to use yielding gripper fingers to adjust the position of the object while being gripped in order to avoid damages of the object.

[15] has shown in experiments that the form closure grip requires a minimum of 7 contact points for gripping any three-dimensional object. Comparing the form closure grip to the force closure grip, it can be stated that the form closure grip reaches more stable grips, and a rotary movement of the object is nearly impossible.

2.3 Basic Types of Grippers

Further to the above classification according to the physical principals, grippers can also be characterised by their mechanical complexity:

The *parallel jaw gripper* has at least two fingers which can be moved towards each other along one axis (cf. Figure 4). Usually, the fingers can be moved independently from each other in order not to shift the object, but they are only able to perform simple operations like open and close. Thereby, a longitudinal, or a side movement is impossible. A parallel jaw gripper has two degrees of freedom. A speciality of the parallel jaw gripper is that its fingers are able to grasp inside and outside with a variable length of fingers.

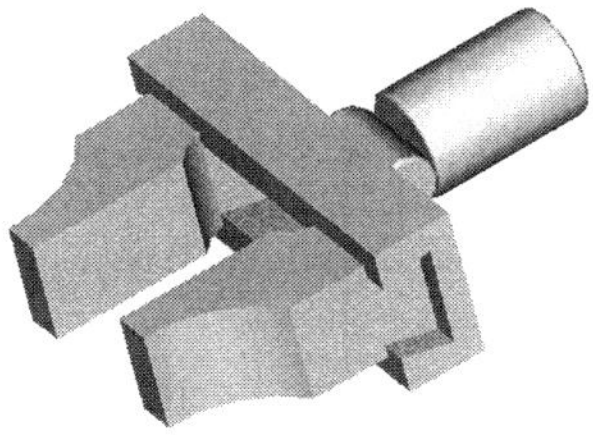

Figure 4. Model of a parallel jaw gripper

While the parallel jaw gripper is based on the model of the thumb and index finger of the human hand, *multifingered grippers* aim to imitate the complete human hand. They are designed to perform multiple tasks and the technique of these grippers is more complex in comparison to parallel jaw grippers. Multifingered grippers have 3-4 fingers and normally every finger can be moved independently of each other in longitudinal axis, in transverse axis and in normal axis, i.e. each finger has at least 3 DOF. Thus, the whole hand has up to 9 to 12 DOF. Some grippers are also able to perform a rotation over one axis, so these grippers have 12 to 16 DOF. Multifingered grippers with high flexibility and the ability to grasp different kinds of objects are called *dextrous grippers*.

The *human hand* is by far the most flexible complex gripper. It allows to adjust gripped objects, and thus to regrasp them without deposing them. Furthermore, the human hand is highly-elastic and has tactile functions. The skin is a very soft surface and prevents the human hand from damaging objects. It are exactly these functions which are required for the healthcare application and it is usually desired to imitate them for having a flexible gripper, thus making the human hand the ideal model of a gripper. However, "research and development leading to the realisation of a fully autonomous and multifingered hand has been going on for three decades. Yet none can be found in an industrial application. This is largely because we do not fully understand the fundamental mechanics of multifinger grasping." [11]

2.4 Gripper Control and Sensors

Similar as for the robot as a whole, the gripper must fulfil high *safety requirements* for health care and thus needs a sophisticated control system. The system must ensure a safe interaction of the gripper with the objects and the environment and has to be able, for example, to recognise a gripper breakdown in order to ensure the safety of the robot. An unproblematic restart by the users from any level of shutdown must be possible – without them being programmers. Also, it has to be considered that the user might be disabled, so that an automatic starting unit for restarting the gripper could be necessary. A voice recognition unit for controlling the gripper is sensible for users, who need to control the gripper by giving simple commands like: open, close, right, left, etc. Depending on the task the robot is to perform, a manual control to steer the gripper must be possible for enabling the highest flexibility.

Controlling the gripper requires a significant amount of information about the object to be grasped coming from different types of *sensors* [7]: Range sensors are used to measure the distance to the object. Force sensors detect the weight of the gripped object or the collision of the gripper or the object with other objects. Tactile sensors, placed e.g. on the fingertips, recognise the contact of the gripper with the object and can also determine the direction and size of the object. Slip sensors are recommendable if the object must be regrasped without deposing it.

In addition, sensors are required to define the position of the gripper in the room. In the first place to define the absolute position in the room, e.g. with the feedback system of the robot, and in the second place to define the distance to other objects in the room. Moving 'obstacles' like persons and other instabilities in the environment have to be safely identified. Moreover, sensors are needed to control and steer the velocity of the gripper while moving.

A visual based system, which uses at least two cameras in order to obtain a stereoscopic view, supports the user in steering a mobile gripper through an unknown environment and to identify the geometry of unknown objects and their location in space. The two cameras must be able to self calibrate in order to generate always a sharp 3D-picture. Thus, the gripper is enabled to avoid obstacles.

Finally, the control system must be able to recognise and inform the gripper when tasks were done by the user in contrast to the original planning e.g. when the user closes the refrigerator door himself instead of waiting for the robot. It must not happen that this leads to an unstable situation or breakdown.

2.5 Selecting Grippers for Healthcare Versus Manufacturing

Grippers for mobile robotics in health care need to be different compared to grippers in industrial systems. While industrial robotics is concentrating especially to develop fully automated work processes, grippers in healthcare should help humans in their daily work. Thus, the goals are dissimilar from each other which puts different demands on the skills of the robot and the gripper.

In health care, for example, the weight of the objects is in many cases not known in advance and sensors are necessary for measuring the weight as information for the control system. Normally, the load-bearing capacity for daily objects lies under 1 kg and the position accuracy is usually not very high. Furthermore, acceleration and velocity of the mobile unit and the gripper can also be lower (and should be for safety reasons).

The *selection of the suitable gripper* starts by deciding on the tasks to be performed by the gripper. Most industrial grippers can only perform simple pick and place operations, and this only for one special part. But with the help of fingers, it becomes possible to grasp with the same gripper different geometrical objects and also more complex parts. Additionally, the position and orientation of the grasped object can be rearranged within the gripper, and thus the time consuming re-grasping of the object is not necessary. A gripper with three fingers can grasp 90% of all possible shapes that can be grasped with the human hand. Thus, multi-fingered grippers are usually the preferred selection for health care applications.

However, as the *mechatronic complexity* of these grippers is significantly higher, their design, manufacturing and programming requires more resources and high qualified operators and the potential failure rate is higher. This is the reason why multifinger grippers are hardly used in industrial production and parallel jaw grippers or specific tools have became the most common type. For healthcare applications, however, the flexibility and adaptability of the gripper are more important than e.g. performance in production or mean time between failure (under the condition that the failure has no impact on safety issues).

Modularity has been introduced as an important concept in robotics and allows to use different specialised grippers for dedicated tasks. The grippers are designed specifically for picking or handling one type of object (which is reflected mainly by their form for taking advantage of the form closure grip). The manipulator is equipped with a standard interface, thus enabling the robot to change quickly between different grippers and also tools like e.g. drilling devices etc. However, this requires dedicated space for storing the grippers or tools and is of limited relevance for mobile robotics and health care, but more interesting for industrial robots as e.g. described in [14].

2.6 Examples of Existing Grippers in Mobile Robotics

This section provides a short description of different existing grippers. Most of them are still on research level today and have not achieved an industrial break through yet. The examples are not limited to the health care sector but show also grippers from other sectors.

The *Two to Six Finger Parallel* gripper by *GMG-Systems* is a flexible industrial gripper with a modular approach. The gripper has a rectangular design and moves the fingers parallelly along a straight line (without longitudinal shift). It can grasp inside and outside with a variable number and length of fingers. The gripping force is spread over the acting fingers, and differs between 190-1030 N dependent on the finger position. The unit weighs 490g and 100g per finger.

The *234-Gripper* by *J.P Baartman* is a prototype with four fingers and 2 DOF [1]. The gripper consists of two perpendicular parallel jaw grippers. The first mechanism contains two fingers moving to opposite directions on one axis. The second mechanism is similar and its axis is placed perpendicular, which enables the gripper to grasp different objects (e.g. squares, triangles, circles outside and inside) with a maximum size of 50 mm^2. The gripper weighs 3.4 kg. In order to grasp objects with a defined number of contact points, the fingertips are designed as spheres. Thereby, and with all fingers moving at equal velocities, parts are not shifted during the grasping process. The fingers are driven by a self-locking spindle, which is connected to a brushless DC-motor. The perpendicular force is limited to 30 N, and the grip force up to 200 N. In order to hold parts in a stable position, the coefficient of friction has to be at least 0.5.

The *Salisbury Hand* is a dextrous hand with three identical fingers, each having three links and three joints to operate a chosen object (Figure 5) [11]. Each finger has 3 DOF, so that it amounts to a total number of 9 DOF. The Salisbury Hand is mostly used together with a PUMA 760 robot arm. The fingers are controlled by four electric motors and a system of pulleys and tendons. The tendons are made of Teflon coated tension cables, which run over the finger joints, and also over the wrist joints. DC servo motors, which are assembled to the forearm drive the tendons and wind and unwind them on capstans. In order to ensure a safe grip, force sensors are placed in different parts of the hand: at the actuators, joints, wrist, and fingers. The fingertips have a spherical shape. Tactile array sensors are used to obtain information about the contact with the object.

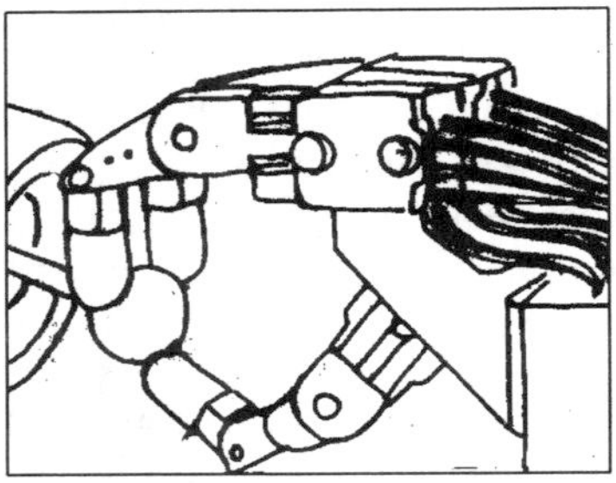

Figure 5. The Salisbury Hand

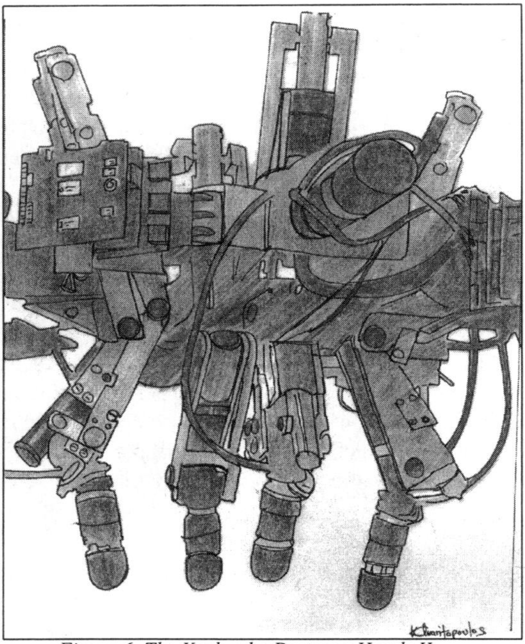

Figure 6. The Karlsruhe Dextrous Hands II

The University of Karlsruhe has a long history in robotics research. The *Karlsruhe Dextrous Hand I* [12] is a three fingered dextrous robot gripper with three DOF in each finger so that this hand has an absolute number of 9 DOF. Its successor, the *Karlsruhe Dextrous Hand II* [6] has four fingers with three DOF per finger, so that this hand has a total number of 12 DOF (Figure 6). Each finger consists of three joints which are driven by a DC motor. Both hands have sensors in each finger tip, which give information about the contact between finger and object. A hierarchical control system architecture, including a sensor data pre-processing layer and a task planner is used to avoid loosing the object. Both hands are able to grasp various objects of various size, and weights with a human like dexterity. In hand II, grasped objects can also be adjusted between the fingertips without deposing them.

The *UTAH/MIT Dextrous hand* is also composed by four fingers, but their orientation is different from the Karlsruhe Hand II. Three fingers are situated at one site of the hand and the fourth at the opposite side, thus acting as a thumb. Each finger has 4 DOF so the hand has a total number of 16 DOF.

By using antagonistic[2] tendons which require a system with 32 polymeric tendons and pneumatic actuators, the hand becomes very anthropomorphic. Each joint is actuated by two pneumatically driven tendons. These pneumatic actuators with the help of 32 force sensors (one for each tendon) can generate forces up to 12 kg. The fingers are arranged on the palm in a manner similar to the human hand. The control is performed by an analogue controller for each of the 16 DOF.

The *Nursing Robot* by *Johann Borenstein* was one of the first working robot systems in health care [3]. It is able to fetch a glass of water and to pour it. It can also operate electrical appliances or replace a cassette in a video recorder and thus is specifically designed for service tasks in a hospital environment. The robot is equipped with a manipulator and has 7 sensor systems integrated. The gripper is equipped with force sensors to ensure proper handling of objects. A video camera is attached with the arm in order to detect the target objects. The arm has 5 DOF.

An *autonomous wheelchair* with a manipulator and gripper was developed by the *Institute of Automation at the University of Bremen (IAT)* for elderly and disabled people [10]. The wheelchair is primarily intended to assist paraplegic[3] persons. The manipulator can handle a glass and transfer it to the user's mouth, for supporting him to drink. The gripper can also grasp a spoon, or a fork and move it to a position where the person can have a meal. The manipulator is controlled by computer vision for identifying objects and steering the gripper to the objects. The mobile basis has three DOF, the robot arm (MANUS) with a parallel jaw gripper has another 6 DOF and with the lift unit, the system has 10 DOF.

The researchers at IAT came to the conclusion that only a visual based system is able to control the wheelchair in an unknown room. By using two cameras, a stereoscopic vision could be generated. But till now, scene interpretation is still an unsolved scientific problem which makes it necessary that the user must support the system by specifying the object to be gripped.

---

2 one who opposes against another

3 someone who is unable to move the lower part of the body

3. Manipulators on Health Care Robots

The following section presents examples of existing manipulators for health care robots. Similar as for the grippers, they are mostly the result of research work and not yet in day-to-day operation.

3.1 Introduction

In this section, we define health care robots, as robots that can assist disabled and elderly persons in carrying out all day living tasks. Health care robots exist in several forms. The main difference between these systems is their ability to operate in a structured or an unstructured environment. The objective of the robotic aid is in general to *assist* the user to function with a maximum of autonomy in his/her environment. This may be interpreted in different ways, such as:

- To be autonomous in the execution of a specific task;
- To be autonomous at a specific working place;
- To be able to function in daily life with less human assistance;
- To be able to function for a number of hours without human attendance.

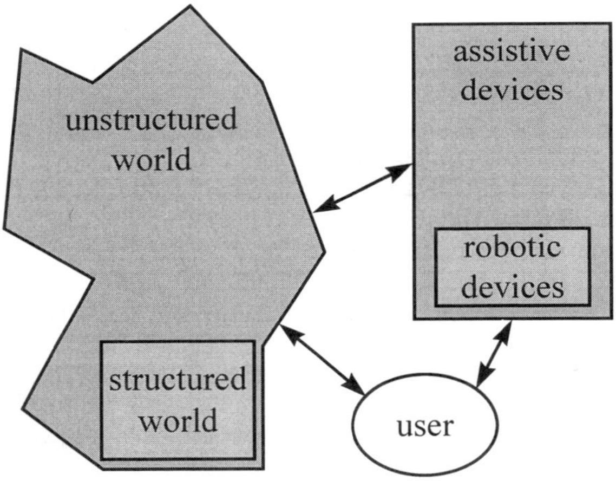

Figure 7. Environment of a user of assistive technology

The environment of the robot user can be modelled as shown in Figure 7. The user has the ability to control the environment, depending on his physical and the technical aids which are available. Focusing on robotic aids, three different concepts can be distinguished:

- Workstations
- Wheelchair mounted manipulators
- Mobile manipulators

The primary usage of fixed *workstations* is for operating in structured environments. Although workstations can move objects to pre-programmed locations very well, problems arise when a user wants to move objects that are outside the working area of the manipulator. Two types of workstations can be distinguished: single task manipulators and multi task manipulators. Single task manipulators can execute one pre-programmed task, such as eating. During the execution of the task, the manipulator will carry out several pre-programmed motions (e.g. pick up a spoonful of potatoes, or pick up a spoonful of carrots), but these motions all belong to one single task (eating). An example of a single task workstation is the HANDY1, described below. Multi task workstations are more flexible. Several tasks can be executed, such as eating, placing a book on a pre-programmed location etc. The drawback for this increased flexibility is the increased size and price of the manipulators. An example of the multi-task workstations is the RAID, manufactured by OxIM Ltd.

Wheelchair mounted manipulators benefit from the possibility to move the robot to the location where a specific task should be accomplished. Naturally, this puts high constraints on the dimensions and weight of the manipulator, since it must, for example, be possible to pass through doors without having to detach the manipulator. The most widely used wheelchair mounted manipulator is the MANUS manipulator, which is manufactured by Exact Dynamics in the Netherlands. Currently, users are part of the control loop in wheelchair mounted manipulators, which puts an extra cognitive load on the user. User evaluations, however, show that this extra load is not experienced as a problem.

The *mobile manipulators* are the most complex group. Although not used in home-situations yet, prototypes are available. Examples are MOVAID (SSSA, Pisa) and ROMAN (Munich), which are both operational in research laboratories.

3.2 Single Task Workstation: HANDY-1

The HANDY-1 robot was originally designed as a single task robot to assist in eating. It has since then been upgraded with other tasks such as make-up and teeth brushing adopting the same working principle. The concept of the HANDY-1 robot is to provide a low-cost robot with a simple user interface that puts very little demand on the user (see Figure 8).

The eating task was originally designed for children with cerebral palsy and the aim was to use the robot as a training device that forces the user to actively move and use the head and mouth for eating while the robot presents the food in front of the user. During eating, the robot works in the following way:

- Food is placed on a special designed tray with five separate areas.
- The robot has pre-programmed motions that manipulate a specially designed spoon that takes food from the tray. In addition, a special gripper function allows the user to access a mug for drinking.
- To operate the robot, the robot has a scanning LED that indicates different pre-programmed robot motions. These motions take either food from the tray at specific positions or drink from the mug.
- The robot is activited by pushing a simple switch at the time when the led is indicating the wanted motion or task.

- The robot executes the task by presenting the food in the proximity of the user's mouth.

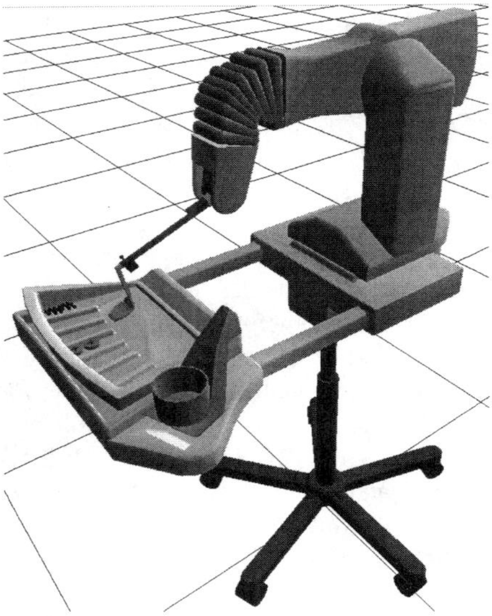

Figure 8. The HANDY-1 robot

When the user has "taken" the food, another push on the switch starts the led scanning and the eating procedure can continue.

Originally the robot was intended to be used as a training device for teaching children to eat by themselves. For children with cerebral palsy it proved to be an efficient method. The robot is also in use by disabled end-users for assisting them to eat unattended. Based on the same principle, other tasks have been developed including putting on make-up, teeth brushing, shaving, and game playing. To perform these tasks, the tray must be changed by a carer. The controller automatically detects the new task to be done. The HANDY-1 is a low-cost system that emphasis simplicity in all aspects. This is shown by quite limited performance in payload, reach and flexibility in operation. On the other hand, it has shown successful in a number of installations for the specific tasks described above.

3.3 Workstation: Raid

RAID is a workstation, developed in the TIDE telematics programme, which aims to assist disabled persons in office environments. It is based on an RTX workstation mounted on a track for increasing its workspace. Typical uses include the manipulation of books, paper documents, computer media, drinks, telephones, audio equipment and similar items. For accomplishing these tasks, dedicated grippers are developed, which can be mounted on the robot arm. The arm is controlled by means of a Microsoft Windows based user interface program.

3.4 Workstation: ProVar

A similar environment exists in Stanford (CA), where a Puma 260 robot arm is used for assisting disabled persons in a vocational environment. A special user-interface is designed for training and remote diagnostics purposes. Using this web-based interface, potential users can control the workstation in a virtual 3D-world. If they see that in this environment the task is carried out properly, they can activate the identical task using the real robot. A picture of the 3D interface is shown in Figure 9.

Two virtual characters are introduced: Pinocchio and Jiminey. Pinocchio serves as the assistant of the therapist or the end-user, whilst Jiminey is responsible for carrying out the designed motions. Currently this robotic system is under development at the Rehabilitation R&D Center, VA Palo Alto Health Care Systems. It is not clear when this manipulator will be commercially available.

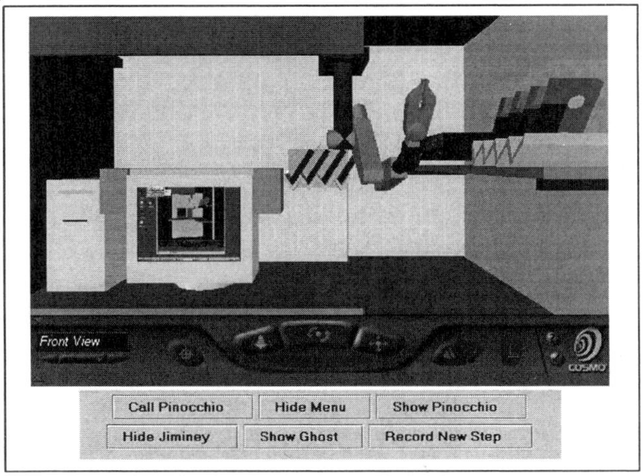

Figure 9. The 3D ProVar user interface

3.5 Wheelchair Mounted Manipulators: MANUS and Asimov

At the time of writing of this book, MANUS was the only commercially available wheelchair mounted manipulator. It is in use by over 150 end-users. It consists of a total of 8 degrees of freedom, including the opening and closing of the gripper, and the lift of the entire manipulator by means of an external motor. Figure 10 shows an image of the manipulator.

The manipulator can be controlled by means of a special input device, such as a joystick, a keyboard or a tongue-switch. Depending on the capabilities of the user, the input-devices can be tuned. In this way, with a minimum of physical and cognitive load, the user has the ability to control the manipulator.

The arm of Manus is rather slim. This is achieved by placing all electronics in the main shaft. No electronics exist in the arm itself. Disadvantage of this mechatronic architecture is that the friction and backlash of the arm is quite high. This reduces the absolute positioning accuracy strongly. However, since the robot is mostly used as a tele-operation device, this lack of accuracy is not very harmful: if a user sees that the manipulator is positioned too much to the right, he or she can displace the gripper towards the required position. Autonomous (pre-programmed) tasks are less straightforward to accomplish, due to this limited accuracy.

Asimov also is a wheelchair-mounted manipulator. The Asimov concept is based on a modular approach originally developed for electrical wheelchairs. The basic features are based on a lightweight arm with a distributed controller and drive system throughout the arm. By adopting this principle, the arm design allows adaptation to user needs as there are no transmissions between the links. The structure is made of carbon reinforced polymer material and aluminium alloys to reduce weight. At this stage, the robot is a design product and has only been tested under laboratory conditions.

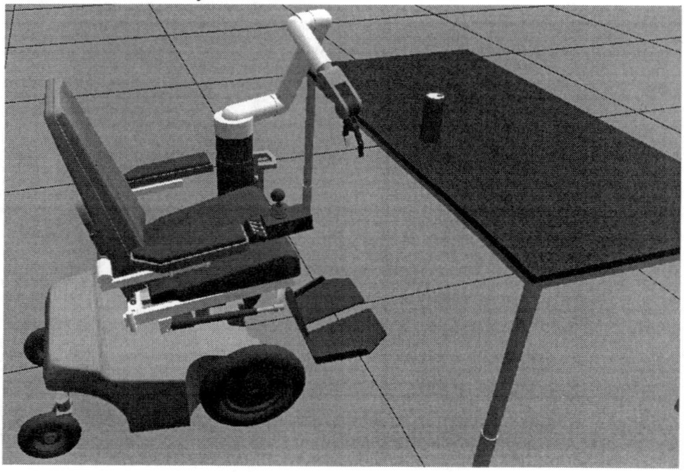

Figure 10. The MANUS attached to a wheelchair

3.6 Mobile Manipulators: MOVAID

The MOVAID mobile robot is composed of a four-wheel mobile base and a robotic arm. Mounted on the first link of the arm is a pan-tilt head supporting two television cameras, and a laser localisation system which is composed of two parts: an on-board rotating part which transmits a laser light, and an omnidirectional infrared receiver. Active beacons are positioned in the room and they receive the laser light and answer back its identification code. These messages are processed in order to reconstruct the position and orientation of the robot.

The end effector used is the three-fingered, two-degree of freedom, MARCUS hand equipped with tactile sensors. It was designed as a prosthetic device and it possesses great gripping capability in terms of set of graspable objects, size and grip force.

Ultrasound sensors are used for obstacle detection. An active bumper around the vehicle halts the system in case of collisions. The vehicle used as a mobile platform for the MOVAID system is the Electric Pedestrian (by INSERM – Unite 103, Montpellier, France). The arm used, is the 8 degree-of-freedom DEXTER arm, which was purposely designed to be part of a robotic mobile system for service applications in hospital and domestic environments.

The MOVAID prototype was installed in a residential site for disabled people in Italy, where it was tested and evaluated by a sample of end-users for an overall period of six months. As a general result, the system was enthusiastically accepted especially by severely motor disabled users and by those with poor or no functionality of upper limbs. Based on the lessons learnt from the MOVAID project, current developments are focussing on the concepts of modularity and integration into a smart home environment.

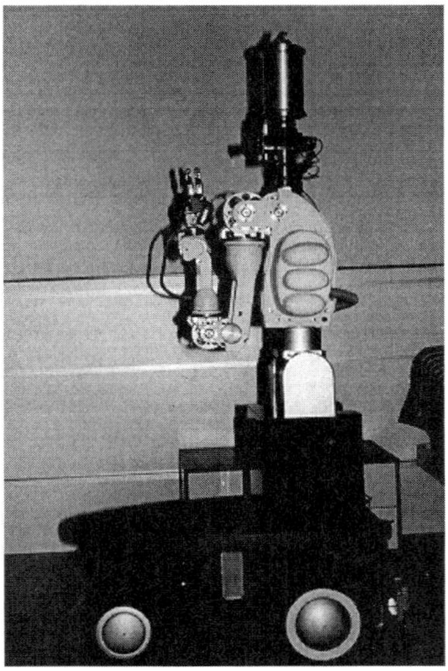

Figure 11. MOVAID

4. Conclusion

This chapter has outlined the state-of-the-art of manipulators and grippers. The main components and characteristics of manipulators have been described and evaluated with respect to their applicability and relevance for mobile health care robots. Links and revolute and prismatic joints have been introduced as the building blocks of manipulators. Different types of drives and sensors have been presented. The programming of robots and manipulators has been explained with the characteristics of on line and off line programming and the presentation of robot oriented and task oriented languages and their basic features.

The theory of grippers has been based on the description of the grasping process and the explanation of grasping constraints. The form and force closure grip have been introduced and principles of parallel jaw and multifingered grippers have been analysed. The major issues in gripper control and different types of sensors used have been outlined. The specific requirements of grippers in health care have been compared with those in industrial applications. Various examples of existing grippers have been presented.

The state-of-the-art of existing manipulators has been presented by distinguishing three different concepts: workstations, wheelchair mounted manipulators, and mobile manipulators. For each category the specific characteristics have been discussed. Different examples for each category have been presented.

5. References

[1] Baartman, J.P., Automation of Assembly operations on Parts: Dissertation Delft 1995

[2] Bolmsjö G., Topping M., Heck H. (et al), RAIL – Project status and Technical Developments. In: G. Anogianakis et al (Eds.): Advancement of Assistant Technology. IOS Press 1997, pp. 24 – 28.

[3] Borenstein J. and Koren Y., Motion Control Analysis of a Mobile Robot, *Transactions of ASME, Journal of Dynamics, Measurement and Control*, Vol. 109, No. 2, 1987, pp. 73-79.

[4] Craig J.J., *Introduction to Robotics: Mechanic and control,* Addison-Wesley. 1988

[5] Engelberger J. F., *Robotics in practice: management and applications of industrial robots,* AMACOM, Division of the American Management Association, Inc. 1980. New-York.

[6] Fischer T. and Seyfried J., The new Karlsruhe Dextrous Hand II., *International Symposium on Intelligent Robotic Systems*, Stockholm, 1997.

[7] Fischer T., Sensor Sytem for Controlling a Multifingered Gripper on a Robot Arm, *International Conference on Intelligent Robots and Systems* 1998.

[8] Fu K. S., *Robotics: control, sensing, vision and intelligence,* McGraw-Hill. 1987

[9] Klafter R.D., Chmielewski T. A., Negin M., *Robotic Engineering: an integrated approach,* Prentice-Hall. 1989.

[10] Kollmann J., Lankenau A., Bühlmeier A. (et al), Navigation of a Kinematically Restricted Wheelchair by the Parti-Game Algorithm, *Proceedings of the AISB Workshop on Spatial Reasoning in Mobile Robots and Animals*, Manchester 1997, Technical Report Series UMCS-97-4-1, Department of Computer Science, Manchester University, 1997

[11] Lucas S.R., Robot Hand-Arm Co-operated Motion Planning. *PhD thesis*, The University of Melbourne, Department of Mechanical and Manufacturing Engineering, 1997.

[12] Magnussen B. and Doersam T., The Karlsruhe Dextrous Hand, a Three Fingered Robot Gripper, *Proceedings of the European Control Conference (ECC)*, Rome, 1995

[13] Pollard N.S., The Grasping Problem: Toward Task-Level Programming for an Articulated Hand. Technical Report 1214, MIT Artificial Intelligence Laboratory, 1989.
[14] Rembold D., Fischer T., Müller M. and Wörn H., A flexible manipulation system for handling a large variety of objects. IEEE, *EAMRI Rensselaer's International Conference on Agile, Intelligent, and Computer-Integrated Manufacturing (CAICIM)*, Troy, New York (USA), October 7-9, 1998, published on CD-ROM.
[15] Somov P., Über Schraubengeschwindigkeiten eines festen Körpers bei verschiedener Zahl von Stützflächen. Zeitschrift für Mathematik und Physik, Vol.42, 1897.

Chapter 11

Manipulator Control Architectures

by Bart DRIESSEN, William HARWIN, Gunnar BOLMSJÖ, Frithjof WEBER

Mobile Robotics in Healthcare
N. Katevas (Ed.)
IOS Press, 2001

Chapter 11

Manipulator Control Architectures

Bart DRIESSEN, William HARWIN, Gunnar BOLMSJÖ, Frithjof WEBER

1. Introduction

Since rehabilitation robots have to operate in the direct neighbourhood of humans, high demands are put on the control performance of the manipulator. The controller must move the manipulator to a destination (not too slow, and not too fast), guaranteeing safe behaviour. The manipulator must be able to operate autonomously for carrying out pre-defined tasks. Think for example at fetching books from a known location, or opening a tap. For fetching objects in a structured environment, this autonomous behaviour is sufficient. However, service robots often work in unstructured, or at most partially structured environments. This means either an end-user, or an intelligent high-level controller (which uses sensors for gaining information about the unstructured environment), will directly control the robot.

In most manipulator control architectures at least three layers can be identified:

- *Low level controllers:* They consist of a set of position controllers, force controllers or impedance controllers. These controllers require high sampling rates (typically 2 ms or faster). Input of low level controllers is a required position, or a required force. Based on measurements (joint positions, exerted force), the drives of the manipulator are controlled in such a way that the control objective (visiting a certain position, exerting a certain force) will be reached. Controllers at this level do not have any knowledge about the objectives of the end-user. The robot acts primarily as a master slave system.
- *Task controllers:* responsible for carrying out a task, issued by the end-user. Real-time requirements are less strict at this layer. Tasks are split in subtasks until the subtasks reach a primitive level, which are understood by the low-level controller. For example the task to pick up a glass can be split in the following subtasks: 1) Go To position above glass. 2) Open gripper. 3) Go Down. 4) Close gripper. 5) Go Up.

All these subtasks can be directly translated into robot commands, which are understood by the low-level controllers.

- *User interface:* minimises the cognitive load issued on the user when asking services from the task level controllers. Therefore, it has to communicate with the end-user and with the task-controller. Especially when the robot is being used as a tele-manipulator, high constraints are put on the design of the user interface.

This chapter gives an overview on widely used robotic controllers. The main emphasise is put on low level controllers and on impedance controllers (a control algorithm which is partially implemented in the low-level controller and partially in the user interface).

2. Manipulator Control Strategies.

The aim of this chapter is to give an overview of these strategies, and to discuss the positive and negative aspects of these controllers. Four control strategies are described:

- Joint control
- Cartesian position control
- Force control
- Impedance control

It is out of the scope of this book to go into the details of manipulator controllers. The interested reader may refer to [2], [6] and [9] for details about low level robot controllers.

2.1 Joint Control

The simplest form of manipulation control is achieved with joint based position control. The motors of the manipulator are considered independent axes, and each joint axis has its own controller often of type PID (see figure 1).

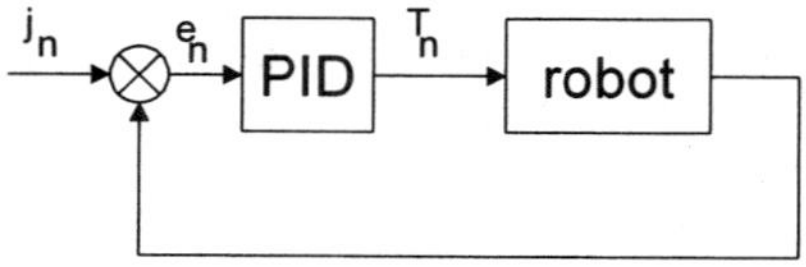

Figure 1. Joint based position control

The PID algorithm is given by the following equation:

$$T_n = k_p \cdot e + k_d \cdot \dot{e} + k_i \cdot \int e dt$$

Several alternatives for the implementation of the PID controller exist (e.g. anti-windup, low pass d-action filtering), but the essence of above listed formula always exists.

Although many manipulators use multi-axis PID joint control, some disadvantages of this control architecture exist. The robot is a highly non-linear system. Therefore, if the PID controller is optimally tuned in one operating point, it might be unstable in other operational points. Gain scheduling algorithms can be used for improving the performance, but this solution is far from elegant.

A more sophisticated model-based joint control scheme, which decouples the non-linear dynamics from the linear dynamics, can eliminate this problem. Suppose the dynamics of the robot are described by the following equation:

$$\tau = M(\Theta)\ddot{\Theta} + V(\Theta,\dot{\Theta}) + G(\Theta) + F(\Theta,\dot{\Theta}),$$

where

τ is the nx1 vector of joint torques,

$M(\Theta)$ is the mass matrix of the robot,

$V(\Theta,\dot{\Theta})$ is the nx1 vector of centrifugal and Coriolis terms,

$G(\Theta)$ is the nx1 vector of gravity terms, and

$F(\Theta,\dot{\Theta})$ is the nx1 vector of friction terms. Then the model based control scheme can be used as shown in figure 2 where,

$$\hat{B}(\Theta,\dot{\Theta}) = \hat{V}(\Theta,\dot{\Theta}) + \hat{G}(\Theta) + \hat{F}(\Theta,\dot{\Theta})$$

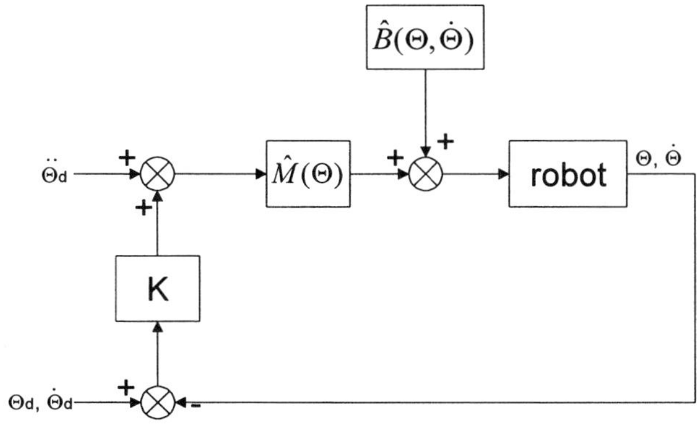

Figure 2. Model based control architecture (computed torque method)

The error equation of this controller is:

$$\ddot{\varepsilon} + K_v\dot{\varepsilon} + K_p\varepsilon = 0$$

It can be seen that this equation does not depend on the parameters of the dynamics of the robot. Unfortunately this situation will be impossible to accomplish, since the compensating models ($\hat{F},\hat{G},\hat{V},\hat{M}$) will always differ from reality, causing model-mismatch depending terms in the error equation. The above listed joint based control schema is also known as the *computed torque method.*

2.2 Cartesian Control

Joint control architectures are rather straightforward to implement, and (since no co-ordinate transformations exist), do not have to cope with singular points. However, if an end-user controls the manipulator only using joint control, it will be impossible to carry out even the simplest tasks, such us picking up a piece of paper, or displacing a (full) cup of coffee. For this kind of tasks, we need Cartesian controllers, which drive the position and orientation of the tool centre point of the manipulator. The position is defined in X, Y, and Z co-ordinates with respect to a certain reference frame. The orientation can be defined in many ways, for example using yaw, pitch and roll co-ordinates, or using Euler angles. In this chapter we define the orientation by three values: α, β, and γ, not considering whether these values are yaw, pitch roll co-ordinates or Euler angles.

A straightforward idea for implementing a Cartesian controller is shown below.

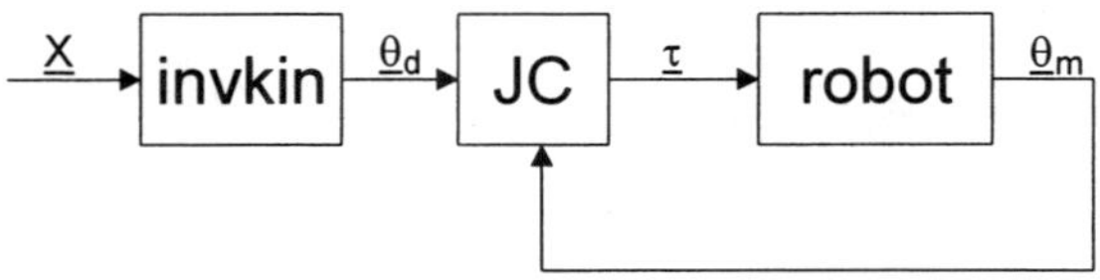

Figure 3. Joint based Cartesian control

Where, JC is the joint controller, $\underline{\mathbf{X}}$ is an 6x1 vector of Cartesian positions, $\underline{\theta}_{\mathbf{d}}$ is a vector of joint setpoints (position, velocity and acceleration), $\underline{\tau}$ is an vector of joint torques, and $\underline{\theta}_{\mathbf{m}}$ is a vector of measured joint positions. **INVKIN** represent the inverse kinematics, which transform Cartesian co-ordinates towards joint co-ordinates.

Problems can arise in the neighbourhood of singular points. At singular points, small displacements in Cartesian co-ordinates result in very large displacements of joint angles. Carrying out motions in Cartesian space at constant velocity will then result in extreme joint speeds, causing any joint controller to saturate. This might cause dangerous behaviour of the robot, since large deviations of the required path will occur. A solution to deal with this problem is to scale down the Cartesian velocity in the neighbourhood of singular point. Another possibility is to invoke a path planner, which simply avoids the singular points. However, this is not always possible, especially when an end-user controls the robot directly as a master slave system (note that in this situation, the robot should follow the instructions of the end-user, who can steer the robot close to or in singular points if he/she wants this).

Alternative Cartesian control schemes exist, such as the transpose Jacobian control scheme or the inverse Jacobian control scheme. The control law for the first controller is:

$$\tau = J^T(\Theta) \cdot K(X_d - X_m),$$

where K is a vector of gains, X_d is a vector of required Cartesian positions, and X_m is a vector of measured (or calculated using the forward kinematics) Cartesian positions. $J^T(\theta)$ is the transpose of the Jacobian (note that for a manipulator $\tau = J^T(\theta)\, F$).

A second well known control scheme is the inverse Jacobian controller, defined by the following control law:

$$\tau = K \cdot J^{-1}(\Theta) \cdot (X_d - X_m)$$

where K is a vector of gains, X_d is a vector of required Cartesian positions, and X_m is a vector of measured (or calculated using the forward kinematics) Cartesian positions. $J^{-1}(\theta)$ is the inverse of the Jacobian (note that for a manipulator $\dot{\Theta} = J^{-1}(\Theta) \cdot \dot{X}$).

Although the inverse/transpose Jacobian controller are intuitively correct, problems arise due to the very non-linear behaviour of the manipulator. Especially in the neighbourhood of singular point, the loop gain of these controllers increases dramatically, resulting in unstable systems. Because of this reason, these control schemes are hardly ever used in practice.

For coping with this problem, a linearising controller can be used, which follows the same approach as the joint based computed torque controller, described above (see figure 4), where

$$\hat{B}_x(\Theta,\dot{\Theta}) = \hat{V}_x(\Theta,\dot{\Theta}) + \hat{G}_x(\Theta) + \hat{F}_x(\Theta,\dot{\Theta})$$

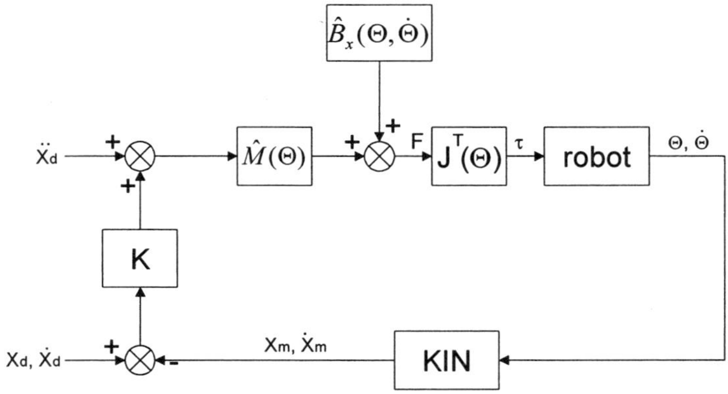

Figure 4. Model based Cartesian controller

In figure 4 the *KIN* block consists of the forward kinematics, for transforming joint angles to Cartesian positions, and the Jacobian, for transforming the joint speed to Cartesian speed. Note again that the performance of above described controller strongly depends on the quality of the robot models used by this controller.

2.3 Force Control

If the manipulator is in contact with its environment, strict position control does not perform anymore. For example, if an end-user wants to move the robot over the surface of a table, but the supplied position setpoint is just below the table, the position controller will try to go through the table in order to reach its required position. If the position controller has some kind of integrating action, the robot will build up maximum forces, which might cause damage.

Force control can be seen as the complement of position control. The robot receives a force setpoint, and the force servo loops make sure that the required force is indeed exerted.

An implementation of a force control servo is shown in the figure below.

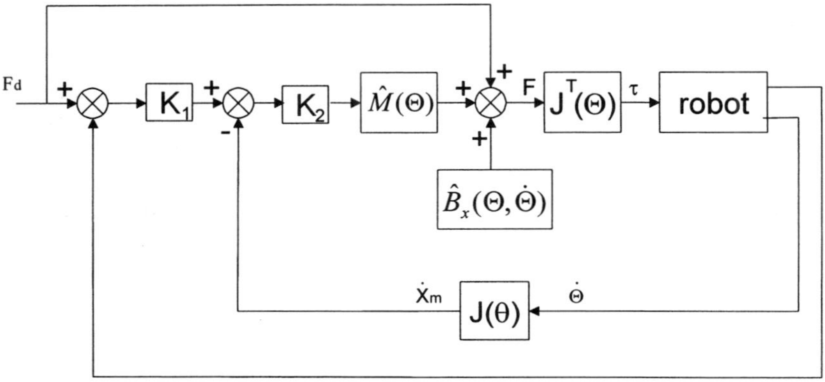

Figure 5. Force control servo

The controller consists of a feedforward link, combined with a feedback loop. If the dynamics of the manipulator are completely known, the feed forward link will produce exactly the required force. However, in practice this situation will never occur, and hence, deviations from the required force exits.

The feedback loop reduces these deviations by feeding the force error to a speed control loop (adding the force error *directly* to the feedforward force often results in unstable controllers). Implementing the feedback loop in this way will cause the interaction force between robot and environment to behave like a spring. The derivation of this control law for a one-dimensional case can be found in [2].

As position controller will degenerate in contact situations, force controllers will degenerate in free moving situations. A compromise is found in hybrid position-force controllers, which control some directions using position control, whilst controlling other directions using force control. Although some nice results are achieved in operating in structured environments with hybrid position-force controllers, in unstructured environments they will not work. The reason for this is that in unstructured environments it is not known which directions should be position controlled, and which directions should be force controlled. In rehabilitation robotics, most applications take place in unstructured environments. A very nice approach for operating in unstructured environments is found in impedance control, described in next section.

2.4 Impedance Control

Hogan proposed the concept of impedance control [6]. He defines interaction ports, as places where objects can exchange energy with each other, e.g. where a robot touches an object. He states that if two objects interact with each other, one object must have impedance causality whilst the other must have admittance causality (Figure 6).

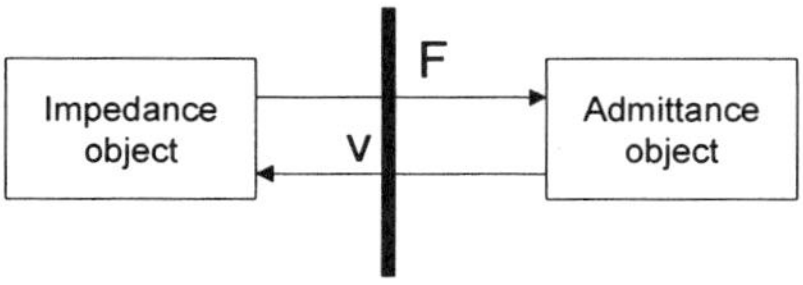

Figure 6. Interacting objects

Impedance objects (e.g. springs) supply *forces* at the interaction port, whilst admittance objects (e.g. masses) supply *velocities* at the interaction port. Most real-life objects have admittance causality, and therefore in order to manipulate objects with a robot, this robot must have impedance causality. This is true for manipulating small masses, however in contact situations with for example tables, the table acts as an impedance, and the robot should act as an admittance. In practice it is not so easy to distinguish impedances and admittances. Therefore it is better to focus on controlling the *interaction* between objects, or in other words, the *relation* between forces and velocities. A simple example is shown in figure 7.

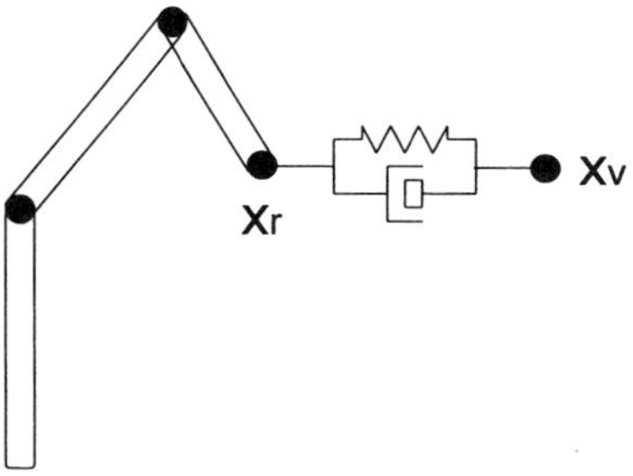

Figure 7. Simple impedance controller

By moving the virtual position X_v, the (virtual) impedance will exert a force on the robot of:

$$F = K(X_r - X_v) + B(\dot{X}_r - \dot{X}_v)$$

The robot will follow the virtual position until an object blocks the robot. The virtual position continues moving and the spring will be stretched, applying higher forces to the robot. A supervisor algorithm must detect this situation, and stop the virtual position from moving. In this way a robot can follow motion, whilst having compliance in forces exerted by the environment. Optionally a force torque sensor can be used for explicitely measuring external forces exerted on the manipulator. More about impedance control will be shown in next paragraph.

3. Control in the Human Machine Interface

Throughout this period there has always been a dual approach to the user interface. Research has either favoured a telemanipulator philosophy or a commanded robot philosophy. The telemanipulator approach has the real attraction of being easy to implement, not necessarily requiring a computer to achieve success, and being easy for the user to understand. It has also inherited a history from the field of upper limb prosthetics where both the myoelectric interface and the Bowden cable interface represent basic telemanipulator-like operation. The disadvantage is that it is a slow interface and can be difficult for the user to use efficiently since there is little way for the person to predict the consequence of individual inputs.

The concept of a commanded robot has always had attractions for potential robot users irrespective of the persons' disability. The ability to command a 'slave' robot to "fetch me a drink" is attractive but is extremely difficult to implement in a way that is likely to achieve success in any but the most highly structured environment. The two most successful commercial rehabilitation robots individually represent these two approaches. The MANUS wheelchair robot is a telemanipulator, whereas the HANDY 1, with interchangeable trays for specific daily activities, is a commanded robot.

There have often been calls for these two approaches to be combined but this has not happened to any significant degree. There have also been calls for rehabilitation robots, and robots in general, to become more tolerant of environmental variations. When a person uses a MANUS robot to lift a glass, in the moments before the glass is actually lifted and the user can get visual confirmation, there is no way to determine if indeed the robot is lifting the glass, rather than attempting to slide it along the surface or push it into the table top. In the same way if the HANDY 1 robot encounters some food that is a little more glutinous than usual, it runs the risk of losing its positional calibration and, as it cycles through the program, it runs the risk of delivering the food just a few tempting centimetres short of the person's mouth, or stalling on the person's teeth.

Thus a robot that can continue to function in the face of environmental changes will have better reliability for the person using it, if this force information can be accommodated at the several layers in the command structure. The interaction between the low level control architecture and the interface layers are now discussed.

Controlling contact force in the user interface

To be successful a robot user must be able to command or co-ordinate multiple degrees of freedom, must get the robot to interact with a stiff environment so that neither the environment nor the robot is damaged, and must interact safely with the robot. This requires not only a complex interface between the human and the machine, but good low-level force control. Currently all commercial rehabilitation robots are based on position control at the joint level and this is a testament to the ingenuity of the users and designers in arranging tasks to tolerate inconsistent or erroneous commands. Only in recent years there has been an impetus to design the required low level control of a robot so that the forces applied to the robot can be factored into the interfaces.

As the human interface is being improved and better control techniques can be employed there is a potential for an assistive robot that has a direct interaction with the person, for example by supporting the individual's arm and attempting to use all possible residual abilities of the person. This approach is evident in rehabilitation devices such as the TIDE funded MULOS project [7], and the ASEL powered orthosis project [4].

Thus we can see that robots are making direct contact with the user and it is now important that the control of contact force is integrated into the human-robot interface. Knowledge of contact force can not only increase the reliability of the combined human-machine system but can also allow additional safeguards to be considered.

Control of contact forces is thus important if a rehabilitation robot is to work effectively in an unstructured environment. Early work on the Spartacus robot by the AEA in France attempted force control in a limited way but only recently has there been a resurgence of interest.

Having the ability to control contact force can not only allow better toleration of discrepancies in the environment but can also be programmed to be an integral part of the user interface. Demonstrations of force control in the user interface have been achieved on both telemanipulator and commanded control modes. RoboGlyph demonstrated a rehabilitation robot language that included commands to move in an environment until the robot touched something allowing objects to be found by feel [3]. Likewise work on a head controlled telerobot demonstrated that force control could be used to enhance a persons ability to interact with a physical environment [8].

Effective force control must occur at a multitude of levels and figure 8 shows how information on the state of the environment, both position and force, should be made available to the user and the intermediate layers. At each layer between the person and the environment it might be possible to reduce the overall cognitive load for the user by processing some information locally at that layer.

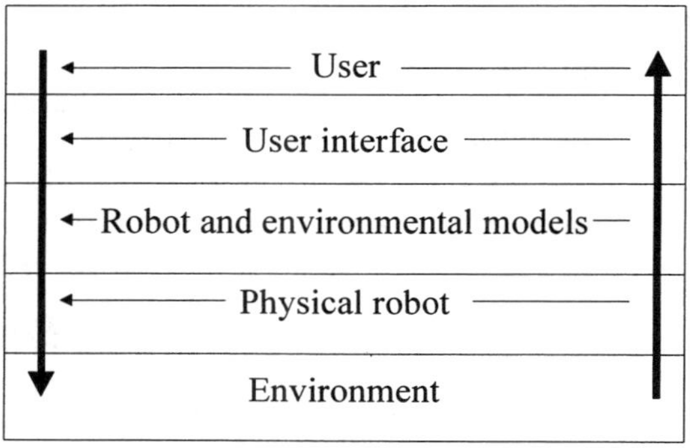

Figure 8. Cybernetics of the user interface

Techniques for impedance control

A new generation of robots is emerging where the control of contact force is an integrated part of the design. The most promising of these concepts seeks to control the mechanical impedance of the robot or mechanism so that it can comply to variations in the environment or varying forces applied by the user.

There are two common approaches. The first is to use a combination of torque/force sensors in the joints or the end effector, and use this information within the controller. The second is to minimise friction in the drive components and predict the forces transmitted by the actuators through the robot structure from measurements of position. The latter approach can use very simple control architectures such as detuning a PD controller.

Figure 9 shows how a simple controller can be detuned to allow a low friction servomechanism to have a programmable compliance.

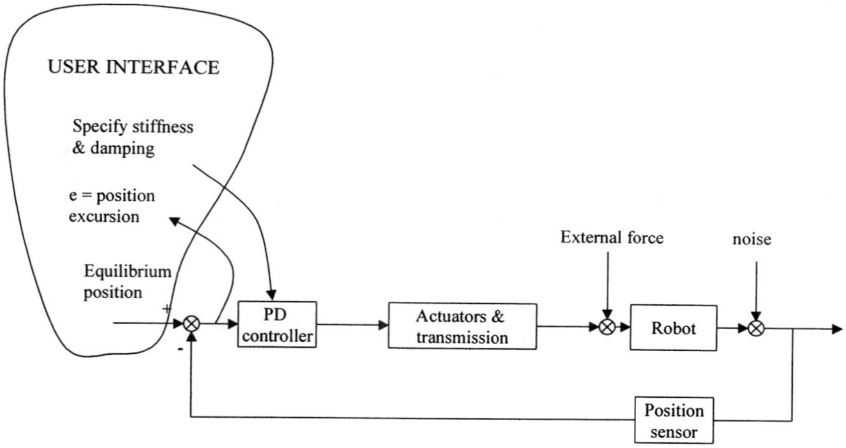

Figure 9. PD based stiffness control based on position measurements

It is important when changing the controller parameters (done within the control loop) to maintain the system stability. But if done successfully a force estimate is available from the servo-mechanism error signal ε. This can either be made by using the programmed stiffness and damping coefficients to predict the force, i.e., or by generating an inverse model of the robot. An enhancement of this concept is to use a model based control architecture as shown in figure 10.

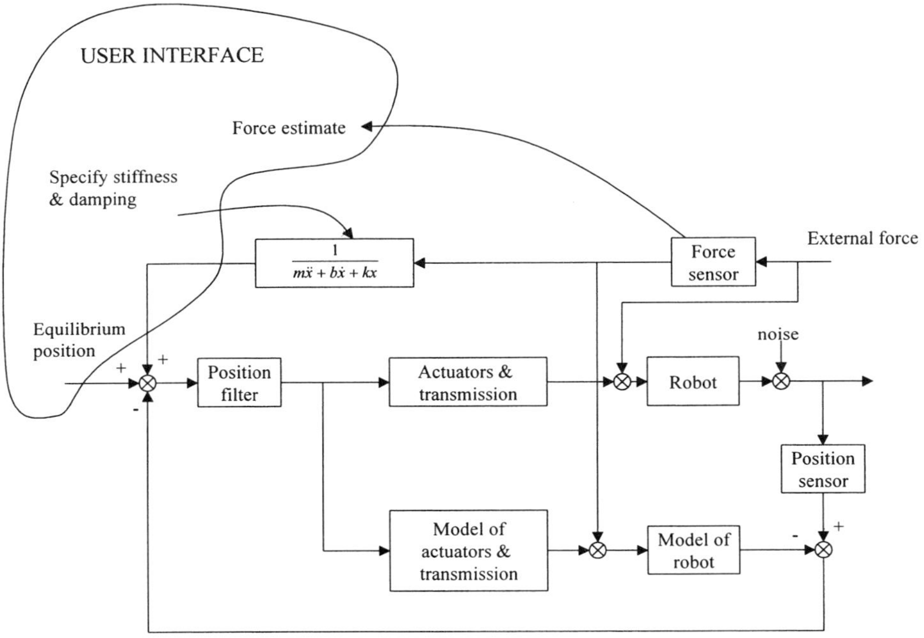

Figure 10. Model based controller

If the model is accurate then no feedback is needed, however, to be useful the robot needs to encounter external forces and this event accounts for unmodelled parameters in the model. The solution is thus to measure this force and introduce it into the controller as shown in figure 10. The inclusion of a force sensor now adds to the complexity and inertia of the robot but has the benefit of making the mechanical design easier since it no longer requires a frictionless transmission. The force sensor also allows force estimates to be used in the user interface thus allowing either a scaled version of the force to be provided directly to the user, or it allows the robot program to identify contact with the environment and take an appropriate action.

Once a decision to use force sensing in the control loop has been made then other configurations are possible. Since impedance control methods are undoubtedly the most useful both from an engineering and from a user interface perspective, two possible impedance configurations are now presented. The first, shown in figure 11, is that of Maples and Becker [4] and maintains stability of an inner force control loop. The outer loop generates a position error signal and this is used to determine the desired force based on a set of stiffness parameters passed to the controller. The second, that of Field and Stepanenko [3], is shown in figure 12 and uses a more complete model of the desired robot mechanical impedance. This claims to offer settings for the apparent mass, stiffness and damping of the robot. Unlike the Maples and Becker approach the Field and Stepanenko controller attempts to get the inner controller to follow a position generated by the filter in response to the programmed impedance and the applied force.

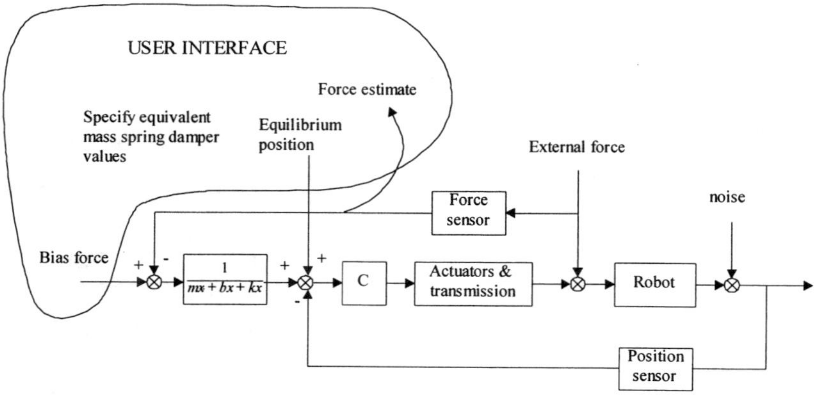

Figure 11. Maples and Becker based controller

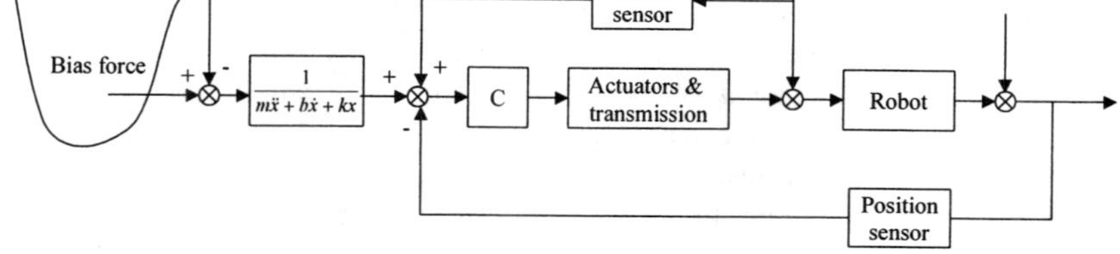

Figure 12. Field and Stepanenko based controller

There is little to choose between these approaches, but the two important points are that control of force is achieved by specifying a target mechanical impedance, and that force and position information is made available to higher layers in the interface.

Discussion

As new commercial rehabilitation robots emerge most will use some form of feedback control. The control architectures described above are only some of those possible for impedance control. But as the robot is incorporated into useful functions such as those demonstrated by the HANDY 1 and the MANUS, the researcher, the engineer and the user can all make use of information that is available in the control loop. To promote expansion and innovation in what is, and is likely to remain, a relatively small field in robotics it is vital that these control loop variables be made available to the higher levels of command and control, up to and including the user.

Several design considerations for new generations of rehabilitation robot now emerge. If both force and position sensing are to be used in the design then some flexibility is afforded in both the mechanical design and the controller design at the expense of overall inertia and cost. If only position sensing is to be used, then the ideal is to minimise friction in the transmission. If this is done and with knowledge of the servo error variable then the higher levels of control and command can make an estimate of the applied force through an inverse model of the robot or an estimate of the controller. It is interesting to note that haptic interfaces used to convey substance in virtual reality applications are essentially robotic devices and most rely on low friction drive mechanisms and position controllers to control force and hence impedance.

Irrespective of the particular solution it is desirable to keep the inertia of moving parts to a minimum. This can be seen from the simple energy equations where, if a robot moving at a velocity ω is suddenly stopped either by the environment or by contact with the user, the energy that needs to be rechanneled or dissipated is of the form $J\omega^2$. Minimising inertia allows higher velocities to be achieved safely and enhances the bandwidth of information flow between the environment, robot and user.

Other considerations are that the actuators need to dissipate heat, in particular when forces are being applied to the robot. Finally we can reiterate the opinion that there is much information in the inner controller that can be used at higher levels as part of the user interface. This information needs to be made available, since in many cases researchers in the field do not immediately have access to the engineers and designers responsible for the original design.

4. References

[1] Chen S., Rahman T., Foulds R., Heredia E., and Harwin W. "A Virtual Headstick for People with Spinal Cord Injuries". *Robotica* 16(5) pp 499-507 (September 1998).

[2] Craig, John J., *Introduction to Robotics: Mechanics and Control.* Addison Wesley Publishing Company, Inc. ISBN 0-201-09528-9. 1989. Second edition.

[3] Field G., and Stepanenko Y., "A new model reference impedance controller for telerobotics", *SPIE 1833 telemanipulator technology*, pp 69-79 (1992).

[4] Harwin W.S., and Rahman T., "Analysis of force-reflecting telerobotic systems for rehabilitation applications" *Proceedings of the 1st European Conference on Disability Virtual Reality and Associated Technologies* pp 171-178 ISBN 07049 1140X (1996).

[5] Harwin W.S., Gosine R.G., Kazi Z., Lees D.S. and Dallaway J.L., "A comparison of rehabilitation robotics languages and software" *Robotica* 15(2) pp 133-151 (1997).

[6] Hogan N., "Impedance Control An Approach to Manipulations: Theory, Implementation, Application, (in three parts)", *Journal of Dynamic systems, Measurement,, and Control.* ASME, March 1985, Vol. 107.

[7] *ICORR97: Proceedings of the International Conference on Rehabilitation Robotics.* ISBN 1-85790-034- 0 (1997).

[8] Maples J.A., and Becker J.J., "Experiments in force control of robotic manipulators", *IEEE Conference*, pp 695-702 (1986).

[9] Richard P. Paul., *Robot Manipulators: Mathematics, Programming and Control.* The MIT Press series in artificial intelligence. ISBN 0-262-16082-X. Ninth printing, 1992.

Chapter 12

Case Studies on Mobile Manipulators

by Bart DRIESSEN, Gunnar BOLMSJÖ, Paolo DARIO

Mobile Robotics in Healthcare
N. Katevas (Ed.)
IOS Press, 2001

Chapter 12

Case Studies on Mobile Manipulators

Bart DRIESSEN, Gunnar BOLMSJÖ, Paolo DARIO

1. Introduction

This chapter presents three mobile manipulators: MANUS, ASIMOV, and MOVAID. Manus is a wheelchair mounted manipulator which is commercially available. At the time of writing of this book, Manus is in use by approximately 150 end-users. Section 2 describes basic aspects of the MANUS. ASIMOV targets the same application area, but is not commercially available yet. Section 3 describes details about ASIMOV and the design process of ASIMOV. The last manipulator described in this chapter is MOVAID. MOVAID aims to supply a mobile base mounted manipulator which can assist end-users semi-autonomously. Section 4 gives technical details about MOVAID. Also results from user trials are described here.

2. MANUS: a Wheelchair Mounted Manipulator

Manus is a wheelchair-mounted manipulator which is currently in use by over 150 disabled persons. It consists of a total of eight degrees of freedom: six for positioning and orienting the end-effector, one for opening and closing the gripper, and one for lifting the entire manipulator. Figure 1 shows a Manus manipulator attached to a wheelchair.

The end-users are severely disabled persons, suffering from muscular dystrophy or cerebral palsy. They can control the manipulator by means of a special input device, such as a joystick, a keyboard or a tongue-switch. Depending on the capabilities of the user, the input devices can be tuned. In this way, with a minimum of physical and cognitive load, the user has the ability to control the manipulator.

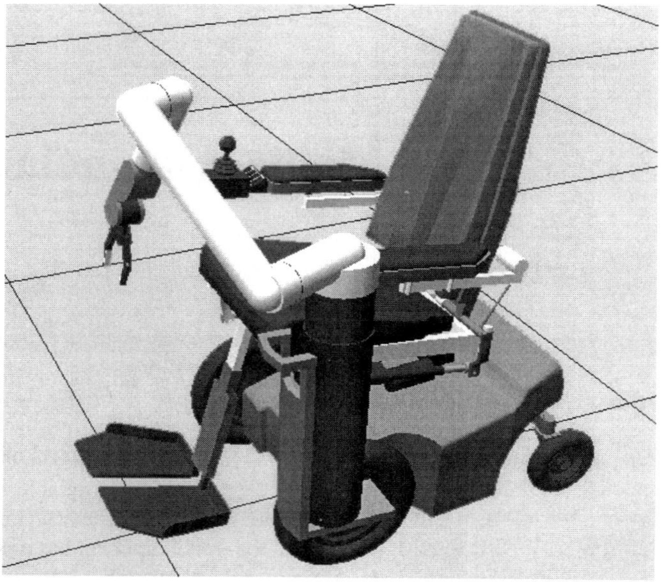

Figure 1. MANUS attached to a wheelchair

This section describes the structure of the Manus manipulator. First of all, the mechatronic structure will be described. Subsequently, the control architecture is shown, and finally the human machine interface structure is explained. At the end of the section, a short discussion about possible improvements is given.

2.1 Mechatronic Structure

Before the development of MANUS, the following requirements were defined:

- MANUS should be slim, so that it can still pass doors when MANUS is connected to the wheelchair
- MANUS should be light weighted, minimising the disturbance on the driving behaviour of the wheelchair
- MANUS should be easy to control with simple input devices such as joysticks, or keypads
- MANUS should be mechanically integrated with the wheelchair
- The control of MANUS by the end-user should be integrated with at least the control of the wheelchair
- MANUS should consume as little power as possible

These requirements resulted in the manipulator that is shown in figure 2. As shown in the figure, the manipulator has 8 degrees of freedom (including gripper and external high/low function). In figure 3, a schematic overview of Manus is shown.

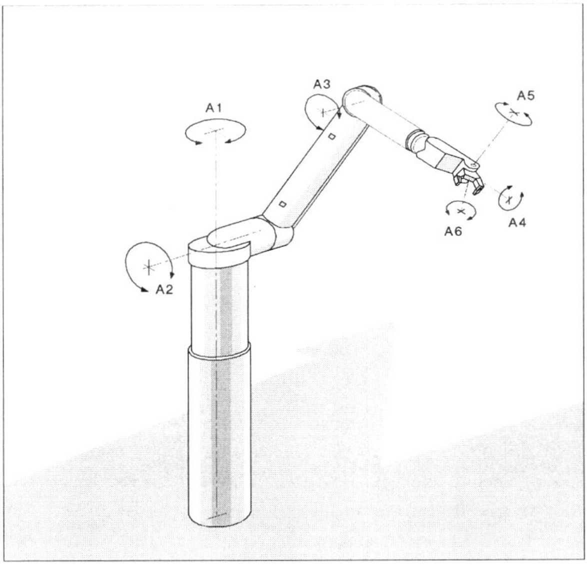

Figure 2. Degrees of freedom of the MANUS manipulator

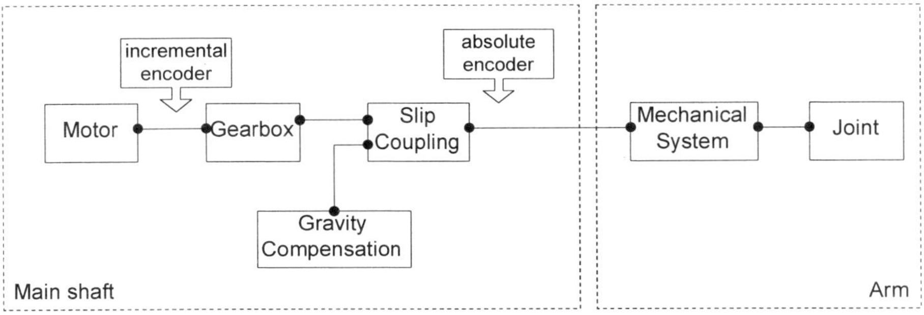

Figure 3. Schematic overview of Manus manipulator

The motors, gearboxes and encoders are placed in the main shaft. The joints are driven by means of a mechanical system of toothed belts, hollow axes, and toothed wheels. Although this set-up reduces the size of the arm significantly, the drawback is that very much friction and backlash exists in the manipulator. In fact, approximately 25% of the motor-power is used to overcome friction. The backlash of the joints is several degrees. Two passive springs compensate for the gravity of the shoulder joint and the elbow joint. These springs are placed at the slow-axis of the gearboxes. Because of the springs, the energy MANUS consumes is strongly reduced (note that MANUS extracts its energy from the same battery as the wheelchair and a respiration device). Slip couplings are placed at the slow side of the gearboxes. In this way it is always possible that someone tears away the MANUS from the end-user in case of unexpected phenomena.

MANUS is equipped with a two-fingered gripper. The gripper is opened and closed via a passive spring. When the end-user closes the gripper, he/she pulls the spring. If the gripper touches an object, the user can continue closing the gripper, resulting in an extension of the spring, increasing the gripper force. No extra user-feedback is given for the gripping force. The fingers of the gripper itself are equipped with a passive canting system which assures that objects are always manipulated using a three point grasp.

For controlling the position of the manipulator, incremental encoders are used. Absolute encoders are used during start-up for initialising the incremental encoders, and for slip detection. No extra force-torque sensors or tactile matrix sensors are currently used.

2.2 Control Architecture

MANUS communicates with the control computer via a CAN bus. For this, a 80592 processor is placed in the main shaft of the manipulator. The control computer is a PC104 system with a 80486 processor card and a dual CAN card. One CAN bus will be used for communication with the manipulator, the other CAN bus will be used for reading the input device (e.g. joystick). Figure 4 gives a schematic overview of the control architecture.

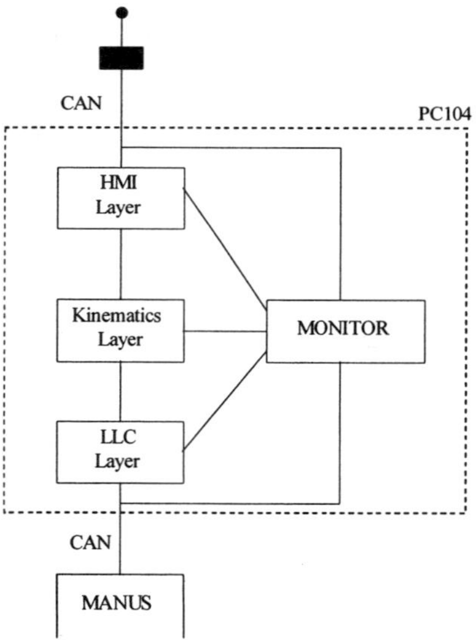

Figure 4. Control architecture

In the *low-level control layer* (LLC layer), the joint controllers are implemented. These joint controllers are implemented as PI controllers with extra feed-forward friction compensation, running at a sampling time of 10ms.

The *kinematics layer* receives high level robot commands (such as move forward, or goto point A), and calculates a path (= sequence of joint setpoints) to carry out the robot commands. The kinematics layer consist of three main elements:

- *the interpolator*, responsible for calculating smooth trajectories between two required positions. In case of direct control (i.e. controlling MANUS with a joystick/keypad in a certain direction), the interpolator makes sure the acceleration during start-up and deceleration during the end of a motion takes place via a smooth profile. Trajectories are calculated in the active user co-ordinates, which can be joint co-ordinates, cylindrical co-ordinates, or Cartesian co-ordinates.
- *the user kinematics*, responsible for transforming the user co-ordinates towards homogeneous transforms.
- *the inverse kinematics*, responsible for calculating the proper joint setpoints for the required homogeneous transform.

A monitoring module observes (and stores) the status of all control layers. A special diagnostics program (running on a separate computer), can communicate with the monitor (via the CAN bus), to detect whether MANUS needs to be revised, or, in case of malfunction, which parts needs to be sent to the manufacturer for repair.

2.3 Human Machine Interface

One of the most important issues in rehabilitation robotics is the design of a user interface (i.e. the program which translates user commands (issued by e.g. a joystick) towards high level robot commands (e.g. move forward, goto point A)). Special requirements for the user-interface exist:

- the interface must be configurable by a therapist,
- the HMI must also be configurable by the end-user,
- the cognitive load on the end-user must be reduced as much as possible,
- it must be possible to operate the manipulator with a wide range of input devices,
- the HMI must be integrated with existing devices, such as wheelchairs or remote control units.

Especially the third point is very important, but also very complicated to accomplish. One must keep in mind that end-users most times can hardly move their hands or fingers, and therefore it is far from straightforward to control a 6DOF manipulator.

For Manus, the HMI layer is set-up in a open, extendable manner. New input-devices can relatively easy be added to the Manus control system. A special configuration program enables therapists to parameterise the HMI for this new input device.

The only way to communicate with Manus is via a CAN bus. At the time of writing of this book, special interface cards were developed to interface with other devices (such as the wheelchair). Using these cards, it will be possible to control Manus using standard joysticks.

3. ASIMOV: a Highly Modular Manipulator for Healthcare Services

The ASIMOV robot is based on a concept that has the principle of modularity in focus. By adopting this principle in the design process, it is possible to arrive in system solutions with a very high flexibility in the general performance of tasks given an unstructured environment and changing or not very tight user requirements. The drawback is that a special design robot for a specific task, such as an industrial robot, in general is optimised for the requirements that are described in a well defined technical specification for a specific task. On the other hand, such robots have limitations outside the given specification and are not easy to adapt, since the robot can be seen as, more or less, one single integrated system. With the principle of modularity, however, customisation is one of the key parameters built into the system that allow for changes of modules and their specific characteristics, including the very basic mechanical configuration of the robot itself. The description in this section will concentrate on the basic principles, developments and characteristics of the Asimov robot, emphasising user and technology.

Robots with a high degree of autonomy is a challenge in robotics research to advance the technology within the health care area. The present status of robot systems, in general those within industrial automation, is that they are more or less used as programmable automatic machines with little functionality compared to the view or idea of robots as they are presented in most motion pictures with autonomous capabilities. However, although the progress in using advanced sensors and controllers is relatively slow, in the real world the basic technology available is advanced enough to create robotics systems that can be successfully used to increase autonomy and flexibility of the robot system. A general trend towards higher degree of autonomy can be seen in new robot application areas coming up including health care and assisting robotics for disabled and elderly people. Nevertheless, most robots used in rehabilitation today have similarities with industrial robots, such as the RT-series robots and SCORBOT which originally were developed for educational purposes and have been used within projects for disabled people [1, 3]. An example of an adaptation of a robot for rehabilitation purposes is Handy-1 which is used to assist in eating [8] and DeVar which uses a PUMA robot for assisting disabled at home or at vocational workplaces [14]. The Handy-1 robot is further developed through improvements in the controller and attachments adapted to the user for specific purposes (shaving, tooth brushing, make up) within the RAIL project [13]. An example of a commercial robot designed to be mounted on a wheelchair is the Manus robot with a relatively advanced design which can be considered to be one of the most successful robots for disabled people of its kind. The combination of wheelchair and manipulator show an increase in interest not only through the manipulator itself, but also through the enhancements of the wheelchair control by providing it with sensors and a control system like any mobile robotic base. The introduction of a controller adds computer resources which can be used for other purposes as well, such as mobile information related functions, which can be expected to add to independence of the user. An example of a mobile robot system with autonomous functionality within the area of health care is the MOVAID project which is a modular robotic system, including both the mobile unit and the robotic arm. A robotic system for health care services is currently under development within the MobiNet project which will integrate innovative design solutions of a mobile base with a robot arm. The robot arm ASIMOV described in this section forms a subsystem within MobiNet and the technology developed can be used for configuring new designs as well as integration to a mobile platform such as an electrical wheelchair. The development of flexible arm/link systems will also have a great impact on adaptable gripper systems, which need a high degree of flexibility in terms of manoeuvrability and dexterity.

3.1 Defining the Functionality

Developments resulting in the ASIMOV concept was initiated from functional requirements as defined for disabled people based on experience from earlier project as well as the experience from the Swedish National Labour Market Board. The overall goal for a robot serving a disabled person is to complement a human assistant and, whenever possible, replace the human assistant for a few hours during the day.

The tasks to be carried out should in principle be manipulative and include picking and manipulate objects between floor, table, book shelve and user. Normal object weight is within 1 kg excluding the gripper. The working range needed is estimated to 0.75 m if the robot arm base is at a height of about 0.7 m (normal table height). Examples of daily tasks for an assisting robot include:

- Control of different equipment by using buttons, such as computer, copy machine, switch lights on & off , kitchen related functions, etc.
- Grasp and pick objects of different size and shape.
- Be able to assist in eating and drinking.
- Pick documents and assist in reading.

Other aspects include safety in using the manipulator, final price and design aspects to reach a high level of user acceptance. Within the framework of the ASIMOV concept, safety has been taken into account, while the last two issues (price and design) have been of minor importance. As a commercial product however, it is of great importance to develop appealing robot devices that provide high value for the money. However, within the area of service and specifically services for physically disabled people, there is a tendency that the price of robot systems take over the whole design process as this parameter is much more critical for success on the market that for traditional industrial robots. For the ASIMOV robot system, we put the economical issue aside and focus on the functionality of the system only, applying the necessary technology.

3.2 System Description

It is clear that any robot to be used by a disabled person will be a challenge in terms of usefulness related both to the manipulative functionality and to the human machine interface. However, the aim was not to identify a user specification and design *one robot* that would fit *any disabled person* but to develop *innovative solutions* that make it possible to *customise* a robot for disabled people on an individual basis. The customisation aspect is important since there are different needs based on both the individual requirements and the disability which in itself may need specific considerations including changes over time.

The basic idea behind customisation is that the ASIMOV design should take into account the different needs that exist in rehabilitation robotics, which in fact defines a working scenario with a set of challenges that include:

- unstructured environment,
- highly different tasks, not specified beforehand,
- users with different skill and different needs concerning the user interface,
- users with changing needs over time.

These issues raise the question of how to realise a highly reconfigurable robot design with a high flexibility in performing different tasks. A general problem with traditional robot designs is that heavy parts such as the drive system, (motors & gear boxes) are placed as close to the base as possible to reduce the necessary torque of the motors. This in turn makes it necessary to include transmissions from the motor/reducer that in many cases goes through the arm. In general, this type of design limits the possibility to rebuild the robot arm to another configuration without extensive work that in principle will generate another robot.

In order to focus on the ability to adapt the design to the user, another concept has been chosen for the ASIMOV robot. Instead of the traditional design, both the drive system and the controller is distributed throughout the robot arm. Due to the weight of the drive system, much care must be taken in the design and dimensioning of the different components. Interestingly, a careful optimised choice of component will reduce the total weight of the robot dramatically, which is also one of the final key parameters. For example, changing the basic concept from base mounted drives to local drives in the links, reduces friction in the transmission and the weight of those components. In addition, the use of planetary reducers instead of harmonic drive type reducers reduce both weight and losses in friction. Finally, for the intended service tasks, structural elements based on carbon reinforced polymers and aluminium alloys can be applied. Within the framework of the design, it was concluded that a systematic approach of module base design should be possible to use in the design of the ASIMOV robot.

To go from concept to reality, further decisions were taken on the design that showed the importance of the modular principle. The motors should be high performance brushless DC integrated with feedback encoders and reducer. These motors have each eleven wires to be connected to the motor drive electronics that generate the control signals and power to the motor. In practice, it is not possible in such case to adapt a modular robot with a custom defined configuration and lead all wires back in the structure to a base controller, especially since we don't even know the number of links and drives beforehand. Instead, the controller for each motor must be placed in the same link structure as the motor. In this way, each link will contain both the drive system and the controller for the motor and the robot system will comprise of a set of link modules with distributed controllers. The final step is to create a method to communicate with all link modules and define a standard mechanical interface between the link modules. The communication is made through a CAN-bus that allows for necessary messages in real time between a host controller and the joint level control that is distributed in the links. In the same way, the power to the distributed controllers must also be taken care of. Applying this technology, a total of four wires (two for the CAN-bus and two for the power) are needed throughout the robot arm independent of the number of motors.

The major benefit of this concept is that in principle it allows an adaptation to the specific user requirements through simplified design and less interrelated couplings between the different subassemblies of the robot arm. The only physical connection that exists between links with drive systems is a communication link that connects each controller and a simple mechanical interface that connects the different links to each other.

Through this design, the system is based on a modular principle that allows for customisation. This means that the manipulating arm consists of a number of self-contained links that can be put together according to the needs of the user. To create this, some basic features are required for the links:

- Each link is considered as an independent module with its own drive system and joint level controller. The drive system is integrated in the links consisting of a careful selection of high performance brushless DC motors. For safety and weight reasons planetary reducers are used that provide reverse motion by hand and low losses in the reducer.
- Each part in the system must be optimised with respect to weight. Design and material of the structure is selected to achieve low mass and high stiffness. In the ASIMOV design most of the components are made of carbon fibre reinforced polymer and aluminium alloys.
- Cables through the robot arm are to be minimised: By using a concept of distributing the joint level control in the links, the local feedback loop is localised to each link. The global control in Cartesian space is facilitated by a host controller that communicates with the nodes through a CAN-bus. This minimises the cables to two wires for the control signals and two wires for the power to the motors.

3.3 The Design Development Process

To be able to design and analyse a complex system such as a robot it is important to use modern techniques where simulations and mechanical design run in parallel with the development of the controller hardware and software. A design method that has been used in the design of the ASIMOV robot is a virtual prototyping method where the design work closely interacts with aspects from the different technical expert fields as well as the user requirements summarised as the functional specification. This allows us to address the specific areas in detail at the same time as we keep the holistic view of the total design process. Thus, a team of experts is able to co-operate in the design process and continuously assess a large number of features by using virtual prototypes and simulation models. A virtual prototyping system, as described in figure 5, consists of a solid modeller and a simulation software. The models created in the CAD system are transferred to the simulation system and the complete mechanism is assembled and simulated. The simulation software makes it possible to analyse and calculate vital engineering information, such as motor torques and inter-link forces. The virtual prototyping method makes it possible to develop and test a large number of virtual prototypes with a minimum of production of physical mock-ups and prototypes, saving valuable development time and costs. Within this project, the software used was PRO/Engineer for the solid modelling and Envision TR for the simulations.

When using the virtual prototyping method the designers are able to explore a wider range of possible solutions without making a single physical prototype until the design is finalised. This makes it possible to explore innovative design solutions that normally would have been rejected at an early stage of the design process. The visualisation of the models in the simulation system makes it possible for people without an engineering background to get a fairly good understanding of the model which is useful in discussions with future users and customers. For the design of a robot that is intended to be used by disabled people, the early and continuous feedback that simulation makes possible is of great value throughout the design process.

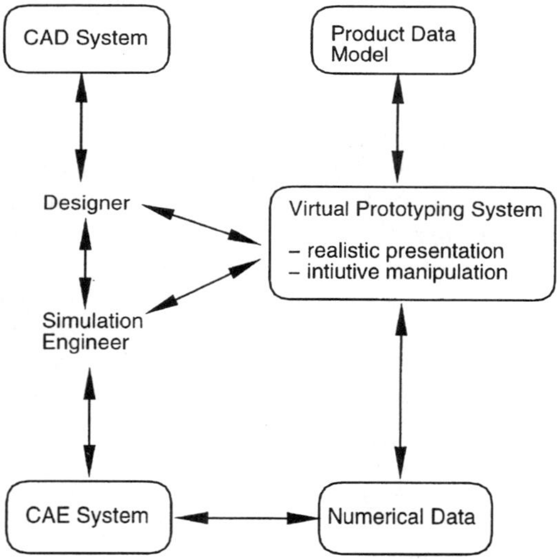

Figure 5. A schematic description of the components and information flow in the virtual prototyping methodology

An early design study of the underlying technology of the Asimov robot, described in figure 6, is a telerobotic arm with 7 joints, primarily designed to be attached to a wheelchair and controlled by a joystick. The modular design approach was modelled and analysed using the virtual prototyping method. The simulation software has also later on been used as a prototyping host controller that synchronise the distributed joint level controllers.

During this work, interaction and discussion with users has led to a quite different design approach concerning the robot configuration and the adaptation to the wheelchair. Basically, it was concluded that it is preferred to have a configuration that is similar to a human arm. The arm should operate in a right hand configuration for people that were right-handed before the injury and vice versa for left-handed people. From this, a new design study was made and a 7-axis ASIMOV robot has the typical appearance as shown in figure 7.

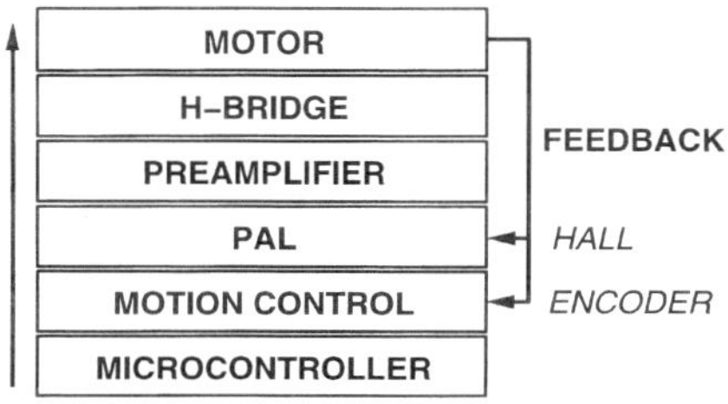

Figure 6. Information flow in the distributed controller nodes in the robot links

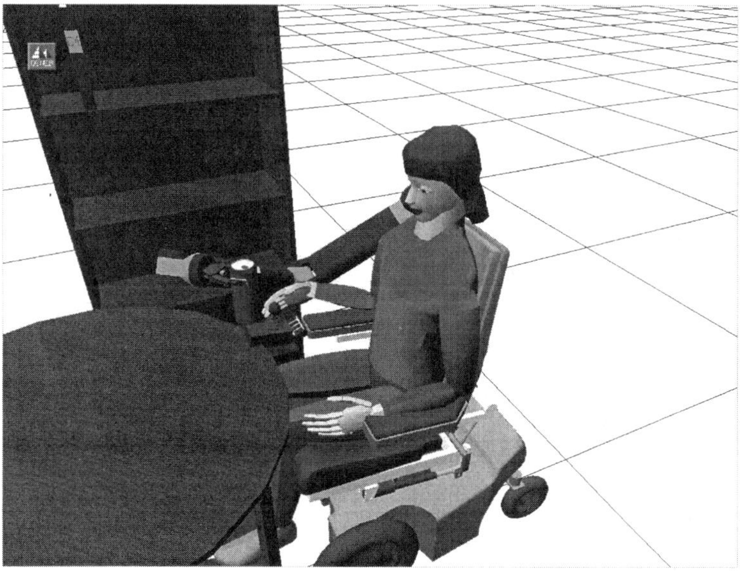

Figure 7. Typical configuration of the ASIMOV robot based on discussions with user

3.4 Control Architecture

Since modular design requires that the motors and the electronics are enclosed into the small space of the robot arm, special electronic circuits have been designed. The principal scheme of the electronic system of the modules is presented in figure 8. Every module contains a microcontroller from Permobil and is connected by the CAN-bus to the main computer. Only four wires are running through the robot arm: two for the power-supply and two for the CAN-bus communication. The motion control unit contains besides a motion generator, also a PID controller and generates pulse width modulated (PWM) signals that run the motor after the commutation order defined by the programmable array logics (PAL) and amplification (H-Bridge). There are some feedback signals from the motor where the hall signal is essential for motor commutation and the encoder signal for the motor positioning.

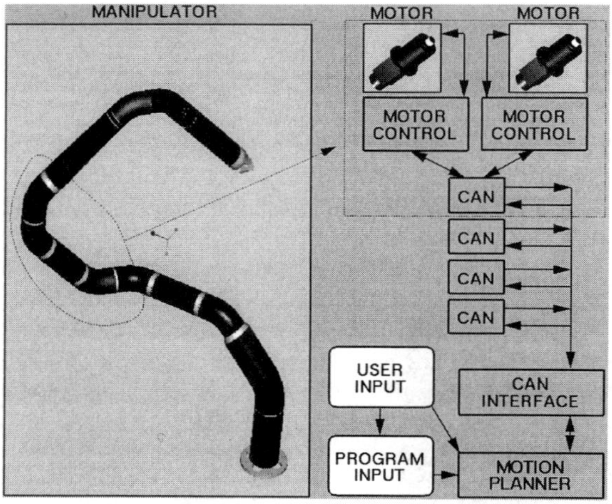

Figure 8. Schematic description of the robot system. One of the modules is highlighted and extracted from the manipulator

3.5 Validation of the Design Using VR-tools

The use of virtual prototyping tools proved to be a successful strategy in order to visually clarify the potential of the ASIMOV robot. After establishing a list of requirements, based on consultation with potential users, a refined model was produced, that should be able to fulfil the user requirements. The models of simulation software, precisely represent the actual geometry, motion and dynamics characteristics associated with the real world system. Envision TR delivers (with the dynamic option) dynamics data such as forces and torques for arbitrary revolute and prismatic joints. While kinematic modelling produces valuable data of how the physical body of the robot should be dimensioned, the dynamics modelling deliver information essential for motor dimensioning, a crucial parameter in the design process.

This information simplified and accelerated the iterative process of the design throughout the project and ensured that great consideration of the user requirements was taken. Furthermore, the simulator was used to generate and perform in real-time the motion control of the physical robot during technical validation and testing. The major problem during the testing proved to be some instability and oscillation. The problem was however temporarily solved by the replacement of the base motor with one of higher torque.

At start, ASIMOV was designed to have 8 degrees of freedom, excluding the gripper, for optimum reachability. At a later stage the removal of one motor was examined in Envision TR and a new and better solution was found, a task that would have required much more time and calculations to accomplish, without the ability of VR-prototyping. The possibility to develop entire motion procedures and working scenarios using simulations and VR-tools showed to be a useful working method for cross-disciplinary teamwork. Fields of interests for ASIMOV are such operations as opening/closing doors, placing/removing a book from a shelf, grabbing a glass and drink from it, etc. A number of successful simulations have been performed concerning this kind of operations [5]. Figure 7 shows an example of such simulation studies during the design and validation process using virtual reality tools.

4. MOVAID: a Modular Mobile Robotic System for Residential Care of the Disabled

MOVAID (MObility and actiVity AssIstance system for the Disabled), shown in figure 9, is a modular mobile robot system for residential care of the disabled is a project partly funded by the European Union in the framework of the TIDE (Technology Initiative for Disabled and Elderly people) research programme from 1994 to 1997, for the development of a semi-autonomous modular robotic system for residential care of disabled and elderly people.

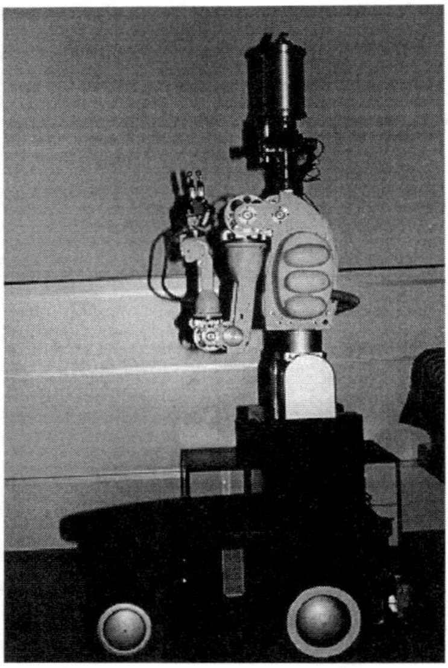

Figure 9. The Movaid

The project was more focussed on the user's satisfaction and acceptance of the robotic assistant rather than on just the efficiency and effectiveness of the device itself. Consequently, potential users helped to define the characteristics of the device at various stages in its development, and then to validate the final prototype on the basis of a user-oriented approach. A strong multi-disciplinary approach to the design was required due to the fact that the challenges were not merely technical, but also involved other aspects, such as acceptability. The design thus included industrial designers, psychologists, and anthropologists.

The goals of the MOVAID project were defined by the envisaged tasks of the robot as required by the needs of the end-user. To find out the needs of the end-user, interviews were carried out with disabled people, their relatives and assistants in three countries - Italy, France, and Switzerland. The questionnaires had questions on the domestic environment, activity at home, aid and assistance received, technical aids, and personal ability. Other additional relevant information such as age, gender, and impairment were also collected. Furthermore the attitudes of potential users towards technical aids was also explored through indirect questions and iconographic research. Three sample tasks were defined to address the daily household activities of cooking, house cleaning, and personal care, as listed below:

- warm-up a dish of pre-prepared food in the microwave oven and serve it at bed;
- dispose of empty packages (or peels) on the kitchen work surface and clean it;
- remove dirty upper and lower sheets from the bed and put them into a container.

These tasks were designed as sample tasks intended to be representative, but not exhaustive, of the capabilities of the MOVAID system. The first task demonstrates the ability to navigate throughout the house, including docking/undocking to fixed workstations, to grasp handles and objects, and to use a microwave oven. The second task mainly shows the ability of the system to recognise shapes and to work with humans. The third task is an example of how the robot can perform a task unpleasant for human carers, thus qualifying the helped/helper relationship.

4.1 The MOVAID System

MOVAID is a distributed robotic system, comprising of a mobile robotic unit with a number of fixed workstations, and of dedicated interfaces for standard kitchen appliances.

Mobile Unit

The MOVAID mobile unit is composed of a four-wheel mobile base supporting a robotic arm and hand. Mounted on the first link of the arm are a pan-tilt head supporting two television cameras, and a Distributed Local Positioning System (DLPS)-based self-localisation system. The mobile base is also equipped with a ring of ultrasound sensors for obstacle detection, which is partially covered by a tray for object transportation. An active bumper around the vehicle halts the system in case of collisions. The male docking system is mounted on the rear lower part of the mobile base. The mobile unit structure is modular, so that the vehicle can be used on its own, as a mobile platform, or the arm can be mounted on a different support (a table or a wheelchair).

The vehicle used as a mobile platform for the MOVAID system is the Electric Pedestrian (by INSERM – Unitè 103, Montpellier, France). The Electric Pedestrian, re-designed to give it a warmer and more pleasant look, is a four-wheel vehicle with two steering front wheels and two driving rear wheels. The electronics for driving the vehicle are located in the lower part, while the main compartment contains the batteries in the front, and the computing unit of the mobile unit (i.e., two PC 104 racks) in the rear.

The arm used on the MOVAID system, is the 8 degree-of-freedom DEXTER arm which was purposely designed to be part of a robotic mobile system for service applications in hospital and domestic environments, such as for the assistance of bedridden patients, transportation and servicing of food and medicines.

In order to ensure the maximum flexibility of operation in a domestic environment, an anthropomorphic approach to the design was adopted. A point to note was that, unlike industrial manipulators, high speed and accuracy of movement were not the goals – instead because the device would be operating close to an elderly or disabled person (as well as relatives and/or carers) the most important consideration was safety. To this end the arm was designed to be light and intrinsically compliant to avoid possible injury to persons in the event of a collision.

Because MOVAID is a semi-autonomous mobile system intended to perform household tasks for elderly or disabled people the characteristics of the arm must respect the constraints imposed by this kind of operational environment. The total weight of the arm and the electronic circuitry for control and actuation had to be kept low; in order to avoid the risk of the robot toppling over, the centre of mass of the arm had to be contained in small space close to the interface with the mobile base. Additionally the space taken up by the arm, either in its stand-by configuration or during normal operation should be limited so as to ease navigation in the home.

The payload of the Arm is about 15 N, and the maximum speed 0.2m/s. The total mass of the arm sub-system is about 35 kg, the total mass of the six degree-of-freedom part (with actuators) about 15 kg, and the mass of the lower arm about 4.5kg. To permit such a low mass the materials of the main components, in particular links and pulleys, have been realised using high resistance aluminium with lighten holes. To maintain the centre of mass near the connecting flange all the eight actuation motors were placed in the proximal links, in particular: motor of the first joint on the mobile base, motor of second joint on the first link, motors of all other joints on the second link.

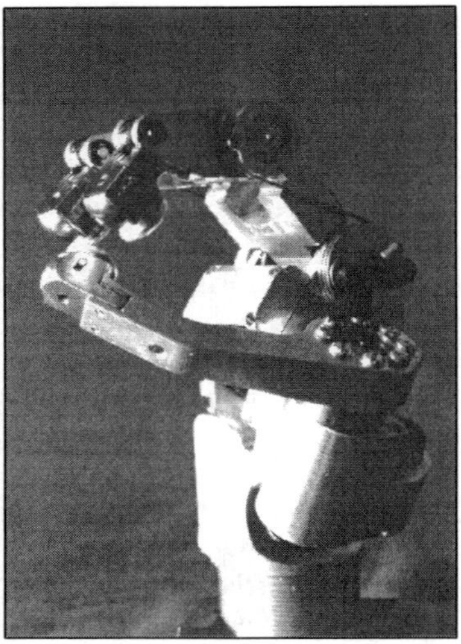

Figure 10. The MARCUS hand

The end-effector of the MOVAID system is the 2 degree-of-freedom MARCUS hand, shown in figure 10. This device was designed as a hand prosthesis and its anthropomorphic configuration allows high flexibility in domestic environments. There are reduction gears in the thumb and fingers with irreversibility mechanisms that make it possible to maintain the grip forces even though the motors are powered off. The prosthesis performs both precision and power grip. The total weight of the hand is 550 g, and the maximum force at the fingertips is 120 N.

The Distributed Local Positioning System (DLPS)-based self-localisation system developed at the University of Genoa allows the mobile base to compute its absolute position and orientation in the environment. It is an active positioning system for indoor applications in multi-robot environments, using a modulated light beam. The system is composed of two parts: an on board rotating unit and a set of active beacons distributed over the operating area (located on the walls at suitable heights). The rotating unit transmits a rotating and modulated beam of light (red laser), and has an omnidirectional infrared receiver. The active beacons are little boxes that receive the beam of light transmitted by the rotating unit and reply with their identification codes. The reply messages from each of the beacons are processed to reconstruct the position and orientation of the robot within the space.

The mobile robotic unit can dock to a fixed workstation through a purposively designed docking system, composed of a special connector for transmission of power and data, and a two degree of freedom mechanical support. This allows connection even at low positioning accuracy. The docking system has been designed so that the female part affixed to the workstation occupies little space. The docking system is also used to correct for any inaccuracies within the absolute localisation system on board the robot. These inaccuracies are due to errors in the position of the beacons, low accuracy of the rotating part, and low accuracy of the odometry.

An Ethernet radio link allows bi-directional data flow between the fixed workstations and the mobile base when the robot is undocked. The fixed workstations send commands to be executed by the mobile base through the radio link, while the mobile base sends back the result of the command executed and the images acquired by the television cameras.

Some photographs of the MOVAID mobile unit, in the demonstrative environment where it has been validated, are shown in figure 11.

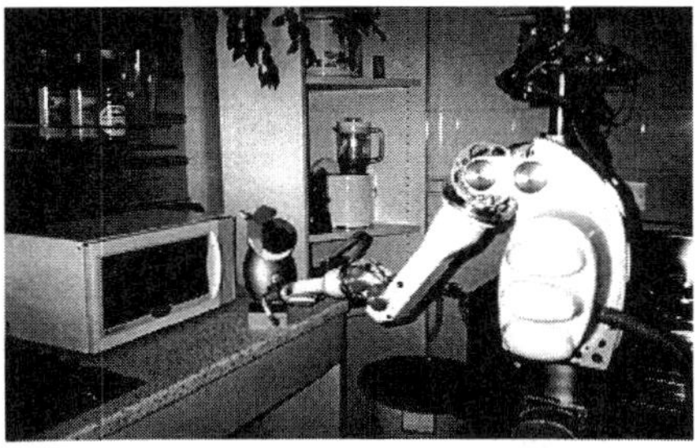
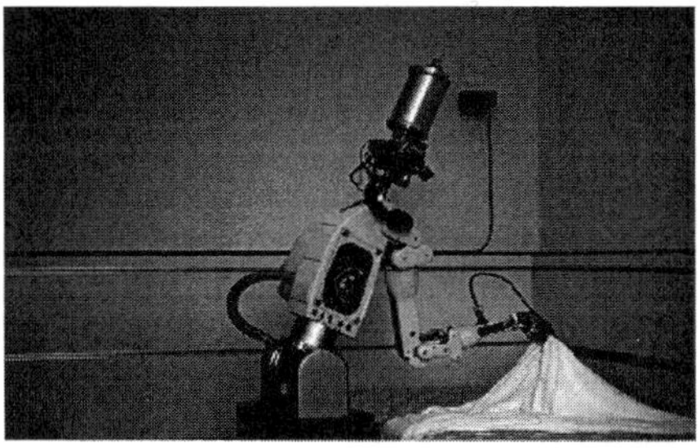

(a) *(b)*

Figure 11. The MOVAID prototype performing the typical tasks in the demonstrative environment: (a) cleaning the kitchen surface; (b) removing dirty sheets from the bed)

Fixed Workstations

The MOVAID fixed workstations are located in the most 'strategic' positions for the robot in the house. For instance, at the validation site there are two fixed workstations: one in the bedroom, close to the bed-ridden user, and the other in the kitchen.

Each fixed workstation is constituted by a PC, which houses the software modules for the system that are not required on-board, namely the supervisory module, the system database, and the graphical user interface. The two fixed workstations are connected into a local network by an Ethernet link, and are connected to the mobile base by an Ethernet radio link. The female sections of the docking system are located near the fixed workstations, one on the bottom of the kitchen furniture and one under the bed.

The fixed workstations permit the user to access the robot through a graphical man-machine interface, which can be used either by means of the standard PC mouse or by a specific human-machine-interface. In fact, an M3S keyboard and mouse emulator allows access to the man-machine interface by means of any M3S input device. The M3S standard, developed through an EU-funded project, allows any M3S output device to be controlled by any M3S input device. The M3S concept is based on the need, expressed by people with disabilities, to own and use an input device that is suited for their functional abilities and personal preferences. Being able to control different devices through one input device avoids the difficulty of acquiring, learning and using new input devices for each possible new assistive device. The MOVAID user can use his/her own M3S input device for accessing the MOVAID user interface, through the M3S mouse and keyboard emulator.

The instructions given by the user are processed by the proper software modules, implemented on the fixed workstations, and then translated and transmitted in the format required by the low-level controllers on board the system.

The Multimedia Man-Machine Interface (MMMI) allows the user to access the MOVAID system, providing tools for required tasks. Moreover, the MMMI provides the user with information on the system status. According to the results of the initial interviews different levels of use were previously defined to better satisfy user needs. In fact, they demonstrate that system autonomy is hardly accepted at home and in personal activities, but on the other hand an assistive robot has to be autonomous in case of emergency for the user. The lower levels of use are characterised by high autonomy for the system and little or no involvement of the user during the execution of tasks. The lower levels are most appropriate for new users or for users who don't want to be involved in the execution of tasks. The higher the level of use, the less autonomy for the system and the more involvement of the user.

The MMMI also provides a continuous flow of visual data, coming from the on-board cameras. Such information is useful both for allowing the user to monitor the robot behaviour, and, mainly, for allowing him/her to help the robot during the execution of tasks. The idea is that the user, seeing what the robot is seeing, could ask for tasks involving observed objects and could help the robot identify objects by indicating them directly on the image received as visual feed-back via the MMMI. Pictures of the MMMI screen layout, at different levels, are given in figure 12.

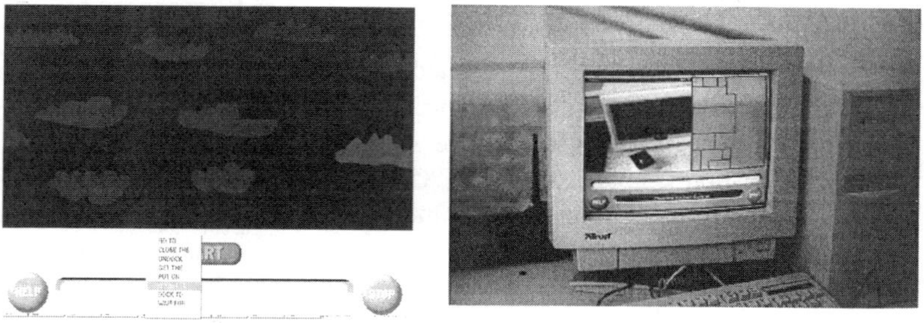

Figure 12. Some examples of the MMMI screen layout

The Supervisory Modules (SM) on the activity workstations plan, schedule and control the execution of all the tasks performed by the system, manage errors and monitor critical situations. The supervisory modules directly communicate with the MMMI, by means of a special synthetic language. The MMMI gives a preliminary interpretation of the input from the user, by translating it into the synthetic language, and transmits user requests to the supervisory level. When a task is requested by the MMMI (expressed in the synthetic language) the supervisory modules interpret this request and produce a sequence of commands for the suitable low level functional module.

The Low Level Functional Modules (LLFM) are the modules allowed to access to the different MOVAID effectors, by invoking a set of Low Level Functions. They translate the Low Level Commands received from the Supervisory Modules into instructions to the Low Level Functions, in the proper syntax and parameters.

The high level Communication Manager module (CM) is responsible for managing communications among the fixed workstation and the low level software modules, by allowing data to be transmitted through the Ethernet Connection, from the workstation core to each low level end-effectors controllers.

Finally, the system Data Base (DB) contains the data that are shared among different modules.

Dedicated Interfaces

The MOVAID project developed dedicated interfaces for two standard products – a microwave oven and an electric citrus press, as shown in figure 13.

Microwaves can be difficult to use by elderly or disabled users because most controls require fine motor control and good vision for their operation. The MOVAID microwave oven interface greatly simplified ease of operation for the target-users, consisting of just 3 functional elements for full use of the oven.

The tools for the citrus press consist of a universal holder, a cutting board and a pressing aid which are used to hold, manipulate, transport, and press the fruit.

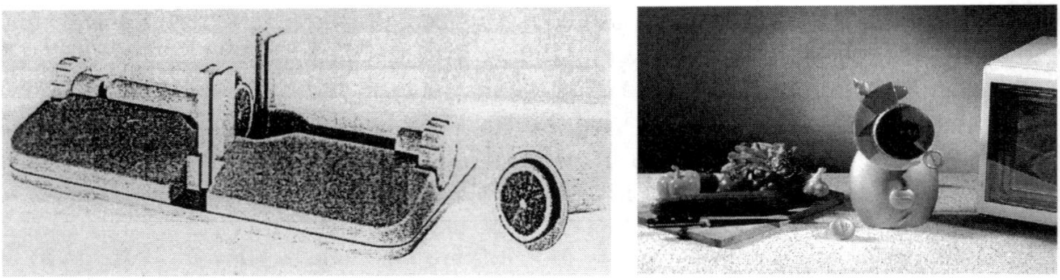

(a) (b)

Figure 13. (a) The MOVAID tools for the citrus press and (b) the MOVAID microwave oven interface

4.2 Validation of the MOVAID System by Users

The MOVAID prototype was installed in a residential site for disabled people in Italy, where it was tested and evaluated by a sample of end-users. The MOVAID system at work in the kitchen with a tetraplegic young man is shown in figure 14.

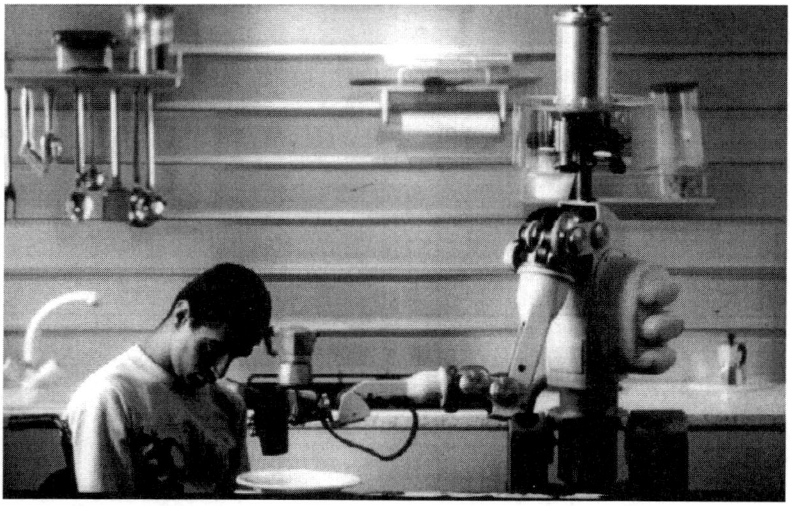

Figure 14. The MOVAID system at work with a disabled end-user

The general aim of the validation of the MOVAID system was to survey the *acceptability* and *perceived usability* of the system, in terms of: system efficiency, system effectiveness, interaction effectiveness, easiness of use, easiness of interaction, pleasure of use, helpfulness, robot behaviour, robot aspect, pleasure of interaction, invasiveness and system autonomy.

The robotic system was proposed to a sample of motor disabled people, with different levels and typologies of disabilities. They were trained to use the MOVAID human-machine interface and to use specific aids for accessing the PC, when necessary. Then, they were asked to request a given task to the robot, at different levels of use of the interface.

Results were collected both by therapists, who observed the users during the execution of the tasks, and by the users themselves, at the end of the trial session. Such data were integrated with other collected through demonstrations of the system (video and photographs) in other sites in Italy and France.

As a general result, the system was enthusiastically accepted, especially by severely motor disabled users and by those with poor or no functionality of upper limbs, while it was evaluated as a helpful, but not strictly needed tool by paraplegic people with full ability of upper limbs. The visual feedback on the screen was confirmed as a comfortable feature for allowing the user to monitor the robot, and the point-and-click mechanism of interaction on the image was in general appreciated and it did not introduce any additional burden to the user's activity.

The aesthetics of the system, although stimulating many comments and suggestions, seems to match the proposed goals of giving the system friendliness and an appliance-like appearance. The system was considered as acceptable in a domestic environment.

The difference in users' attitude between the first phase of analysis of users' needs and this phase of validation is clearly evident. In the first phase, users were proposed something which was almost completely unknown and a generalised sense of mistrust emerged. In the phase of validation, instead, users were asked to evaluate something much more concrete, which they could see while operating (live or in a video). This greatly changed the opinion of users who, in the validation phase, showed a much more positive attitude. Most users felt stimulated to propose new tasks, and many suggested modifications and improvements in relation to their own needs. The substantial change of opinions on a possible robotic assistant before and after the MOVAID experience is shown in figure 15.

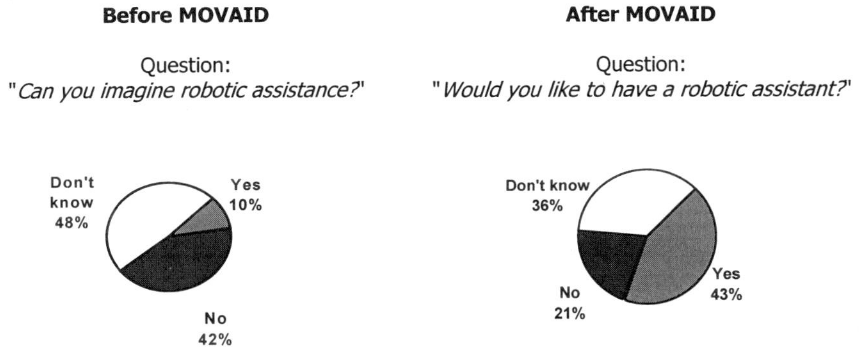

Figure 15. Levels of acceptance of the concept of a personal robotic assistant before and after the MOVAID experience

5. Conclusions

Manus is the only commercially available wheelchair mounted manipulator. Over 150 manipulators are being used, and it is expected that these figures will rapidly grow in 2000. Although the ergonomics of the Manus are one of the main reasons for the success of this manipulator, the only thing it is missing is a certain kind of compliancy in its movements.

A modular robot referred as the ASIMOV robot was designed by the virtual prototyping method and a seven axis prototype based on the modular technology developed has been built. The physical robot showed to be very well correlated to the virtual model. The initial technical validation of the robot proved well to match the basic initial specifications. The weight of the robot is approximately 12 kg and the working range about 1.5 m. The maximum joint speed surpass the specified. It is possible to increase the ratio of the reducers by a factor of four and still preserve the maximum joint speed of 90 degrees/s. Some controller problems that were identified will most likely be solved in the next generation of ASIMOV by the implementation of new control algorithms, modification of some drive systems and the reduction of the size of the robot arm. The power consumption proved to be very low, about 50 W at typical performance, which is quite insignificant in comparison with the power consumption of the rest of the wheelchair.

Although much was achieved by the virtual prototyping approach, there is still need for improvements of the robot concept. Below follows a list of suggestions, based on an interview with a potential user of ASIMOV and experimental results received from the trial run of the robot:

- Reduction of the length of the robot arm by a factor of 2/3.
- Reduction of the size of the electronics. This work is in progress and will allow for smaller link units.
- Introduction of monitoring the current in the motor phases. This enables torque control and software safety control of the robot.
- Study the possibility to increase of the gear box ratio by a factor of 2-3. This will increase the load capacity with minor negative effect on the total weight and speed of the robot.
- Implementation of full modularity and unlimited rotations by introduction of slip ring connectors. At present, there is a limitation in the number of turns to be made.

Other more innovative solutions are the replacement of the CAN-bus with radio communication and the implementation of a "plug and play" strategy, where the modules could be connected and unconnected by a simple operation. The modules would instantly recognize the new configuration, change the kinematic model and update the adaptive control. However, these ideas are for the more future versions and will be studied later on.

Presented here was the MOVAID project as an attempt to propose a robotic solution to the problem of personal assistance to disabled and elderly people. One of the real challenges of the project was to demonstrate that a robotic solution is feasible, not only technically, but especially as a product that can not only improve the quality of life for the target users, but would also be accepted by them. These dual goals of functionality and acceptability required a multi-disciplinary approach to the design. The design team included industrial designers, psychologists and anthropologists.

Potential final users were the focus of the project, and with this in mind a number of disabled and elderly people were involved in project activities from the beginning.

A total of 207 final users from three different European countries participated in the project.

From a technical point of view, refinements to MOVAID will aim to increase performance and reduce costs, by stressing the system modularity and distribution and by relying on commercial components.

6. References

[1] Bolmsjö G., Eftring H., and Neveryd H. Robotics in rehabilitation. *IEEE Transactions on Rehabilitation Engineering*, 3:77 83, 1995.

[2] Dallaway J.L., Jackson R.D. "Raid - a vocational workstation" *ICORR'92* Keele-UK.

[3] Dallaway J.L., Jackson R.D., and Timmers P.H.A. Rehabilitation Robotics in Europe. *IEEE Transactions on Rehabilitation Engineering*, 3:35 45, 1995.

[4] Danielsson C., Holmberg L. "Evaluation of RAID workstation" *RESNA'94* Nashville USA.

[5] Fridenfalk M., Lorentzon U. and Bolmsjö G., Virtual Prototyping and Experience of Modular Robotics Design based on User Involvement. In *Proceedings of the AAATE 99 Conference*, (Christian Bühler and Harry Knops, Editors), pages 308-315, IOS Publishing (1999), November 1999, Düsseldorf, Germany.

[6] Gelin, Rodolphe et. al. "AFMASTER: An Industrial Rehabilitation Workstation" *Proceedings of ICORR99*, pp. 149-155. July 1-2, 1999, Stanford, CA.

[7] Hawkins Paul BA (Hons), Topping Mike BA Cert Ed., "The Design And Development Process For The Handy1 Robotic Aid To Eating And Drinking," *Proceedings of ICORR'97*. April 14-15, Bath, UK.

[8] Hegarty J., Rehabilitation robotics: The users perspective. In *Proceedings of the 2nd Cambridge Workshop on Rehabilitation Robotics*, Cambridge, UK, April 1991.

[9] Hok Kwee, Ph.D., Quaedackers Jacques "POCUS project: Adapting The Control Of The MANUS Manipulator For Persons With Cerebral Palsy" *Proceedings of ICORR99*, pp. 106-114. July 1-2, 1999, Stanford, CA.

[10] ICAN-Integrated Communication and control for All Needs. EC-TAP project nr. DE4204.

[11] Kazi Z, Beitler M, Salganicoff M, Chen S, Chester D, Folds R. Multimodal user supervised interface and intelligent control (MUSIIC) for assistive robots. In: *1995 IJCAI Workshop on Developing AI Application for the Disabled*. 1995; 47-58.

[12] Tone Oderud, Gemma R. Overboom, J.A. van Woerden. "Experiences from the Evaluation of a Manus Wheelchair-mounted Manipulator". *Proceedings of AAATE97 (Advancement of Assistive Technology)*, pp. 20-23. 19 Sept-2 Oct. Porto Carras, Greece.

[13] Topping M. and Smith J., The development of Handy 1, a rehabilitation robotic system to assist the severely disabled. *Industrial Robot*, 25(45):316 320, 1998.

[14] Van der Loos M., Hammel J., and Leifer. DeVar L., "Transfer from R&D to vocational and educational settings", In *Proceedings of the Fourth Int. Conf. on Rehabilitation Robotics,* pages 151 155, Wilmington, Delaware, June 14-16 1994.

[15] Wagner J.J., van der Loos H.F.M., et al. "ProVar Assistive Robot Interface". *Proceedings of ICORR99*, pp250-254. July 1-2, 1999, Stanford, CA.

[16] Web: http://home-1.worldonline.nl/~dynamics. 2000-05-16.

[17] Woerden J.A., van Nelisse M.W. "Integrated solutions for assistive devices," in *The European Context for Assistive Technology; Proceedings of the 2nd TIDE Congress*, Paris, Assistive technology research series, vol. 1, p. 387-392.

Chapter 13

Sensing Strategies for Mobile Robots

by Fernando MATÍA, Nikos KATEVAS, Fabrice WAWAK, Gerard LACEY

Mobile Robotics in Healthcare
N. Katevas (Ed.)
IOS Press, 2001

Chapter 13

Sensing Strategies for Mobile Robots

Fernando MATÍA, Nikos KATEVAS, Fabrice WAWAK, Gerard LACEY

1. Introduction

The chapter begins introducing navigation sensors for mobile robots, including both odometry sensors (strongly related with locomotion systems) and other navigation sensors such as proximity sensors, lasers and vision systems. The sensor calibration problem is also addressed.

Following, a set of proposals for the integration of heterogeneous perception methodologies is presented, together with sensor fusion and sensor redundancy techniques. They will be useful for localisation and mapping tasks, which will be discussed in the following chapters. The concept of virtual sensing is also introduced as an appropriate way to supply sensor information to the navigation module in a standard format.

Finally, the selection, configuration and placement of sensors are discussed. This analysis concludes with the development of generic methodology that would be a proposed guideline for researchers on how to select configure and place sensors on a mobile robot.

2. Navigation Sensors

Lets assume a highly sensitive robot. This robot could be equipped with some of the following perception devices:

- A set of encoders for incremental location estimation,
- Bumpers for collision detection,
- Proximity sensors such as ultrasound (sonars) and infrared sensors,
- Floor detectors, internal sensors such as battery charge sensors,
- Security sensors such as microphones, smoke, temperature and movement sensors,
- Vision based sensors, etc.

We will review these and other related sensors that could be chosen in the design of a mobile robot.

2.1 Odometry Sensors

Dead reckoning systems is the abbreviation of *deduced reckoning of sailing days*. When the locomotion system are wheels, they are called *odometry* systems. The method enables calculation of the position given the travel time, the direction and the velocity (fixed). The origin of odometry systems may be found in the first automobiles. Conventional solutions at that stage offered accumulative errors, although present methods are very similar.

The problem statement is as follows: we want to obtain the position at k+1, from the position at k. This means that we need to know the linear and angular displacement increments, $\Delta d(k)$, $\Delta\beta(k)$, at instant k. Starting from the wheels movement, it is clear to see that they both depend on the wheels configuration. This aspect will be discussed on Chapter 14 where we will deal with localisation issues. But, in general forward and angular motions may be calculated as a function of each wheel movement:

$$\Delta d(k) = f_d(\Delta d_1(k), \ldots, \Delta d_n(k), \Delta\beta_1(k), \ldots, \Delta\beta_n(k))$$
$$\Delta\beta(k) = f_\beta(\Delta d_1(k), \ldots, \Delta d_n(k), \Delta\beta_1(k), \ldots, \Delta\beta_n(k))$$

where n is the number of wheels. The linear displacement $\Delta d_i(k)$ may be measured by a sensor as $r\,\gamma_i(k)$, with r being the wheel radius, while the angular displacement $\Delta\beta_i(k)$ may be measured directly. In both cases angular positioning sensors are required. The most well known angular positioning sensors are potentiometers, synchros and resolvers and optical encoders.

Potentiometers produce a voltage $u_0(k)$ proportional to the turn angle: $\gamma(k) = [2\pi/u_{REF}]\,u_0(k)$. They are fabricated from carbon, ceramic plastic or a ceramic-metal mix, and supply a discontinuous measure due to they physical construction. Their advantages are the ease of interface as well as their very low cost. Among their disadvantages are that they get easily dirty, are very sensitive to electrical noise and their medium accuracy.

Synchros transmit angular information through electromechanical systems, while resolvers are a particular case of synchros. In both cases, the voltage is proportional to sinus and cosinus of the angle.

Optical Encoders may be classified in incremental and absolute. The first ones measure angular velocity and infer relative position, while the latter directly measure angular position and infer velocity. In incremental optical encoders, a light source generates wave pulses, where period is inversely proportional to speed. In fact it may be considered a single channel tachometer encoder. Phase quadrature encoders use a double channel, so resolution increases. An electrical circuit detects which wave leads, and so they measure the rotation sense. They have four possible states, and the circuit supplies a number of lines in a three bytes counter. A third channel C may exist, which is activated at an origin position. The three ports may be read from a user program.

While from encoder line counts, forward and angular wheel displacement may be deduced, another utility that some mobile robots need is homing. A special mechanism is used to locate wheels at a home position. The principle is that rotating wheels turn clock-wise slowly until the origin is found (using a capacitive or inductive sensor that will be described later). Then the wheel rotates anticlock-wise a bit to compensate inertia (as printers do).

Absolute optical encoders are based on a binary code disk. There are appropriate for very low speeds, giving back a code for each absolute position. Medium resolution is 1,000 counts per revolution. Grey code disk is a special one in which only one bit changes at each step, and so ambiguities are eliminated.

Finally, in order to calculate the effective movement of the wheels, the effective turning radius must be evaluated. This is due to the own weight of the robot, that produces an effective radius (r') less than the real one (r), r'< r, and that indeed may not be equal for all wheels.

2.2 Velocity and Acceleration Sensors

Velocity sensors are less common sensors, because speed may be obtained from location. Velocity sensors use movement as source of energy (this means that they are passive sensors). They may be classified in two groups: linear velocity sensors (LVT) and angular velocity sensors. In LVT it is more difficult to measure, so usually we transform the problem into an angular movement.

Examples of angular velocity sensors are the tachometer and the tachometric generator. A tachometer is a proximity sensor that measures the pass frecuency of a rotatory element. It uses an exciter that accurately divides the wheel (e.g. in 60 divisions), and finally, the discrete signal is changed to analogue. The tachometric generator gives a proportional voltage to axis speed, working as a conventional electrical generator.

Acceleration sensors measure absolute acceleration by using a couple tender-mass. From strength and mass acceleration may be derived (Newton law). The main types of acceleration sensors are the following ones: piezoelectric, drags, capacitive and servo-accelerometers.

Velocity and acceleration sensors measure neither absolute nor incremental location from the wheel's movement. Sometimes they are used as an odometry system complement. Two examples are Doppler navigation and inertial navigation.

Doppler navigation has its origin in nautical and aerial applications for velocity measurement in respect with earth. Irradiated energy reflects on a surface (ocean floor of earth surface) which is moving in respect with the emitter. The speed is obtained as $v=v_D/\cos\alpha$, where v is actual speed and v_D is measured speed and α is the phase difference. A higher frequency is received in the closer region, so it must be filtered to extract the main frequency. The best solution should be to use four sensors situated at 90 degrees each. The main advantage is that their use avoids slipping problems, terrains with low uniformity or vehicle roll due to weight balancing. Their disadvantages are their high price, which makes them impossible to use in robotics applications, and errors due to vertical movement of the vehicle in respect with the floor. If the floor moves (water), the sensor indicates movement with the vehicle stopped.

Inertial navigation was initially thought for airplanes. Later on it was adapted for missiles and submarines. It consists of a gyroscope, oriented with respect to a fixed axis. If the path follows one of the edges, it gives the acceleration error. Integrating twice, the position error may be obtained. A gyroscope maintains a consistent orientation of the three accelerometers. Their advantage compared to doppler sensors is that they avoid slippery problems and problems introduced by terrains with low uniformity or vehicle roll due to weight balancing. Their disadvantage is that they do not work with constant velocity.

2.3 Navigation Sensors for AGVs

Automatic Guided Vehicles (AGVs) are the simplest mobile robots, since they move following a prefixed path. No human operation is needed, and a host computer may coordinate the movement of vehicles. In comparison with mobile robots, the latter are more flexible, because AGVs cannot deviate from the planned path. Usually they follow some landmarks in the floor, by using one or some sensors located in the front or under the vehicle.

The most common sensors used by AGVs are audio or radio wire, optical sensors, magnetic sensors, odour and heat sensors. In wire guided AGVs, there are two sensors in the front of the vehicle. The difference between incoming signals from them centres the vehicle. Accuracy is 0.5 cm. If the signal disappears, the AGV stops. Initial installation is expensive but sensors are cheap. An example is the bridge joining Sạn Diego and Colorado.

When using *laser sensors* in AGVs navigation, then AGVs are called *Laser Guided Vehicles* (LGVs). The use of laser in navigation increases the accuracy to 0.1cm and most importantly requires no severe intervention with the shop floor. Laser sensors need to locate beacons placed in the vicinity of the workspace, but do not require the use of buried elements (e.g. wires).

Optical guidance is an alternative to wired guidance. Applications include low-structured environments where more flexibility for path modifications is needed. Some types of methods are used: a high contrast between the floor and the line, a reflective tape, or a chemical film that iluminates when it is iradiated with ultraviolet light. Most of the sensors allow the vehicle to follow left or right hand of the tape. This allows selection of the appropriate path when a bifurcation is present. Among their advantages is that they are passive sensors and that measurement is not interrupted if the line is broken. The disadvantages are that they deteriorate with time (and so they need maintenance), that dirt and objects may hide the line, and that, if chemical tape is used, it is not visible (they need careful maintenance). In some cases, more than two sensors may be used, so turn commands may be easily implemented to allow the vehicle to return to a path.

In *magnetic guidance*, a magnetic tape in the floor is used. Robot sensors are based on the Hall effect. They need low maintenance, tape interruptions are not a problem, and length is unlimited. Again, several sensors may be used, so some of them measure the path and others detect branches on it.

Odor and *heat guidance* sensors try to emulate ants guidance systems. A piezoelectric sensor measures heat energy emitted by the floor. The vehicle carries two capacitive elements: one generates positive voltage, and the other negative voltage. Turn is so proportional to the voltage difference. A metal piece can be added as cover to avoid any external interference. These sensors may be also used for human detection in security applications. A disadvantage is that they cannot be used when hot water pipes are present.

A solution to this problem is a film of alcanfor diluted in alcohol. Alcohol evaporates, and the vehicle must follow the alcanfor odour, which is not dangerous for humans. Sensors are based on a quartz glass with silicon that absorbs alcanfor molecules. Outputs of both oscillators are compared to drive the vehicle, while fresh air is introduced to eliminate interferences with other flows.

Intermittent guidance is another method that is based on the use of wireless systems. This method is needed when the environment frequently changes, in cleaning tasks, or when modification of the floor is not feasible. The advantages are more flexibility and more autonomy. A hybrid case may consist on an AGV that follows a virtual path using odometry, but that, from time to time, localises itself by using a grid on the floor.

2.4 Proximity Sensors

While AGVs are designed to navigate in more or less structured and predefined environments, autonomous mobile robots are designed to navigate with on-line path planning and obstacle avoidance. In order to do this, they need proximity sensors.

Proximity sensors enable the measurement of presence, distance or movement, in units that may vary in the range from millimetres to meters. There are two main types of proximity sensors: *active sensors*, that emit energy (radio directional and ranging), and *passive sensors*, that capture energy from objects, for example a CCD (coupled charged device). Proximity sensors may be classified in: tactile, electric and magnetic, reflection, optical, and infrared light.

Tactile sensors may behave like an antenna (when contact is made, the circuit closes), or like a bumper. Magnetic and electric sensors may be classified in magnetic, inductive and capacitive. Magnetic sensor behaviour is like a switch. In the presence of a magnetic field (for example, closed door) a flow is originated. When the sensor approaches it (i.e., over a mobile robot); a polarity is generated and the attraction between the two poles closes the circuit. It is based on the Hall effect, so voltage = material constant · flow density · current / thickness.

Inductive sensors are used to detect metal at short distances. A ferrite core is affected by an oscillatory field. If an object enters the field, a current flow is induced on it. This originates a magnetic field, which modifies original impedance. When the object is too close, oscillations disappear. *Capacitive sensors* are similar to inductive ones. They detect both metals and dielectric materials. They work at short distances. When an object approaches it, the capacity changes.

Reflection sensors compare the difference between emitted and reflected energy. Two types may be distinguished: microwave and ultrasound. Microwave sensors work at large distances (1-50 m) and they emit in the microwave spectrum (GHz). If an object reflects enough energy, the receptor changes its status. Ultrasonic sensors are the most common sensors for indoor applications. They are also called *sonars* (SOund NAvigation and Ranging). They emit in the ultrasonic region (20-200 KHz), so people cannot hear it. Their main features are the following:

- They detect the closest distance to objects
- Due to the low speed of sound, the same membrane may act as emitter and receptor (this can be configured)
- Received signal amplitude is inversely proportional to time: $d = (s \cdot t)/2$
- They are used for a range of a few meters
- They must be calibrated for a determined range
- The measurement values drift with temperature changes
- Dispersion angle is proportional to sensor diameter $\theta = 1.22 \cdot s / (w \cdot 2r)$
- If w is fixed, a point emits energy in all directions (θ = infinite)
- If r increases, oriented wave lines are attenuated

There are important drawbacks in their use. Their most typical error sources are changes in propagation speed, reflection problems, inclination (the solution is to increase the dispersion angle; the use of more sensors increases the resolution, but computing time increases), roughness, and reception of the echo from another sonar (the solution is to shoot them alternatively, or to shoot sets of them at the same time). Their advantages are their low price (we can have a set of them) and the easiness of use. Their main disadvantage is their low reliability due to several error sources.

Optical sensors are photoelectric devices for proximity measurements. Their range is from centimetres to meters. They are another example of active sensors. They can work in four configuration modes: opposition, reflection, diffusion, convergence, and opposition. Any object in between breaks the flow. An application example may be intruder detection.

Reflection mode consists on detecting beacons in the walls. Diffusion is used for obstacle detection. They are faster (speed is equal to speed of light) if compared with a typical configuration of 24 sonars that need more than a second to report the corresponding measurements. But it does not return a measure of distance. In convergence mode, they only sense in the intersection area. This may be used for floor detection.

Infrared light sensors measure phase-shift, instead of time (speed of sound is low). They allow the measurement of distance as well as speed and direction of a mobile obstacle. The phase-shift may be obtained electronically multiplying emitted and received signals and averaging along many cycles. Usually they are used to measure short distances: 1-5 m or less (< 2MHz). To measure distances, a ring of infrared sensors is usually used. They measure intensity of the received signal. The result is inversely proportional to the square root of distance

2.5 Laser and Vision Sensors

Laser telemeters (also proximity sensors) are a special case of optical sensor. They are known as *laser radars* or "*lidar*" (light direction and ranging). Energy is emitted at impulses and distance is derived from the time of flight. They may be used as laser altimeters, for obstacle avoidance or for vehicle detection in highways. They supply speed and height.

Rotary lasers are based on the rotation of the wave 360 degrees at more than 1 or 2 rpm, and a mirror at 45 degrees. This avoids the problem of hidden areas. They often work in conjunction with reflecting beacons. They measure angular position.

Scanning laser range finders combine the lidar with the rotary lasers by providing both range and angular position to the detected object. They do not need reflecting beacons and therefore are useful as they can be used in unstructured environments. Some systems have 360-degree coverage, while the most use 180 degrees. They are most commonly used in localisation and mapping applications [5], however they can also be used without a map for generalised landmark recognition [8].

Vision systems use one or more cameras to capture an image of a scene. There are two major classifications of vision systems: *passive* and *active*. In passive vision a static CCD camera observes a scene. If more than one camera is used to capture the scene from many viewpoints it is called stereovision. Active vision is where the camera is moved as a direct response to the demand for more information. The path of the camera provides the necessary extra information for the task at hand.

Passive vision systems are able to extract the presence of landmarks, detect movement in the scene. When a single camera is used it is difficult to estimate the distance to objects. Distances to objects in the scene can be estimated by exploiting knowledge about the environment such as the expected size of recognised objects and their location in the image. However this requires the system to be trained on the selected features and it is consequently inflexible.

If two or more cameras are used (stereovision) we can triangulate on any feature that can be uniquely identified in both images. Stereovision triangulation methods, discovered by Erastothenes, Alejandria (276-194 b.c.), need an adequate illumination, and dead areas exist (where features are not visible in both cameras). Such triangulation requires that the distance between the cameras and their relative orientations be know with very high accuracy. This is achieved by performing exhaustive camera calibration.

Structured lighting systems (laser lines or patterns of lighting) may be used in conjunction with static cameras to measure the height of objects in a scene. The camera measures the degree to which the objects in the scene deform the projected light pattern. This deformation can be used to measure the height of objects around the robot such as kerbs and steps for a mobile robot. This technique has the limitation that sunlight can wash out the effect of the projected light. As with the stereovision system the relative distance and orientation of the light source and the camera must be known with high accuracy in order to produce the height measurement.

Omni-directional vision systems are another important subgroup of specialised vision systems. In this case the single camera is pointed at a curved mirror, giving it a 360-degree view around the robot. An example of images can be seen in Figure 1 along with an image of an omni-directional camera on a robot.

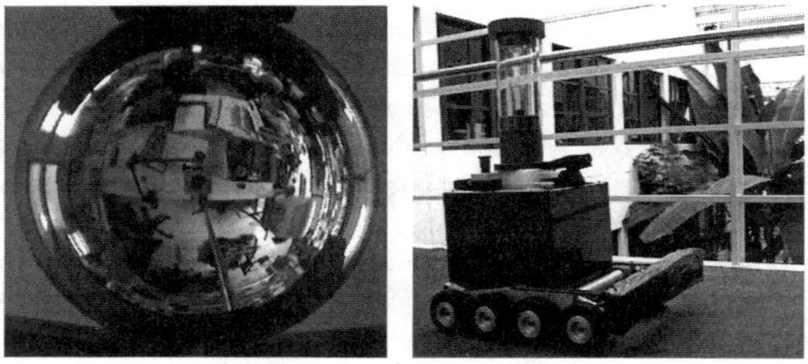

Figure 1. Omni-directional Image and camera

The images from omni-directional cameras can be used for localisation and mapping as in [11] or can be unwrapped to provide a panoramic images for human interpretation as shown in Figure 2.

Figure 2. Unwraped Omni-directional Image

Active vision systems are a relatively new concept in vision systems. The camera(s) are able to move on high-speed pan-tilt platforms. The movement of the camera(s) is driven by the need to track particular image features or gather specific information. The systems are often modelled on the binocular human vision system where the eyes focus on small areas and move rapidly from feature to feature building up a full picture of the scene.

Vision systems may be used for different applications, from localisation and mapping to face and gesture recognition. The vision systems research is very large field and a wide variety of approaches and techniques are used in the construction of systems. The cost of visions systems hardware is falling rapidly and new techniques are being developed in response to the greater processing speed available. As a consequence we can expect to see vision systems play a much more significant role in the future.

2.6 Special Sensors

We include here sensors that may be used for specific missions, such as cleaning, transport, inventory (bar code checking), security missions, vigilance, dangerous tasks, nuclear waste inspection, and bomb detection and removal. In the design, it must be taken into account that the final aim of a mobile robot is to interact with humans while carrying out a useful task. In security applications these sensors must be able to detect fire, smoke, movement, gases, or radiation, and must work in the most adverse situations, like low visibility or high temperature.

Security sensors may be classified in acoustical detection, vibration sensors, presence sensors, motion detection, and acoustical detection. An example of acoustical sensor is a microphone with an amplifier adjusted to the medium. Any sound that overpasses this level is detected. Vibration sensors are useful for detection of movement located at wheels level to detect floor vibrations (like footsteps). Any vibration makes the flow deviate and so received energy decreases. They are cheap and simple.

Presence sensors are based on sonars. A ring of 24 sonars may detect changes in distances. Any unexpected measurement will report the distance to the intruder, while the number of the sensor will supply the angle with respect to the intruder. Motion detection sensors may be optical or infrared (passive). They are based in changes in received light level, and they detect movement, not presence.

Movement may be detected by using a vision system and specific image processing algorithms, or with sonars. In the second case, proximity sensors, distributed covering the contour of the robot, give relative movement. Alarm must be confirmed with several sensors, and sensor noise and wrong functioning must be taken into account.

3. Integration of Perception Methodologies

3.1 Sensor Fusion, Integration and Calibration

The main algorithm for sensor fusion, and perhaps the one that provides more accurate results is the well-known Kalman filter. Figure 3 shows the Kalman filter scheme.

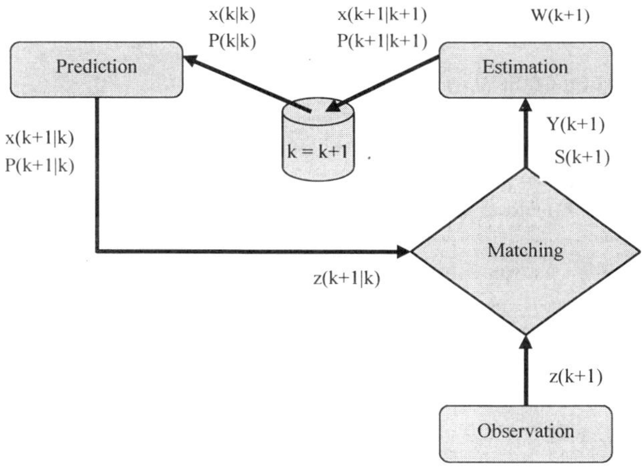

Figure 3. Kalman filter scheme

Lets define,

$x(k)$: state array (robot oriented position)
$P(k)$: state uncertainty matrix
$z(k)$: measurement array
$H(k)$: observation matrix
$w(k)$: observation noise
$u(k)$: velocity commands
$v(k)$: kinematics noise
$R(k)$: covariance matrix for $w(k)$
$Q(k)$: covariance matrix for $v(k)$

And let there be:

$$x(k+1) = F(k)\,x(k) + G(k)\,u(k) + v(k)$$
$$z(k) = H(k)\,x(k) + w(k)$$

Then, the algorithm has four steps as follows,

1. Prediction: Initial prediction of the position at instant k+1 with the information available at instant k just using the kinematics model,

$$x(k+1|k) = F(k)\,x(k|k) + G(k)\,u(k)$$

The calculation of the position uncertainty matrix estimation,

$$P(k+1|k) = F(k)\,P(k|k)\,F^T(k) + Q(k)$$

And the prediction of the sensors measures,

$$z(k+1|k) = H(k)\,x(k+1|k)$$

2. Observation: An actual array of measurements $z(k+1)$ is obtained from the sensors.

3. Matching: Calculation of the measurement innovation Y and its covariance matrix S at instant k+1,

$$Y(k+1) = z(k+1) - z(k+1|k)$$
$$S(k+1) = H(k+1)\,P(k+1|k)\,H^T(k+1) + R(k)$$

4. Estimation: Calculation of Kalman filter gain,

$$W(k+1) = P(k+1|k)\,H^T(k+1)\,S^{-1}(k+1) + R(k+1)$$

And estimation of the corrected position and its covariance matrix at instant k+1 with the total information available at instant k+1,

$$x(k+1|k+1) = x(k+1|k) + W(k+1)\, Y(k+1)$$
$$P(k+1|k+1) = P(k+1|k) - W(k+1)\, S(k+1)\, W^T(k+1)$$

Initial R(k), Q(k) and P(k) matrices must be fixed experimentally, taking into account the error of sensors and models. Their diagonal elements represent uncertainties on state or measurement values. It may be said that the Kalman filter provides sensor integration in the sense that the observation array z(k) may contain data from any kind of sensing device, indeed redundant information provided by two or more sensors.

The Kalman filter may be also used for sensor calibration. In fact, any recursive algorithm, such as the gradient approach, able to minimise the error between the actual measures and the simulated measures with the present parameters, may be fine. Parameters to be calibrated may be classified into intrinsic and extrinsic. The first ones are those that may not be measured by direct observation. The second ones are those that may be obtained approximately by direct observation. For instance, in the case of a camera, the focal distance, the distortion and the optical centre location are intrinsic parameters, while the position of the camera is an extrinsic one.

The way in which Kalman filter may be used for sensor calibration is just to use as state vector x(k) the parameters to be calibrated, instead of the mobile robot oriented position. The prediction step provides again simulated measures at the present state (i.e. with the present parameters). The observation step provides a set of sensor captions taken at different robot locations, rather than being taken while the robot is moving as usual (where the Kalman filter was used for localisation, i.e. position estimation and mapping). Figure 4 shows an example of data taken from a laser at different distances from a room corner, together with the simulation (straight lines) of the same measurements at the same locations.

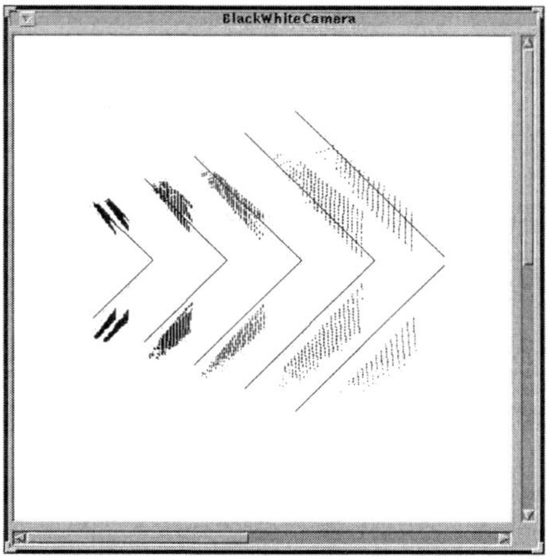

Figure 4. Calibration of a laser system

The best feature of the algorithm is that the same procedure may be used to calibrate any kind of sensor (proximity, vision, etc), just replacing the dimensions of the x(k) and z(k) arrays, and so of the corresponding matrices, accordingly.

3.2 A Generic Perception Framework for Virtual Sensing and Sensor Redundancy

The use of a generic perception module will be described along the next two chapters. Figure 5 shows its internal composition. It easily allows both sensor and model fusion for navigation, localisation and mapping. Sensor fusion is done at the observation stage, were data from different sensors (lasers, cameras, proximity) may be integrated. The way in which that integration is carried out may be just the Kalman filter, fuzzy logic, or any other probabilistic approach. In fact, the use of the Kalman filter explicitly allows to manage sensor redundancy by decreasing the possible errors provided by different measurement sources.

Measures that are not available at any instant will not be integrated into the filter. Furthermore the models of both the robot kinematics and the sensors are combined at the prediction stage.

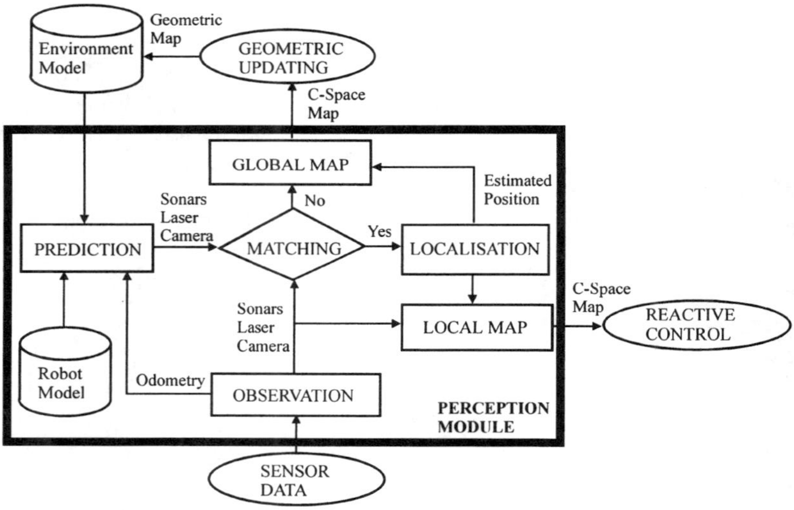

Figure 5. Perception framework

As has been stated above, localisation and mapping issues will be discussed in further chapters. Nevertheless, the navigation module in charge of avoiding obstacles also requires accurate sensor data. Conventional navigation algorithms employ directly proximity sensor information, perhaps with a simple filtering algorithm just to avoid noise. Nevertheless, the integrated perception framework already introduced has enriched information that contributes to the elimination of errors from different sources (the sensor data and the models), and so it may be used to provide better information to the navigation module (reactive control module in the figure).

For instance, instead of using instantaneous filtered values from proximity sensors, a more reliable local map that has a continuous shape of the obstacles in the surrounding of the robot may be used to "simulate" distances to obstacles (see discussion about local and global mapping in the chapter about mapping).

Another application of virtual sensing is to apply the same navigation algorithms to mobile robots with different contour shape. Although the locomotion system also affects the kinematics, and so the movement control parameters, in most cases (small mobile platforms), the use of a local map instead of instantaneous measurements allow to (again) "simulate" virtual proximity sensors located over our robot. The physical sensors only exist in the original platform were the navigation algorithms were designed for. The only special care that must be taken is that the map must be built quickly enough so that the provided information is recent, but, at the same time, the erroneous measurements are removed quickly.

3.3 Sensor Fusion and Primitive Sensor Model

Sensor fusion implies sensor modelling and a method to represent the environment. The model used influences the reliability and the accuracy of the representation although it is not the factor influencing those values. The section proposes a general purpose model that may be used for simple as well as complex sensors as those were presented in the sections above. The model is employed to analyse the sensor fusion cases. The model is called *Primitive Sensor Model (PSM)* and it was introduced in [6].

The Primitive Sensor Model describes in a simplified way the action of a virtual sensor represented by its primitive model. For the simplification of the presentation occupancy grid is used for the environment representation (3D to 2D representation). By the use of PSM the actual sensors employed by the robot may be modelled in the three-dimensional space with their virtual equivalents. PSM is considered as a conical sphere sector a° wide, with a total range of r_t cm and an optional blind zone of r_b cm ($r_t \geq r_b$). The axis of the conical sphere sector is considered identical to the central sensor (e.g. acoustic, optic) axis of the actual sensor head or the portion of it modelled. The PSM can be placed anywhere w.r.t. the robot's local coordinating system, but only its projection on the occupancy grid plane is considered. The blind zone range r_b defines the areas where sensors readings are not considered reliable thus their projection on occupancy grid are not taken into account. Hence PSM's active range lies between r_b and r_t. The primitive sensor model returns a detection range r as the one-dimensional measurement of an obstacle at distance r cm from model's origin on sensor's central axis. The model does not provide any angular information concerning the detected obstacle which can be at any point within the model coverage but at distance r from the origin. Thus, for each sensor reading r, the primitive sensor model interprets that there is: i) free space from r_b to r, but within the sensor coverage, ii) blocked space at distance r from model origin - within sensor coverage -, and iii) unknown space elsewhere. This modular model definition can result to PSM's footprints on the occupancy grid as circles, ellipses, squares or sectors of the above or other complex geometrical shapes, depending on PSM's parameters and placement. PSM reminds models used for ultrasonic sensors. Although special propabilistic [3] sensor models presented e.g. for ultrasonic sensors used in mobile robotics navigation, the simplicity of PSM makes it suitable for model accommodation of more complicated sensors as laser range finders or even optical sensors. Thus several primitive models with properties configured appropriately, could be combined to synthesise sensors of higher complexity. One the other hand the simplicity of the sensor fusion procedure remains.

The footprint of the proposed PSM used is shown as case (a) in Figure 6. The PSM paramer of the example is a = 90°, $r_b = 0$ and $r_t \geq 0$. The model is placed in such a way that results a footprint of an 90° wide angle at 0,a of the *x-y* coordinate system attached to the occupancy grid and at $\pi/4$ w.r.t. x-axis. In Figure 6 the white colour is representing cells that are reported by the sensor model as free of obstacles, while black cells indicate blocked areas and grey cells are representing areas that cannot be considered either as free or blocked.

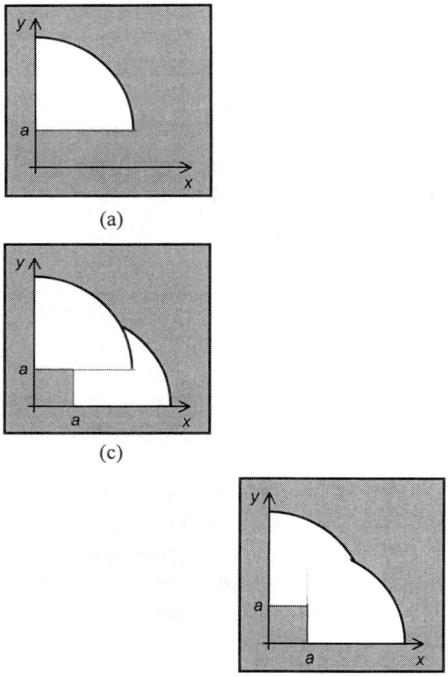

Figure 6. Sensor fusion cases using the primitive sensor model

Let consider the case where two PSMs have an overlapping area, as in the case where two sensors PSM_1 and PSM_2, with identical characteristics are placed at *(0,a)* and *(a,0)* respectively. In addition, let assume that the sensors are both reporting the same range value, translated that the sensor detects an obstacle at the given range *r*. The cells of the occupancy grid laying on the arc segment of radius equal to the reported value are considered as blocked while all cells belonging in the interior of the angle are marked as free. If one considers a method that updates first the cells corresponding to PSM_1 and then cells corresponding PSM_2, the result on the occupancy grid is shown in Figure 6 (b). Considering the reverse update ordering of PSMs, the result is shown in Figure 6 (c). Another alternative could be that the print procedure gives priority and updates first the cells that were characterised as free indepentently to the PSMs they correspond to, and then - in the same manner - the cells to be marked as blocked. The result is shown in Figure 6 (d) for the example of PSM_1 and PSM_2. The reverse (blocked first, free follow) is shown in Figure 6 (e).

The main differences in the above mentioned approaches can be commented as follows: The cases (b) and (c) are favouring particular PSMs, assigning specific priorities to their readings. Intentional priority assignment is applicable in particular cases where enhancement of a sensor contribution is a demand due to its high reliability. Case (d) reflects on the grid the worst guess, when all sensors are treated equally and the worst obstacle report is taken into account. If we consider sensors with identical reliability degree and assume the same ability of detection in all linear and angular ranges, then case (d) will never reflect a real situation. This is because in case (d) the reliability of the first sensor in detecting free cells, is questioned by the reliability of the second sensor in detecting blocked cells, while both are sharing the same reliability degree under the power of assumptions defined above. Coping with the fact that in real applications, detailed environment information by the means of one-to-one correspondence of available information with the environment status will not be available due to the cost of data acquisition and data manipulation, one has to fuse the information available considering it as an abstraction of reality. This is performed in the last sensor fusion case (Figure 6 (e)). The last approach recovers from false alarms introduced by distant obstacles in overlapping areas. Arcs like those shown in Figure 6 can be produced by one or more obstacles placed anywhere on the arc at distance r from the most right of the arc to the most left edge. Considering a case like (d) a false alarm which would be caused in the overlapping area, because blocked cells in this area would have caused a shorter range report to both sensors than the one reported. It is obvious that these arcs were produced by obstacles detected somewhere outside the shared area of responsibility. Depending on the number of sensors employed and independently from their angular resolution the method of case (e) can fuse effectively the information acquired and represent accurately the environment. The same is applicable when modelling complicated sensors e.g. their angular resolution may be correlated to the angular intervals between several PSMs used to model them. Thus, one can achieve an angular resolution equal to the angular PSMs intervals assuming equal sensor distribution in all directions. On the other hand, the linear resolution perpendicular to the detection axis, cannot be further improved as it decreases as far as the range of detection increases (for each measurement).

4. Selection, Configuration and Placement

The selection of the sensors to equip the robot is an important issue. However, researchers and system integrators underestimate the importance of sensor placement on the robot and focus more on the selection.

There are four factors that influence the decision where to place the sensors on the robot:

1. the *sensors* themselves
2. the *shape* of the robot
3. the *kinematics constrains* of the robot
4. the *navigation strategy* used

The sensing principle (as well as the band of frequencies of the phenomenon being measurement - light, ultrasound, microwaves etc.) and the properties of the sensor itself (resolution, accuracy, reliability, range etc.) are factors that have to be considered. Redundancy of information might or might not be desired. Thus, placement of two sensors observing the very same portion of the workspace might be considered as an activity to assure redundancy (if those sensors are basing their measurements on an independent phenomenon) or waste of sensorial resources (if the previous is not the case, or redundancy is not a system demand). The sensing principle is posing constrains on the actual position of the sensor w.r.t. the robot body or the workspace. E.g. an ultrasonic sensor placed on the floor level within the sound lobe is useless, because it will report the same value all the times - the range at which the floor is detected. Given that the above problems are resolved, one may consider the problem of placing the sensors w.r.t. the robot's coordinates.

Full symmetry of the robot shape simplifies the problem e.g. circular shaped robot imply that cocentrical placement of sensors would be a safe decision. The importance of the issue becomes evident if one considers non-symmetrically shaped robots. In those cases it is empirically proven that not all positions on the robot might be treated equally. The "corners" at parallelogram shaped robots concentrated the attention of the researchers. Figure 7 (a) and (b) gives a proof of that. Figure 7 (a) depicts the Active Kinematic Histogram [6] of a square shaped robot (80cm x 80cm), which is shown on the left, while Figure 7 (b) depicts in white the Active Kinematic Histogram of a parallelogram shaped robot (131cm x 82 cm), which is also shown on the left. The importance of the robot "corners" is clear when one considers the potential rotation that the robot might perform by the center of rotation. In such a case the robot would collide with the obstacle overhanging in the obstacles histogram.

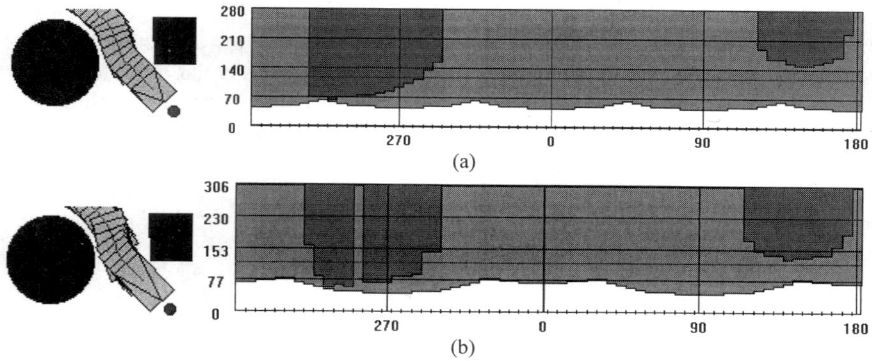

Figure 7. Active Kinematic Histograms of square and parallelogram shaped robots

In the case of the square shaped robot the robot's AKH maintains the symmetry between each of the four quadrants in polar space. In the case of the parallelogram shaped robot this symmetry is lost. However, the symmetry remains between the two semicircles. In more complex shapes the symmetry is lost completely. Losing symmetry the heuristic rules become invalid. The information on the points of interest remains in the robot shape represented in the AKH. A one-to-one correlation between points of interest and AKH values is: the higher the value of the robot AKH the higher the collision risk at a potential rotation. Given that the AKH represents information in polar space, the angular positions of the peaks on the robot's AKH should be interpreted by the system designer as a demand for incrementing the angular resolution at the positions of interest. Therefore, the values of the robot's AKH gives a relative measure of the angular resolution required at all points of the robot periphery.

However, both of the above factors have to be crosschecked with the kinematics constrains applied on the robot and the navigation strategy used. The kinematics are embedded in the AKH but the reader has to take into consideration that many AKH's may be dynamically constructed during the robot motion, as the AKH is constructed by the instantaneous rotation center which is not a fixed point w.r.t. the robot's coordinate system. On the other hand, the kinematics constrains give valuable information regarding the sensors' placement. There is no need to observe a direction in which the robot will never move in e.g. in a car-like robot the side motion on the axis of the rear wheels is not allowed, therefore sensors may skip these directions.

Last but not least comes the navigation strategy. The strategy might need to overrule some of the decisions made based on the above, but the analysis should document the reason for that. In all cases, the navigation strategy might conclude in addition of sensors or an increase of the angular resolution e.g. side motion direction might be observed by an additional set of sensors because the strategy needs to foresee the side space in advance.

5. Conclusions

After many years studying planning and control technologies, researchers have realised that the main preoccupation must be perception, and integration of incoming information from heterogeneous perception systems. In fact, the purpose of the perception module is to provide an adequate information about the environment to the modules of planning and control.

Perception is a process that aims to interpret the information coming from sensors in order to estimate a model of the real world. One of the major areas of research that ensure such a process is computer vision. But during the past decade, a strong advance in sensor technology has allowed a new generation of sensors. The problem is to elaborate an appropriate physical model of each sensor, to ensure a good interpretation of the information. Spatial information is a fundamental requirement for mobile robotics technology.

For the construction of a robust spatial model, an integration framework has to be established allowing to confront the information coming from different sensors. Basically, three frameworks are used for the integration of spatial information. First, the measures themselves can be used. But with that technique, integration is made quite difficult especially due to the heterogeneity of the sensor data. Geometric maps or occupancy grids can be used to homogenise data representation. These topics will be discussed in Chapter 15 (mapping). With that framework, the sensor measures expected free and occupied areas of the environment.

There are basically two steps in sensor integration. The first one, multisensor fusion, aims to integrate at a given instant the piece of information brought by each sensor. The second one, sequential integration, updates the previous world model with the updated information brought by the next step. The most crucial information needed to ensure this second step is a good estimation of the position of the robot. It is essential to know exactly where to integrate the new information in the previous model. Here is the link between the perception and localisation issue. Localisation issues will be discussed in a further chapter. The perception framework is constructed through the Kalman filter.

6. References

[1] Dorst, L., M. van Lambalgen and F. Voorbraak, *Reasoning with Uncertainty in Robotics*, Springer-Verlag, 1995.

[2] Durrant-Whyte, H.F., *Integration, Coordination and Control of Multi-Sensor Robotic Systems*, Kluwer Academic Publishers, 1988.

[3] Elfes, A., *Sonar-based Real-World Mapping and Navigation*, IEEE Journal of Robotics and Automation, Vol. RA-3, No. 3, pp.249-265, 1987.

[4] Everett, *Sensors for Mobile Robots. Theory and Application*, A.K.Peters, Ltd, 1995.

[5] Forsberg J., U. Larsson and A. Wernersson, *Mobile Robot Navigation using the Range Weighted Hough Transform*, IEEE Robotics and Automation Magazine, March 1995, pp. 18-26.

[6] Katevas N., and S. G. Tzafestas, *The Active Kinematic Histogram Method for Path Planning of Non-Point, Non-Holonomically Constrainted Mobile Robots, in Advanced Robotics,* the International Journal of the Robotics Society of Japan, Special Issue on Intelligent Mobile Robots, 1998, Vol. 12, No. 4, pp. 373-395.

[7] Katevas N., *Intelligent Autonomous Mobile Robots - Contribution to System Architecture and Path Planning*, Ph.D. dissertation, National Technical References.

[8] Lacey G. *Adaptive Shared Control of a Robot Mobility Aid*, in Field and Service Robotics, John Bares (Ed), CMU, Pittsburgh, August 1999.

[9] Rembold, *Stereovision Systems for Autonomous Mobile Robots*, Intelligent Autonomous Systems, 1995.

[10] Wawak, F., Matía, F., Peignot, C. and Puente, E.A.. *A Framework for the Integration of Perception and Localisation Systems over Mobile Platforms*. In “Progress in System and Robot Analysis and Control Design”, 1998.

[11] Winters N., J. Gaspar, G. Lacey, and J. Santos-Victor, *Omni-directional Vision for Robot Navigation*, in Proceedings of the 1st International IEEE Workshop on Omni-directional Vision (OMNIVIS'00) at CVPR 2000, South Carolina, USA, June 2000, (to appear).

Chapter 14

Mobile Robots Localisation

by Fabrice WAWAK, Fernando MATÍA, Nikos KATEVAS, Gerard LACEY, William HARWIN, Stanislao LAURIA

Mobile Robotics in Healthcare
N. Katevas (Ed.)
IOS Press, 2001

Chapter 14

Mobile Robots Localisation

Fabrice WAWAK, Fernando MATÍA, Nikos KATEVAS, Gerard LACEY, William HARWIN, Stanislao LAURIA

1. The Localisation Issue in Mobile Robotics Applications

Vehicle localisation is a key requirement in mobile robotics. The expansion of sensor technology enables the manipulation of extensive environmental information. Without position estimation, only an instantaneous perception and a basic reactive control is possible, banning the possibility of path planning. Note that in the literature, the problems of perception and localisation are often disconnected. In this chapter it should be kept in mind that the localisation issue is working integrated with perception.

In the design process of a localisation system, it is necessary to decide the kind of sensors to be used, the localisation method to be implemented, as well as the accuracy that is required for position estimation. Sometimes, the method just needs to provide identification of the room where the platform is, but more often, an accurate estimation of the position in the room is needed.

The chapter is first going to describe with some detail the devices that are able to estimate the position of the platform. Following, different localisation methods will be described. Typical localisation methods are usually classified in two essential categories, the *absolute localisation methods* and the *relative localisation methods*.

Absolute localisation methods aim to determine the absolute position of the mobile robot. One of the most well known and standardised systems is the *Global Positioning System* (GPS). The absolute positioning is characterised by the fact that such a system gives an estimation of the mobile robot position with a bounded error due to the imprecision of the technology used for the positioning.

On the other hand, relative localisation methods make use of an incremental system to update an initial position. A representative system based on a relative positioning is the dead reckoning system. The main drawback of a relative localisation system lies in the fact that such a method accumulates the imprecision. Hence, the error of the position of the mobile platform increases continuously without a bound. To overcome that problem, a step that refines the position estimation is added. The purpose is to continuously control the error of the position keeping it into an acceptable interval. An approach is to make use of information by another sensor type. That new information provided, is matched to a world-model and the position given by the dead reckoning system. The platform position is then estimated. This method is limited by the accuracy of the world model.

2. Specific Devices for Localisation

Devices for localisation are classified into two main groups: incremental and triangulation devices. Incremental devices are based on dead reckoning. The new position is estimated from the previous one and a measurement of the platform displacement. Triangulation devices are able to crosscheck drivers spatial information sources to locate the platform. Both techniques and their limitations are discussed.

2.1 Dead Reckoning and Kinematic Systems

Dead reckoning is the abbreviation of "*deduced reckoning of sailing days*". When the motion method (kinematic system) is wheel-based, they are called *odometry* systems (*see also* Chapter 13). The *configuration* (a 2D oriented point) describes the *position* and *orientation* of the robot w.r.t. the global reference frame.

Lets suppose that $\mathbf{x}(k) = [x(k)\;\; y(k)\;\; \theta(k)]$ is the robot configuration at instant k. Localisation based on the odometry system consists on obtaining $\mathbf{x}(k+1)$ from $\mathbf{x}(k)$ and linear and angular position increments, $\Delta d(k)$ and $\Delta\beta(k)$, between instants k and $k+1$. The estimation of the new position results:

$$x(k+1) = x(k) + 2\,\Delta d(k)/\Delta\beta(k)\,\sin(\Delta\beta(k)/2)\,\cos(\theta(k) + \Delta\beta(k)/2)$$
$$y(k+1) = y(k) + 2\,\Delta d(k)/\Delta\beta(k)\,\sin(\Delta\beta(k)/2)\,\sin(\theta(k) + \Delta\beta(k)/2)$$
$$\theta(k+1) = \theta(k) + \Delta\beta(k)$$

that may be approximated taking into account that $\Delta\beta(k)$ is small:

$$x(k+1) = x(k) + \Delta d(k)\cos(\theta(k) + \Delta\beta(k)/2)$$
$$y(k+1) = y(k) + \Delta d(k)\sin(\theta(k) + \Delta\beta(k)/2)$$
$$\theta(k+1) = \theta(k) + \Delta\beta(k)$$

If we focus on the kinematic system, the previous position increments, $\Delta d(k)$ and $\Delta\beta(k)$, may be calculated from the wheels movement, and so related with the encoder values studied in the previous chapter. There exist several kinematic systems (*see* Chapter 7), which possess different manoeuvrability. The most typical ones are:

- Differential steering
- Ackerman steering
- Synchro drive
- Tricycle drive
- Omni-directional motion

In the case of *differential steering*, the vehicle has drive and castor wheels. The two drive wheels have a fixed position, while the castor wheels have free movement. Here, two optical encoders are enough, supplying $\Delta d_1(k)$ and $\Delta d_2(k)$. R(k) is the curvature and *a* the drive wheels separation. It is clear that:

$$\Delta d_1(k) = \Delta\beta(k)\,[\,R(k) - a/2\,]$$
$$\Delta d_2(k) = \Delta\beta(k)\,[\,R(k) + a/2\,]$$

and so

$$\Delta d_2(k) - \Delta d_1(k) = \Delta\beta(k)\, a$$

Then

$$\Delta d(k) = \Delta\beta(k)\, R(k) = \Delta d_1(k) + a\,\Delta\beta(k)/2 =$$
$$= \Delta d_1(k) + [\Delta d_2(k) - \Delta d_1(k)]\,/\,2 = [\,\Delta d_1(k) - \Delta d_2(k)\,]\,/\,2$$

$$\Delta\beta(k) = [\Delta d_2(k) - \Delta d_1(k)]\,/\,a$$

The advantage of differential steering is its high accuracy (in theory). Its disadvantages are that floor rugosity must be uniform, angular motion produces high errors and that *a* is an uncertain parameter. It has problems with steps (i.e. floor rugosity) as well as with slippery floors. Tracked vehicles are an extreme case of differential steering kinematic system, where it is impossible to eliminate slipping and therefore odometry is not useful.

Ackerman steering uses two steering wheels. Turning a bit more the external wheel than the internal one eliminates slipping. This locomotion system is characterised by the fact that perpendicular lines in both wheels intersect at the back edge. From the angle of the external wheel θ_E it is possible to obtain the angle of the internal one θ_I:

$$\tan\theta_E = L / h$$
$$\tan\theta_I = L / (h - a)$$
$$h = L / \tan\theta_E = L / \tan\theta_I + a$$
$$1/\tan\theta_E - 1 / \tan\theta_I = a / L$$
$$\cot\text{an}\,\theta_E - \cot\text{an}\,\theta_I = a / L$$

were *h* is the curvature of the external wheel and L is the separation between both edges. The angle of a virtual wheel (*see also*, bicycle model in Chapter 7) located in the middle of the directional edge may be deduced from the angles of both wheels:

$$\tan \theta_E = L / h$$
$$\tan \theta_C = L / (h - a/2)$$
$$h = L / \tan \theta_E = L / \tan \theta_C + a/2$$
$$\text{cotan } \theta_E - \text{cotan } \theta_C = a / 2L$$
$$\text{cotan } \theta_C = \text{cotan } \theta_E - a/2L = \text{cotan } \theta_I + a / 2L$$

were θ_C is the angle of the virtual wheel. The main advantages of this system are its accuracy and easiness of information maintenance. It is mainly used in outdoors applications. Inaccuracies are introduced in cases of high slippage (when more than two edges are used, existence of more than one intersection edge as wheels runways are concentric circumference arcs).

Linear and angular displacements $\Delta d(k)$, $\Delta\theta(k)$, may be obtained from back wheels movement $\Delta d_1(k)$, $\Delta d_2(k)$ and forward angle $\Delta\theta_C(k)$ as follows:

Right wheel: $\Delta d_1(k) = \Delta\theta(k) [h(k) - a]$
Left wheel: $\Delta d_2(k) = \Delta\theta(k) h(k)$

so

$$\Delta d_2(k) - \Delta d_1(k) = \Delta\theta(k) a$$

and

Virtual wheel: $\Delta d(k) = \Delta\theta(k) [h(k) - a/2]$

Taking into account the expressions from differential steering, it comes out that

$$\Delta d(k) = [\Delta d_1(k) + \Delta d_2(k)] /2$$
$$\Delta\beta(k) = [\Delta d_2(k) - \Delta d_1(k)] / L$$

or

$$\Delta\beta(k) = \tan \theta_C(k) [\Delta d_1(k) + \Delta d_2(k)] / 2L$$

In the first case two encoders are enough, while using the virtual wheel three encoders are necessary (but the third one may be used to decrease the error of the others).

In synchro drive kinematic system, three or more wheels are mechanically coupled. Wheels turn and move forward at the same time:

$$\Delta\theta_1(k) = \Delta\theta_2(k) = \Delta\theta_3(k) = \Delta\theta_4(k) = \Delta\theta(k)$$
$$\Delta d_1(k) = \Delta d_2(k) = \Delta d_3(k) = \Delta d_4(k) = \Delta d(k)$$

Two encoders are enough since $\Delta d(k)$ and $\Delta\theta(k)$ are directly measured from encoders. Its advantages are wheel synchronisation, high accuracy, and that motors generate the same torque at every wheel. Its disadvantages are that the driving belt may generate errors, wheel friction with floor is high in turns, and that angle errors appear when forward movement does not exist.

In *tricycle drive*, the solution is identical to that for the Ackerman steering case:

$$\Delta d(k) = [\Delta d_1(k) + \Delta d_2(k)] / 2$$
$$\Delta\beta(k) = [\Delta d_2(k) - \Delta d_1(k)] / L$$
$$\Delta\beta(k) = \tan\theta_C(k) [d_1(k) + \Delta d_2(k)] / 2L$$

The main advantage is its high simplicity. Disadvantages are that the centre of gravity moves forward in inclined terrains with loss of stability, and that angle errors may appear when forward movement does not exist.

Omni-Directional motion refers to the case when wheels are free move in any direction. The equations for a three wheel-based system follows:

$$v_1 = v_x + wR$$
$$v_2 = -v_x \sin 30 - v_y \cos 30 + wR$$
$$v_3 = -v_x \sin 30 + v_y \cos 30 + wR$$

It is highly manoeuvrable, however it tends to slip and have low efficiency.

2.2 Triangulation Devices

A triangulation device is a sensor, or a set of sensors, which allow the estimation of its position by measuring some landmarks in the environment. Several examples will be discussed. The first one is the case of a triangulation system based on the detection of passive landmarks in a known environment. The landmarks are chosen so that they may be recognised by both their colour and shape (red colour and circular shape in the following example). The camera must be colour with pan and tilt movements, so it may be oriented towards the beacons.

An improvement of this system may be achieved, by using natural landmarks in indoor environments, such as windows or doors. The triangulation needs at least three landmarks to behave as an absolute positioning system, so more than three beacons must be located at each room, to allow the camera to reach at least three from any point of the room.

The second example is a system that detects reflecting landmarks, also distributed along the walls of the room. In this case the beacons are built with the same material as traffic signals (diamond gray), (they are able to reflect infrared laser light). A rotating system is designed to guarantee that the laser beam is continuously rotating at constant speed.

A laser emits light towards a mirror that reflects it horizontally. When the light finds a reflecting surface, an echo is received. The integrated hardware is able to calculate a value for both the angle of the landmark and the number of landmark, based on a barcode-like labelling. This method may be used continuously while the robot is moving. Again, with at least three landmarks the system may give an absolute position.

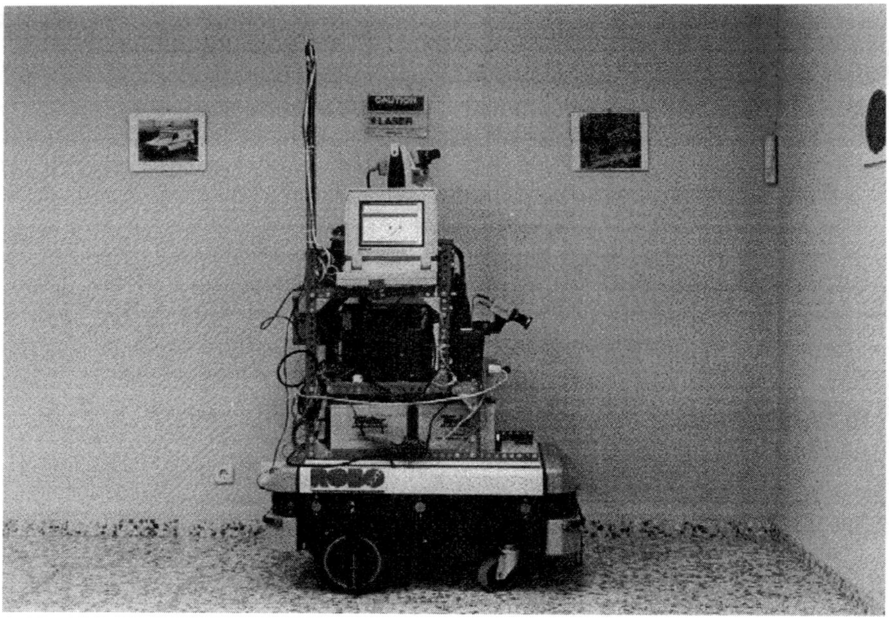

Figure 1. Landmarks in the room

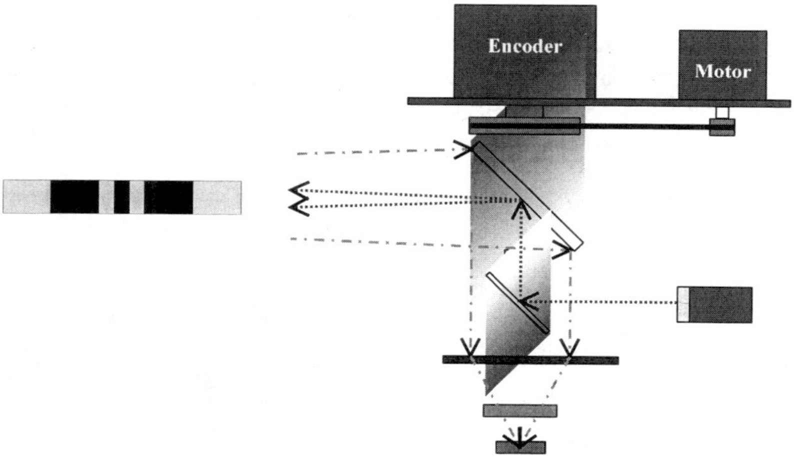

Figure 2. Laser navigation system

3. Localisation Methods

The core idea of localisation methods is to supply an estimation of robot position based on sensor information that is not *a priori* specifically designed for localisation purposes, but used as position estimators. The localisation methods are classified following two criteria: *spatial availability* and *time availability*. Figure 3 illustrates both classifications. The horizontal axis presents time availability from continuous to discrete. This means that the methods are classified following the frequency at which position estimation is possible. The vertical axis represents space availability, that is to say the area where the estimation is valid.

These notions are relative. The notion of time availability depends on the updating cycle of the whole mobile system and the notion of space depends on the dimension of the universe of the mobile platform. Four classifications could be defined: continuous, discrete, global and local.

A continuous localisation is a method able to provide the position at each updating cycle of the mobile system. That specific localisation mode is sometimes called on-line localisation because the estimation of the position is possible in real-time. On the contrary, a discrete localisation is a localisation that estimates the position at only some specific instances. We include here the methods that require haulting the robot motion.

Localisation methods can be classified into global and local methods. The first category provides absolute position, (also called *triangulation methods*). They make use of the same operating principle of triangulation devices. Local localisation systems provide the platform position relative to a subset of the universe. They provide a relative estimation with respect to a previous one.

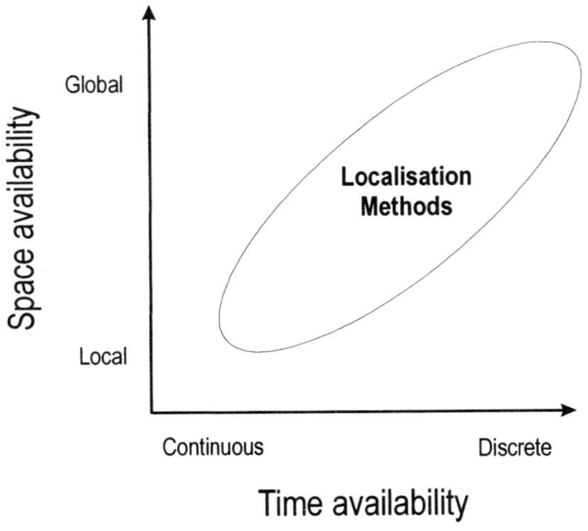

Figure 3. Classification of localisation methods

The previous classifications should also be used to classify the specific devices described. What is added in the methods described here is *a priori* knowledge –generally some kind of description of the environment– enabling a matching between different sources of information. The type of *a priori* knowledge required could also be a way to classify the methods.

Of course, co-operation between different kind of methods, in order to balance the limitations of each method, is possible. We will show some examples, as well as some experimental results.

3.1 Global Positioning Techniques

A global localisation system is characterised by the fact that there is no need to have *a priori* estimation of the platform position. The *a priori* knowledge required is the absolute position of some references (active or passive beacons that are also called landmarks for vision applications) into the environment. These methods are based on trilateration or triangulation techniques.

The trilateration technique estimates the platform position knowing the distance of the platform from the beacons. The common geometric trilateration technique applied in 2D space is illustrated in figure 4. Theoretically, the distances R_1, R_2 and R_3 from beacons B_1, B_2 and B_3 are enough to determine the absolute position *P*. The position *P* is the intersection of the three circles C_1, C_2 and C_3. That technique is transposable to the 3D space. An application example of that technique are the Global Positioning Systems (GPS).

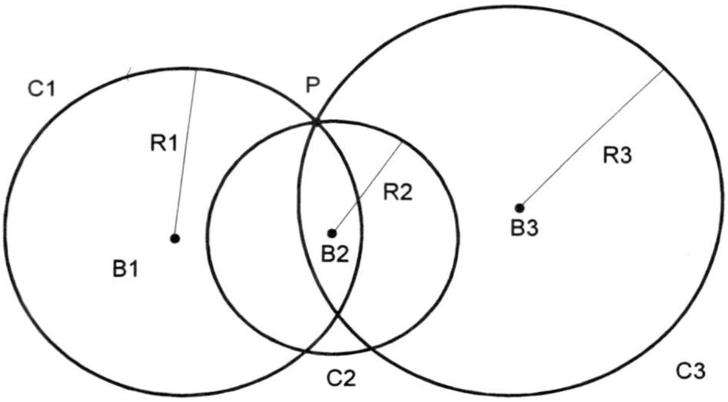

Figure 4. Triangulation from the distance for the platform to some beacons

A triangulation technique estimates the position of the platform knowing its orientation with the beacons. The common geometric triangulation technique in 2D space is described in figure 5. Theoretically, the angles θ_1, θ_2 between beacons B_1, B_2 and B_3 are enough to determine the absolute position *P*. The position *P* is the intersection of the circles C_1 and C_2, circles that constitute the constraint conditioned by the chords (B_1,B_2) ,(B_2,B_3) and the angles θ_1 and θ_2. An application example of that technique is a vision system that is able to localise the direction using some landmarks.

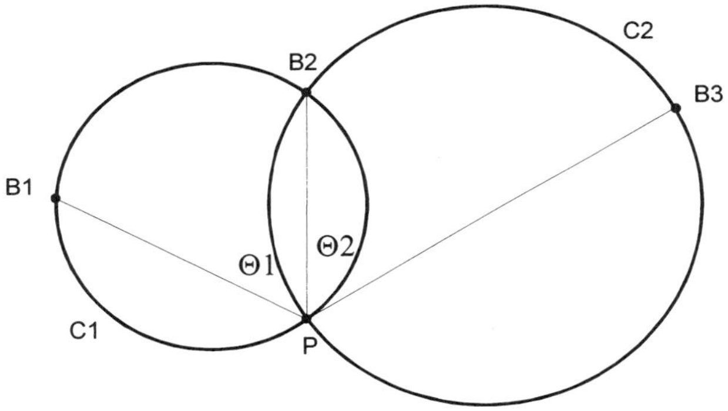

Figure 5. Triangulation from the direction of the platform with beacons

But before being able to apply both previous techniques, two problems have to be addressed: how to distinguish between different landmarks, and how to manage the excess information when more than three landmarks are present.

3.2 Incremental Localisation

In this case the *a priori* knowledge required is a previous estimation of the absolute position. This estimation may be obtained using the kinematic model of the vehicle. This information is not accurate due to the fact that physical characteristics are difficult to model, but may be used as an initial estimation. This *a priori* information is combined with incoming information from external devices (in this case measuring errors).

Both error sources may be compensated in the following way. First, the kinematic model predicts the position of the vehicle. Using sensor models, we can predict their measures at that position, and compare them with the incoming sensor data. Finally, if the difference between them is small, a Kalman filter, or, if the system is non-linear, the extended Kalman filter, may be used to estimate the new location as the estimated one is corrected proportionally to this error. The Kalman filter equations can be found in the previous chapter.

The Kalman filter performs a recursive integration of new information coming from the sensors of a system to estimate its state. An *a priori* knowledge about the system dynamics and noise characteristics is required.

The Kalman filter is based on the calculation of a weighted average of the system state. That weighted average is manipulated through covariance matrices which are a direct indication of the error of a variable. So there are three important covariance matrices in the Kalman filter that represent the *a priori* knowledge about it:

- the P matrix, that is the covariance matrix of the system state (i.e. the error of the state estimation),

- the R matrix, that is the covariance matrix of the sensors measurements (i.e. the noise of the sensors measurements),
- and the Q matrix, that is the covariance matrix of the system dynamics (i.e. the noise of the kinematic system).

In order to relate the Kalman filter with localisation systems, the system is defined as the mobile platform & the system's state as the robot configuration.

Figure 6 illustrates a general localisation module. From the geometric map, the sensors models & odometry, a sensor data prediction is produced. A matching between the prediction and the real sensor data sorts out the data for the estimation of the platform position.

Location estimation with different sensors have in common the *a priori* knowledge characterised by the *P* matrices, that indicate the error of the platform position, and *Q*, that indicates the noise of the odometric system. A matrix *R* represents the noise of each sensor system. In that way, an estimation of the position can be realised by all the different sensors. The next section is going to stress the link between the methods realised through matrix *P* and explains how to integrate heterogeneous sensors into the localisation module.

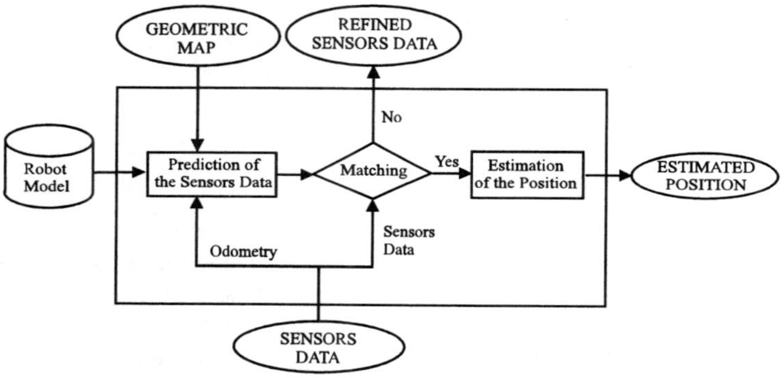

Figure 6. Localisation Module

4. Implementation Examples

4.1 Continuous methods

In these methods, the localisation algorithm is computed at each cycle. This means that accumulative errors are not present. Examples of sensors that may be used are ultrasonic, active vision systems and rotating lasers. As mentioned above, in the category of the relative localisation methods, a dead reckoning method gives an initial estimation of the position.

But, to reduce the accumulation of the uncertainty due to that technology, different sensors may be used.

A first method realises a matching between the information coming from ultrasonic sensors and a modelling of that type of sensors. Here we usually speak of local methods, because, first, it is not easy to calculate the absolute position from the information they supply, and second, sensor accuracy is not high enough for absolute positioning. An ultrasonic sensor measures the time needed for an ultrasonic pulse emitted by the sensor to come back due to a reflection on an object. That time is converted into a distance representing the distance of the closest object detected by the sensor. Because of the spherical divergence of the sound, an ultrasonic sensor is usually modelled by a beam of a conical shape.

In order to predict the distance given by an ultrasonic sensor, we utilize a world model placed with the sensor model. Figure 7 illustrates the concept. Now, the robot localisation is performed by finding the position of the robot that performs the best matching with the value given by the real sensor.

Another method uses the same kind of matching by an infrared laser system. The active vision system is composed of a source that emits a laser beam parallel to the ground in front of the mobile platform, and a camera with a special filter that is able to detect laser infrared light. Hence, the camera image displays lines drawn by the laser beam on the obstacles detected.

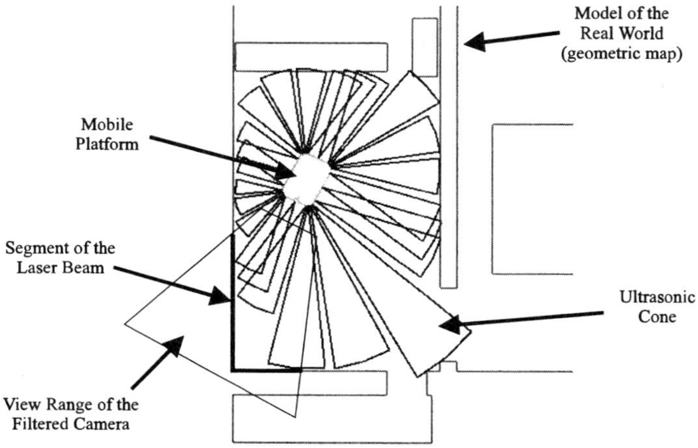

Figure 7. Sonars and Active vision Modelling

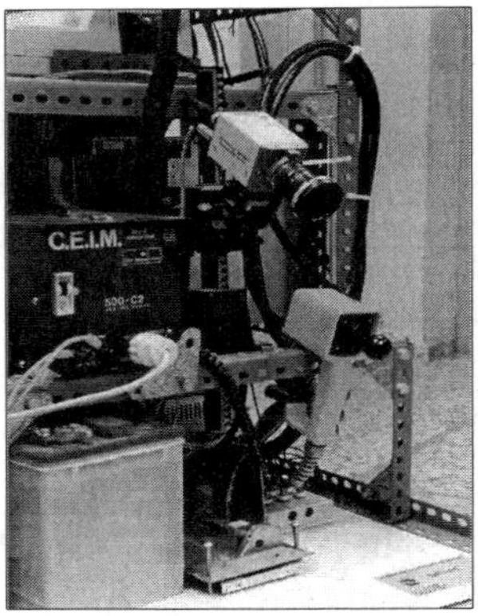

Figure 8. Infrared laser and b&w camera

To model the information given by such a system, the idea is to determine the zone seen by the camera into the model of the real world. The field of view is too small to implement an absolute positioning system. The segments (determined by the shape of the obstacles) in that zone are extracted (see figure 7). The localisation step here has to achieve the best matching between the segments extracted by the model and the lines seen by the camera, therefore estimating a position for the sensor model, i.e. a position for the mobile platform.

In the case of the rotating laser, both global and local methods may be applied. By using landmarks independently, they are distinguished using the initial position estimation (local method). In this case, measures may be integrated recursively using the Kalman filter. By using at least three landmarks, a global localisation system can be realized.

Another method inspired by map-based positioning is an approach in which the robot uses a laser range finder to create a map of its local environment. This local map is then compared to a map previously stored in memory. The sensor is a rotating laser scanner mounted 120 cm. above ground on the mobile robot. Although the laser scans a sector of 180 degrees, it provides 360 range measurements (one measurement/0.5°), stored in a PC. In order to have a complete 3D data set the laser has been mounted vertically, rather than the standard horizontal position, on a rotating platform. As a result, each data acquisition, providing a *vertical slice* of the environment (a scan from the ceiling to the floor), can be syncronised with the rotating platform and robot movements with great accuracy. In these tests, it has been decided to produce 60 different vertical slices, one every 6 degrees.

With this approach a 3D set of data from the sensor is obtained. Hence, it is possible to obtain the same dynamic and static features for both the latest and the previous maps. Then, the *Range Weighted Hough Transform* (RWHT), so far used for feature extraction with traditional 2D data in non dynamic situations, is used here for the first time with a 3D set of data in order to handle dynamic situations. Finally, the system is able to detect free corridors where the robot can move in order to reach the final target.

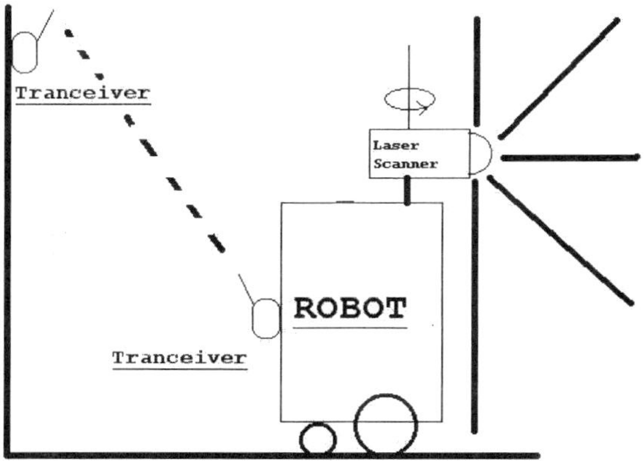

Figure 9. Raser Range Finder

Figures 10 and 11 show respectively a typical 3-D set of data and a single vertical slice. In particular, each vertical scan has been partitioned as *upper wall* and *lower wall*. In this way, it is possible to select only a stripe nearby the ceiling (i.e. the *upper wall* section), where it is unlikely that any change has occurred since the previous complete 3D scan, giving a *static* map. The *lower wall* section can be defined by excluding the data corresponding to the floor, the ceiling and the *upper wall* sectors for a *dynamic* map.

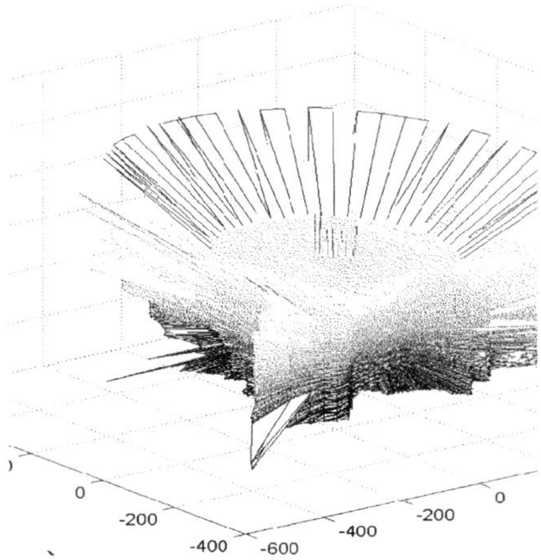

Figure 10. Example of a room 3D laser scan

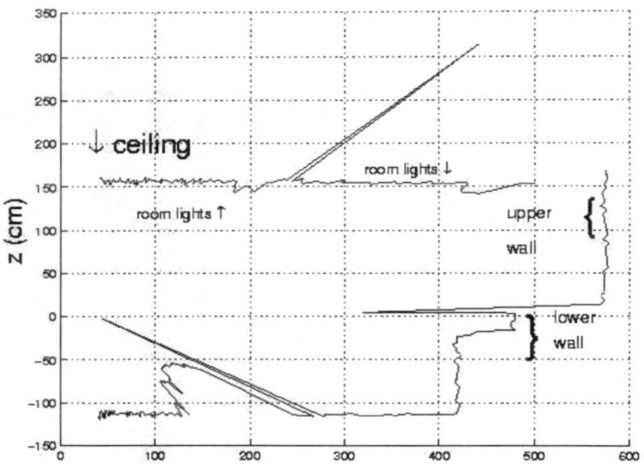

Figure 11. Example of a vertical laser scan

4.2 Discrete Methods

In these methods, the position of the platform given by the odometry system is improved only at specific moments. In the first approach that we are going to present, the landmarks are artificial, and have been designed so that they are easy to identify. In the experiment being described, they are a red circle with a radius of 10 cm into a white square of 25 cm (see figure 13), and the robot is equipped with a conventional colour CCD camera with pan and tilt movements.

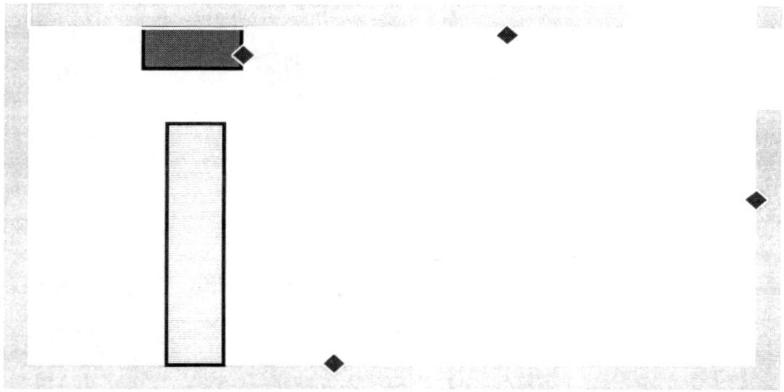

Figure 12. Reflectant beacons position

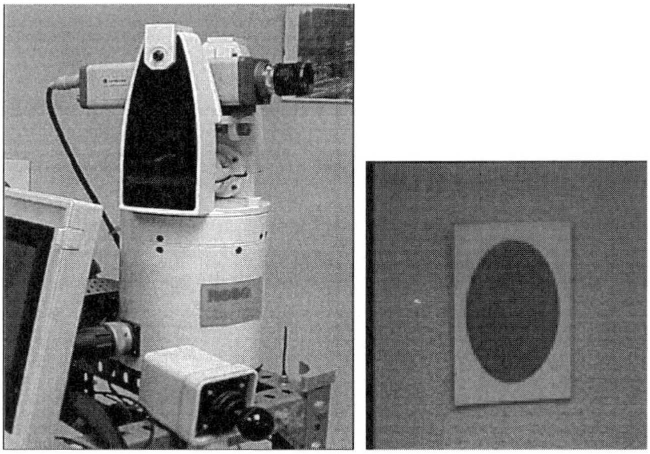

Figure13. Pan and tilt camera and artificial landmark

Based on: i) the prediction of the mobile robot position produced by the odometric system, and ii) the fixed position of the passive landmarks, the mobile camera performs a search in the environment for landmarks on specific points. If a landmark is found, the exact angle between the mobile camera and the concerned landmark is extracted from the position of the landmark within the image of the camera. Finally, a triangulation estimation calculates the estimated position of the mobile robot. The localisation can be done by triangulation with three landmarks, but also with one landmark if the robot is moving.

The algorithm for the first case, which corresponds to the discrete case, has several steps. First of all, the mobile tower supporting the colour camera is positioned using coordinates (Y_l, P_l). Then, with the colour image of the mobile system, (dY, dP) the deviation of the landmark from the image centre, has to be estimated to adjust the previous direction evaluation.

The image processing consists of both segmentation and featuring operations. Colour identification is realised with a three component threshold operator that allows discrimination of quite good accuracy for red pixels. After this, the presence of the landmark is confirmed with the projected histograms, *Hu* and *Hv* of the image respectively onto the u and v axes of the image. Due to their disposition in the environment, only one landmark is visible in the image. So, the landmark can be identified as the greatest peaks of the histograms. The co-ordinates (u_l, v_l) of the landmark centre are defined as the centres of gravity of the greatest peak in the histograms *Hu* and *Hv* respectively. Then, the directional shifts (dY, dP) are estimated with the calibration matrix of the camera:

$$dY = \text{atan}((u_l - u_c).du/f)$$
$$dP = \text{atan}((v_l - v_c).dv/f)$$

where (du,dv) are the dimensions of a pixel, (u_C,v_C) the optical centre and f the focal distance.

The use of an *omni-directional vision sensor* is another example of discrete localization method. This allows the use of the global positioning method that gives an answer to the problem of the narrowness of field of view in conventional cameras. A panoramic mirror, like spherical or hyperbolic mirrors is placed, in front of the camera. In this way, the image provides a global vision of the environment allowing the observation of 360 degrees with only one image.

Recent applications with this kind of device have underlined its efficiency facing the problems of remote surveillance, teleoperation, navigation or environment modelling. Here we propose to use it for localisation. The omni-directional vision system proposed in our experimentation is a mini black and white looking-up CCD camera. In front of the camera, a spherical mirror is placed, centred on the optical axis of the camera (figure 14). The light rays are reflected on the mirror before reaching the camera.

The localisation method we are dealing with is an absolute localisation based on a triangulation technique. As already stated above, usual triangulation techniques need to know *a priori* the absolute position of the whole set of landmarks. The vision system has to provide the direction of the landmarks, yaw-pitch coordinates (Y_l,P_l), relative to the robot. If at least three landmarks are identified, the triangulation method is able to estimate the platform position. The landmarks could be specific landmarks put into the environment (artificial landmarks), or landmarks already existing in the environment (natural landmarks).

In this way, the localisation task could be realised in two phases. The first phase is a rough-seeking in the environment of what could be a landmark. The second one is a confirmation of the landmark presence and the determination of its exact direction. Finally, a triangulation method may be used to determine the platform position. In order to be efficient, the localisation method has to be able to recognise most possible landmarks and provide their relative direction with accuracy.

The image processing performs a segmentation of a black and white image to extract the objects supposed to be landmarks. Figure 15 gives an example of the images that are obtained by the omni-directional camera. The useful information is the information provided by the reflection on the spherical mirror. In the example, the information is represented by the pixels contained in the middle band of the circle. The first phase of the method performs a search of landmarks in the useful zone of the image.

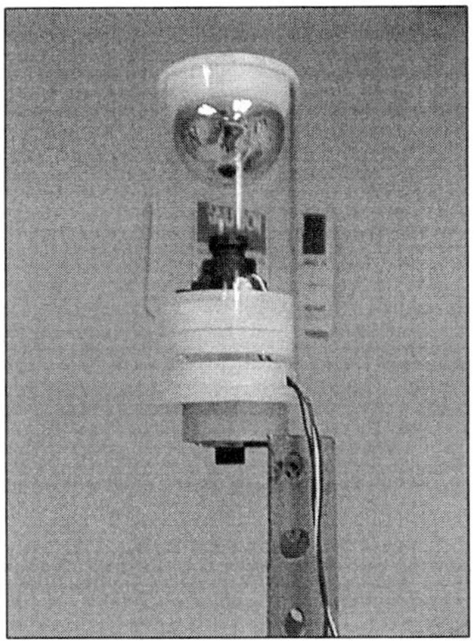

Figure 14. The omni-directional camera

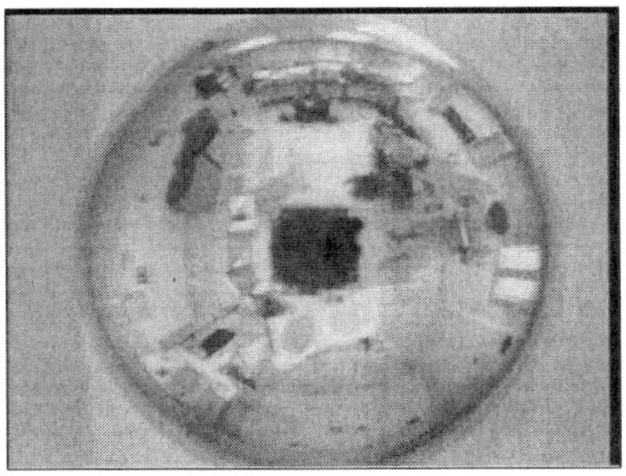

Figure 15. Image from the omni-directional camera

Due to the landmarks nature, the object attributes that we are seeking for are *red* and *elliptical* (perspective view of a circle). From the estimation of the greyscale Equ_{RED} equivalent level of the B&W image of the color reference (R,G,B) of the landmarks, a threshold operator T computes a binary image allowing to identify the first characteristic that is "objects with the colour of the landmarks". The next equation illustrates the digitisation of the image:

$$Equ_{RED} = 0.299\,R + 0.587\,G + 0.114\,B$$

$$T(px) = 1 \quad \text{if } Equ_{RED} - \Delta p < px < Equ_{RED} + \Delta p$$

otherwise

px being the pixel value and *Δp* a tolerance

It is obvious that not only the red objects are extracted due to the non-bijective operation of greyscale equivalent colours. So, after the labelling of the image to distinguish the objects, a featuring operator is used to distinguish the objects according to their geometric characteristics.

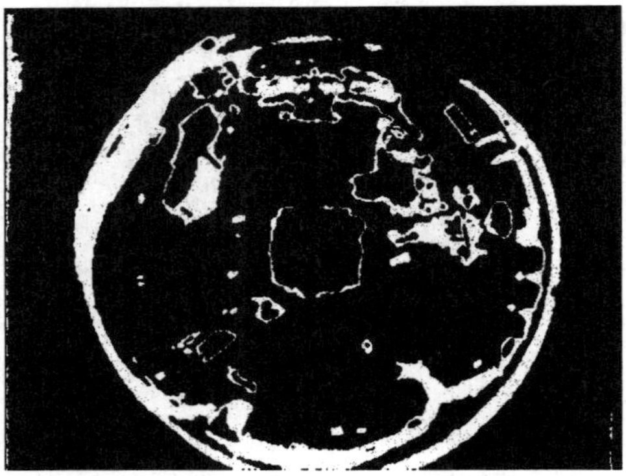

Figure 16. Umbralisation

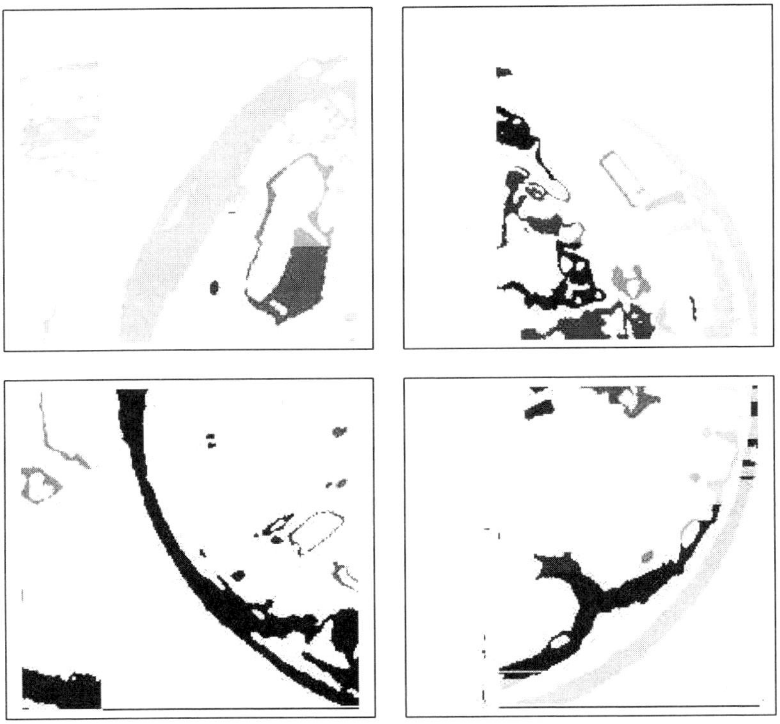

Figure 17. Labelling

In the omni-directional image, the landmarks are pseudo-ellipses because of the distortions and aberrations induced by the mirror. As a first approach, the compactness descriptor *(perimeter)²/area* is used to discriminate the objects.

After identifying the landmark candidates (*see* Figure 18), the centre of gravity of the selected objects gives the position (u,v) of the supposed landmarks into the image. To estimate the direction (yaw-pitch (Y,P)) of each landmark relative to the mobile robot, a model of the optic system is needed. By using this model, the yaw-pitch coordinates (Y_l,P_l) provided by the first step of the method constitute some hypotheses about the landmarks positions.

4.3 Co-operative Methods

The previous section exposed several typical methods of localisation. But the performance of a robot localisation system lies in its ability to integrate the different techniques in a unique framework. Along this chapter, work is focussed in indoor environments, where passive artificial landmarks may be set out. A lot of methods provide a solution making use of an incremental and recursive updating method matching the sensor measures and their models.

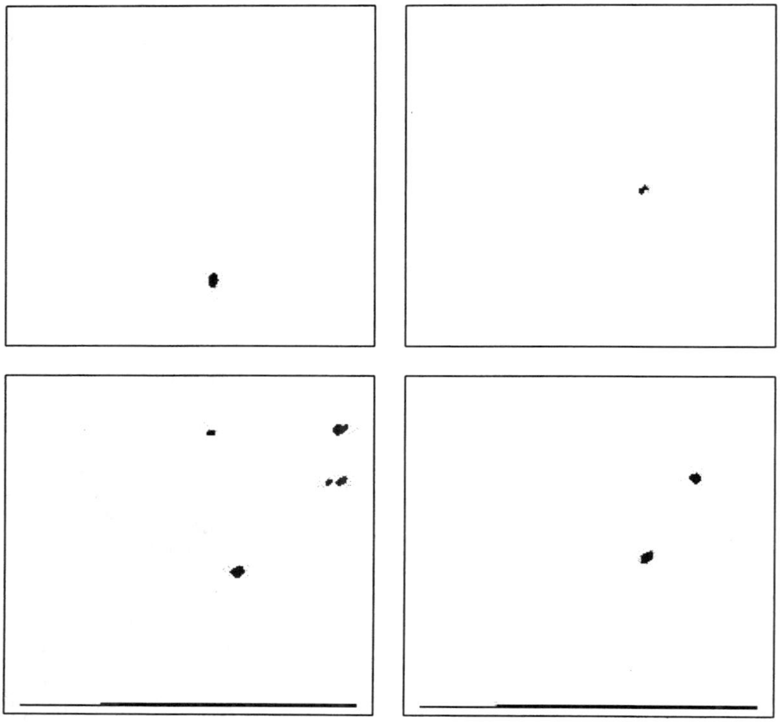

Figure 18. Landmarks Identification

We know that the on-line methods, i.e. ultrasonic and laser methods, make use of a Kalman filter and can share the same statistical resources that are the matrices P and Q. In fact, matrix Q is fixed because it corresponds to the noise of the odometric system. Matrix P is updated at each step by the Kalman filter. The methods collaborate since if one of the methods is not able to localise the mobile platform, i.e. to reduce the matrix P, perhaps the other could to do it.

If both of the previous methods are not able to localise the mobile platform, the P matrix elements increase. A criterion must be specified to use each technique at each moment. The first method proposed here is a co-operation between a continuous and a discrete method (the active vision system and the colour pan and tilt camera).

Suppose that, as stated above, the robot is moving along a room (*see* Figure 19). While a wall (or obstacle defined in the *a priori* map) is close to the front of the robot, the laser system is able to obtain visible segments for localisation. But when the robot is moving in an open area (far to the wall), the laser system is unable to update the position estimation, and so the P matrix increases, this means, the uncertainty increases (the figure represents with ellipses the uncertainty in the position).

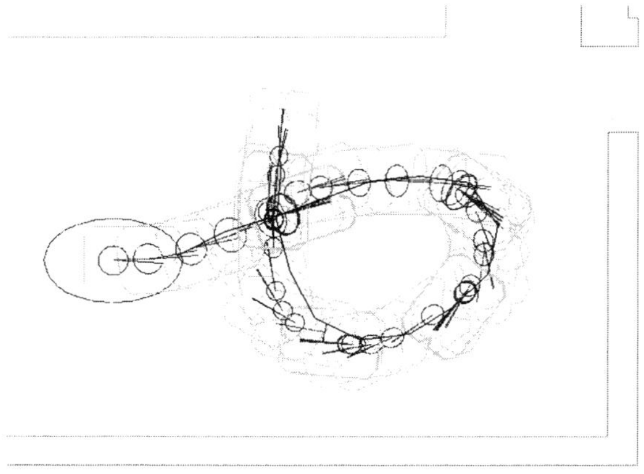

Figure 19. Cooperation between infrared laser and color camera

Here the landmark method intervenes. If a threshold of the acceptable error of the position is crossed, the landmark method stops the platform and performs a localisation algorithm. Once the localisation with landmarks has been completed, matrix P is initialised to a bounded value due to the error of the landmark method. The other methods may start computing an estimation of the mobile robot position based on the latest results.

The main drawback of any relative localisation lies in the fact that a quite accurate initial estimation of the robot position is necessary to start the method. In the previous example, the landmark method is unable to work if it doesn't have a previous estimation of the position. Without it, the camera is unable to find the landmarks. A method could be designed to allow the robot localise itself without that constraint. This may be an absolute localisation method based on two vision systems: a mobile camera and an omni-directional camera. The co-operation between both systems allows to overcome their individual limitations.

The idea of a co-operative system is supported by the advantages of each individual system that is, in one hand, the global vision ability of the omni-directional system and, on the other hand, the precision of the mobile system. In this way, the omni-camera may be employed using a global localisation method as a first approximation, and then the pan and tilt camera, to confirm the presence of each landmark and to provide an accurate localisation. Finally, a triangulation method determines the platform position.

5. Conclusions

This chapter has presented some guidelines for the implementation of a localisation module integrated into a perception system, by using multisensor fusion. The efficiency of the collaboration of different integrated methods of localisation has been stressed. It appears that the main advantage of such a localisation system lies in its ability to integrate heterogeneous sensor information and so to be configurable depending on the environment. Furthermore, the manoeuvrability of the kinematic system also affects the odometry system accuracy, and the way in which the environment is defined. It plays an important role in the selection of the sensors to equip the mobile robot. Some conclusions may be extracted from the section on future developments. To realise the experimentation, we have used an experimental mobile system that is shown in the Figure 20.

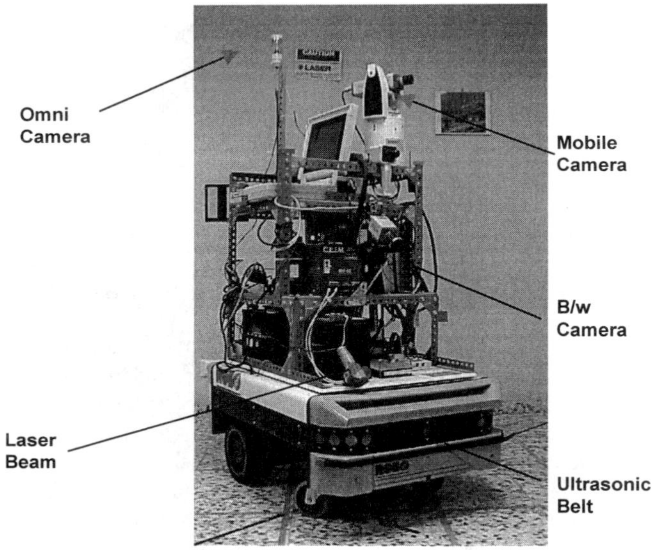

Figure 20. ROBUTER Mobile Platform

The mobile platform has a belt of twenty-four ultrasonic sensors, a laser beam system, a mobile camera and an omni-directional camera. For the laser navigation system, we have a MRV-4 robot from Denning-Branch Int. Robotics (*see* Figure 21).

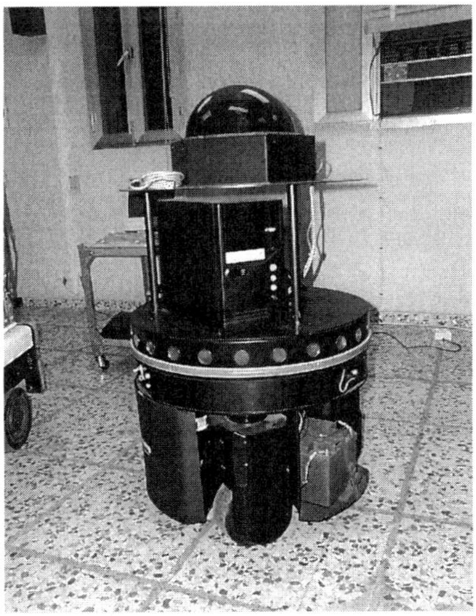

Figure 21. MRV-4 Mobile Platform

With those devices, and following the implementation of the integrated localisation framework, various experiments were realised, in which the robustness and accuracy of the localisation methods were assessed.

In the zones of the environment relatively free of unknown obstacles, the ultrasonic and laser methods are able to localise the mobile robot. More precisely, the ultrasonic system ensures continuously a rough localisation that is reinforced by the laser system at some dedicated moments. If the platform manoeuvres in a zone of the environment full of unknown obstacles, both of the previous methods are not able to localise the mobile robot. After a period of time the accuracy threshold is reached and the landmark method causes a pause of the robot motion in order to perform error correction.

It appears that the localisation with the ultrasonic system is a very robust technique. Due to the geometric characteristics of the ultrasonic belt, the platform is frequently able to detect around it a known pattern of the environment to ensure localisation. The problem of this method is its accuracy. Because of the measurement principle, the method is sensitive to second order echos, especially when the obstacle (the environment feature observed) is not exactly parallel to the sensor. In fact, the best results of that localisation technique are obtained when the mobile platform follows a wall.

The localisation with the active vision system is very accurate in spite of some limitations. The accuracy is limited in particular by optical distortions and image digitisation. But, if the detected pattern of the known environment is close to the platform, accuracy is quasi-perfect, i.e. about the millimetre. The problem of this method is its low robustness. There are two cases in which that sensor system is unable to provide information. Firstly when the camera looks at a free space zone (because no segment is seen in the image). Secondly when there is an unknown obstacle in front of the platform (because no segment is matched). In fact, due to the narrow view range of the camera of the laser system, these cases occur frequently.

Regarding the rotatory laser navigation system, it has good accuracy and reliability. Figure 22 represents the medium values and variances of the detected landmarks angle.

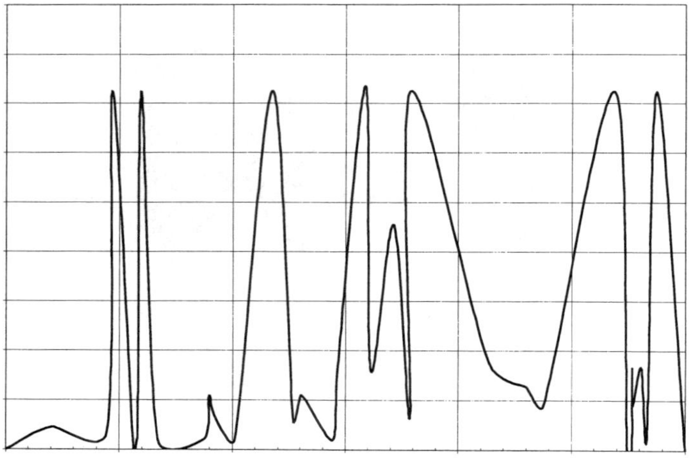

Figure 22. Histogram from laser navigation system

The sensor has its worst performance at -135° & +135°. This may be explained given that in these cases, a metal piece that supports the encoder blocks the field of view. Similarly, the position obtained after localisation has been analysed at different robot locations to calculate medium values and variances. In all cases, the standard deviation has been about 10^{-4}. These values have always been less in orientation than in position.

Furthermore, when the robot approaches too much the walls, the measured values have a lower accuracy. Anyway, the estimated position was never over 3 cm. During the tests, the sensor accuracy is not affected by the fact that the robot is moving.

The landmark method is a robust method. It is able to ensure a localisation despite of unknown obstacles, if the landmarks are not hidden. That last restriction is avoided introducing more landmarks in the environment. The accuracy of that method is quite good and depends on the proximity of the landmarks and of the angle between the camera and the landmarks. The advantage of such system lies in its ability to provide a quite accurate position of the landmarks.

The accuracy is only limited by the pan and tilt system that positions the camera and the digitisation of the image where the landmarks are searched. Such a mobile camera system has to assume a strong constraint due to the narrowness of the field of view. That spread can be about 10 degrees. So if the *a priori* estimation of the robot position is not accurate enough, the system will not locate any landmarks. A subsequent procedure looking for landmarks by arbitrarily moving the camera by the first estimation could conclude consumption of time before any reliable has happened. An immediate solution to compensate that restriction could be to add a remote-controlled zooming system on the camera. But the problem remains insoluble when the robot is completely lost.

As stated above, the accuracy of the landmark's localisation depends on the accuracy delivered by the mobile system. This accuracy sums the error on the landmarks localisation into the colour image and the error on the command of the mobile tower position. The error on the image comes from the digitisation of the image and is estimated by the equations:

$$dy = du/f$$
$$dp = dv/f$$

with (du, dv) the dimensions of a pixel and f the focal distance

The error on the command of the mobile tower position comes from the steps of the motors that ensure the positioning. The error is estimated with the equations:

$$dy = Ny.Ay$$
$$dp = Np.Ap$$

(Ny,Np) and (Ay,Ap) being the number of steps and aperture angles of the yaw and pitch motors, respectively.

In practice, the respective yaw-pitch errors on the image are (0.018°, 0.013°) and on the tower positioning (0.014°, 0.014°). These values are now acceptable for the geometric triangulation method facing the required position accuracy. Due to the fact that the main constraint of this method is that the mobile robot has to be stopped, a good idea is to combine it with any of the previous methods that do not need to do so. This constraint leads to use of the method only for extreme situations when the other methods are not able to localise the robot.

In the omni-directional camera system, the method had to corporate several limitations especially those coming from the optical aberrations of the mirror reflection. Therefore, although such a sensor has low resolution compared to the resolution delivered by the multiple cameras system that would provide similar field of view (one has to use several co-centrically placed cameras to achieve 360^0 coverage), it is very efficient in co-operation with the previous mobile system. With this sensor, the accuracy of an object localisation from its image is not uniform. This phenomenon is due to the distortions and aberrations induced by the optical devices and especially by the mirror reflection. Though, the accuracy can be characterised by (Dy, Dp), the errors on the yaw and pitch measurements respectively. In fact, the imprecision of the calculation comes from the digitisation of the image and can be evaluated from the two following statements:

- the closest the object we want to localise is situated close to the centre of the circular image of the mirror, the more imprecise is the calculation of Y,
- the closest the object we want to localise is situated close to the circumference of the circular image of the mirror, the more inaccurate is the calculation of P.

The estimation of *Dy* on the image gives a result of 0.77^o and an error of one or two pixels could be made with the detection of the landmark into the image. So, the whole imprecision could be 2.31^o. The repercussion of this imprecision on the position is not easy to evaluate because of the non-linear property of that repercussion. But the result is unacceptable by the triangulation method with respect to the accuracy required by our system. In fact, depending on the landmarks configurations and the robot position with respect to that configuration, the imprecision of the estimation of the robot position could be greater than the few centimetres of the cells width tolerated by the data fusion (see the introduction remark). So, in the proposed application, the first estimation of the landmark direction it is sufficient to provide a command of position where the mobile camera is supposed to see a landmark.

This positioning command does not only have to support the omni-directional errors (*Dy,Dp*). Another factor of imprecision is the shift of the relative positions of the vision systems. The sum of these inaccuracies induces a global error of few degrees on the mobile camera position. Anyway, such a global error does not interfere in practice with the good results of co-operation. This is due to the spread of the field of view of the mobile camera of 10° that allows it to see the landmark in spite of the error on the mobile camera position.

As a conclusion of this co-operation method, its efficiency is emphasised and it has been shown that the relative imprecision introduced by the omni-directional system does not necessarily affect negatively the results of the method. It is obvious that the detection methods used here are simple and fault detection is performed, especially with the omni-directional images. But, this constitutes a first approach and more robust methods could be considered later.

As regards the Laser Range Finder, there are various basic types of uncertainty associated to this method. The range measurements from the sensors are noisy and contain large spurious errors. Figure 23 shows the map of the room using only the *upper wall* and *lower wall* sections and it is possible to distinguish the four walls (A, B, C, D). It is clear how, the noise at ground level (i.e. *lower wall* section), such as shelves (walls B and C), obstacles (corner between walls A and B or corner between walls C and A), cupboards (walls C), windows (walls A) and a desk in the middle of the room, can affect the measurements. The robot is positioned in (0,0). Values, in the X, Y-axis, are in centimetres and indicate the distance given by the laser scan.

The RWHT is then applied to both the *upper wall* and *lower wall* sections to obtain a robust and noiseless range of measurements of the environment from each vertical slice (i.e. *UpperData* and *LowerData* respectively). In this way, horizontal 2D layouts of the environment at two different heights (i.e. at approximately ceiling and floor level), with each layout equivalent to a complete *standard* laser scan of the environment, have been obtained with two further advantages. Firstly, each range measurement is noiseless, that is the spurious measurements (e.g. false or missing readings), due to poor sensor performance, have been eliminated with the RWHT method with little computational complexity. Hence, each measurement is giving the *correct* distance between the robot and a flat surface associated to that vertical slice. In figure 24 *UpperData* and *LowerData* are overlapped with the map of the room.

Secondly, the use of two different 2D layouts allows the system to solve the uncertainty in the origin of the measurements (i.e. did the measurement originate from a known feature or is it a new feature or spurious data?). Indeed, the layout at ceiling level is only giving data associated to static objects. In this way, it is possible to extract dynamic changes in the lowest layout

At this point, the RWHT is applied again to *UpperData* and *LowerData* respectively to extract the flat surfaces. In particular, with *UpperData*, walls are detected whereas, with *LowerData*, both horizontal and vertical surfaces (such as tables or walls) are extracted. Figure 25 shows the RWHT histogram for the *UpperData*. The X and Y-axis indicate respectively the orientation and the perpendicular distance from the robot associated with a given flat surface. The first four groups of highest peaks give the desired information about the four room walls. Figure 26 shows the same histogram in two dimensions (i.e. without the Y axis). Figures 27 is similar to figure 26 except that *LowerData* is used instead of *UpperData*.

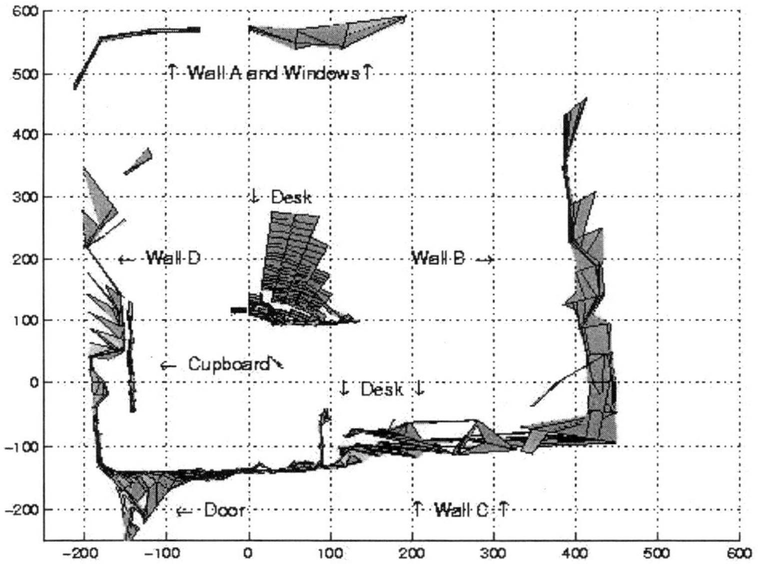

Figure 23. Map of the room using the Lower and Upper sections

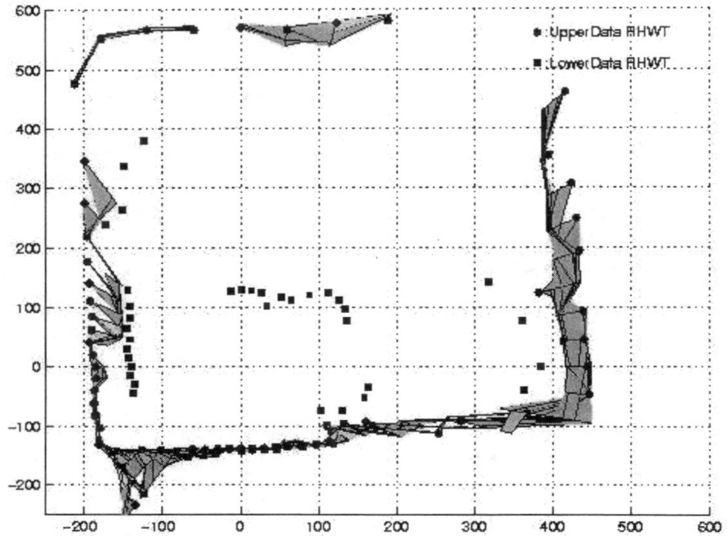

Figure 24. The map and the values extracted from each vertical scan for the Upper and Lower sections (each value has been indicated as a dot)

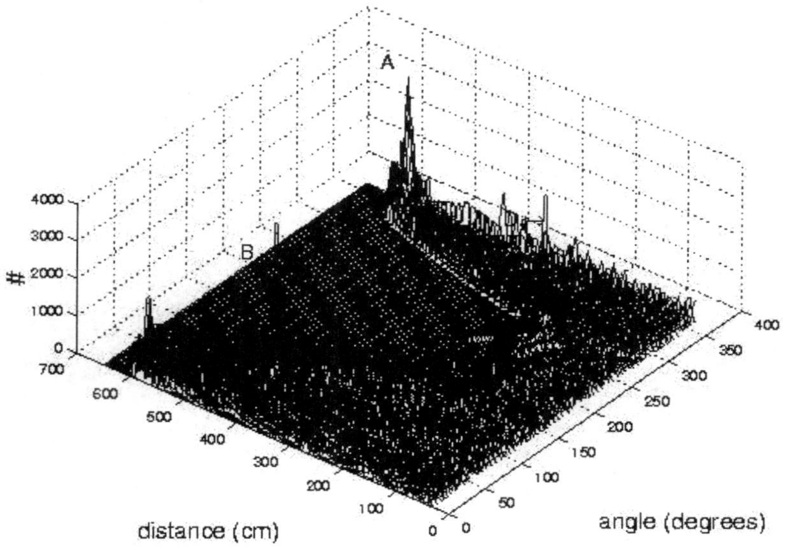

Figure 25. RHWT Histogram for Upper Section. The highest peaks give the direction and orientation associated with a flat surface (i.e. a wall)

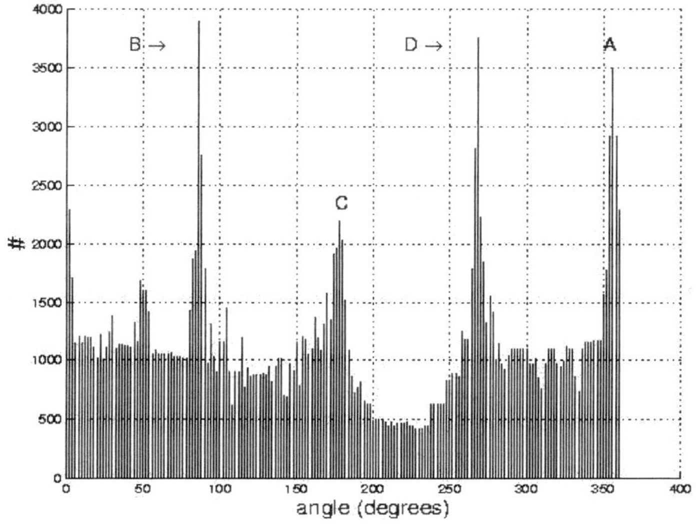

Figure 26. RWHT histogram for Upper section. Projection of figure 25 along the distance axis

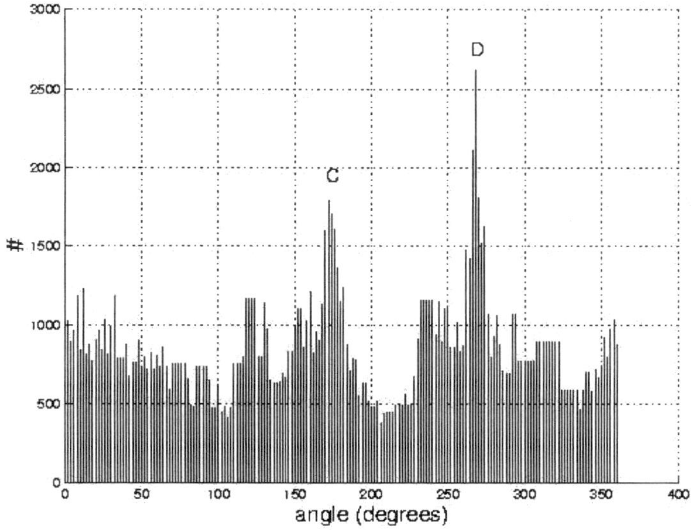

Figure 27. RWHT histogram for Lower section. This is similar to Figure 25 but for Lower section

Comparing figures 26 with 27 it is possible to note how in figure 26 (and then with *UpperData*) the four walls can be detected contrary to figure 27 (and consequently with *LowerData*) where, the presence of objects or dynamic changes in the environment obstructs the wall detection.

Once the walls have been detected, it is possible to calculate the movement relative to latest checked position and obtain the new position comparing the latest static map with the previous static map (obtained in a similar way but in a previous moment). The first step is to establish a correspondence between the latest static RHWT histogram obtained and the previous static RHWT histogram. Figure 28 shows an example when two consecutive maps have been obtained with a robot rotation of 8 degrees anti-clockwise with no translation after the data relative to the first map have been collected. Figure 28 shows in the same graph both RHWT histograms relative to the two different instants in a 2D format (without the distance component), with a resolution of 2 degrees for *UpperData*. As showed in figure 28, comparing the two RHWT histograms relative to the *UpperData*, it is possible to extract the four walls as the highest peaks. The shift between the two histograms is equal to 6 degrees. Figure 29 is similar to figure 28 with the difference that *LowerData* has been used instead of *UpperData*.

A comparison between figures 28 and 29 shows the great advantage of using a static map in this step. Indeed, In figure 28 it is easy to associate for each wall the corresponding peak in each histogram and consequently compute both the distance and angle shifts.

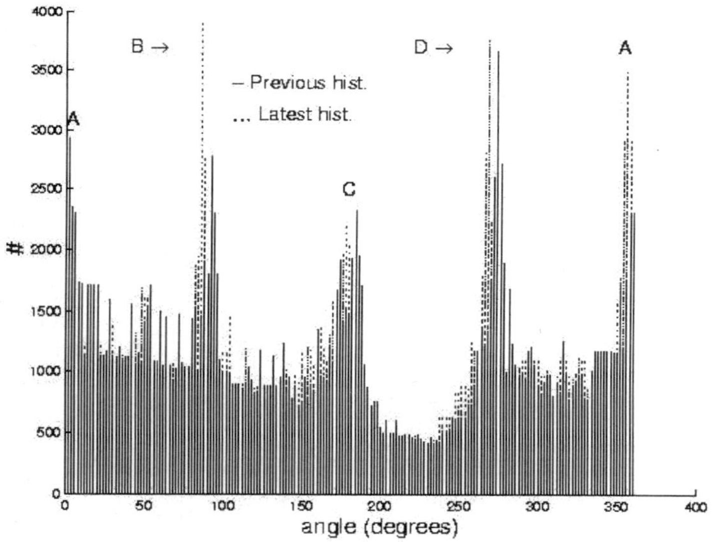

Figure 28. Comparing two different histograms for the Upper Section. In this graph two histograms obtained in two different moment have been overlapped

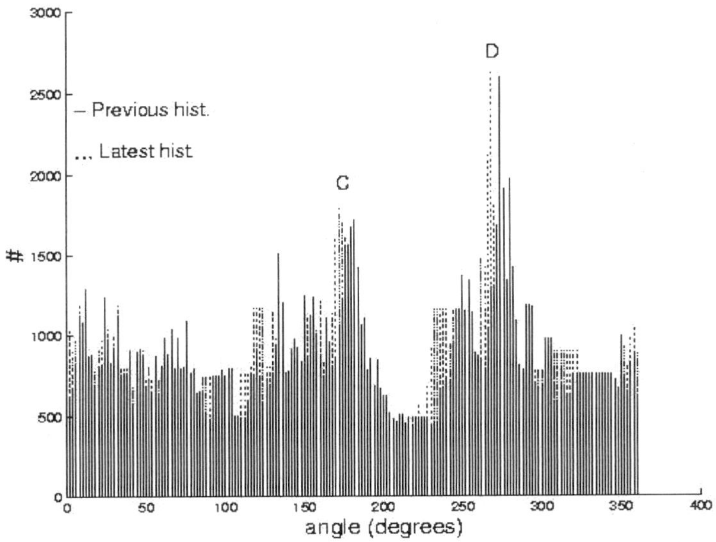

Figure 29. Comparing two different histograms for the Lower Section. In this graph wo histograms obtained in two different moment have been overlapped

Finally, the authors would like to remind that the purpose of the perception module is not just to estimate the position of the robot. Its matching and integration of the information provide a sorting out of the information intended to the next two steps of the perception module that are rough mapping and refined mapping. The rough mapping issue makes use of the integrated information to provide a safety modelling of the environment. The refined mapping issue exploits the information rejected by the matching to update a static modelling of the environment (next chapter focuses in these aspects).

6. References

[1] B. K. P. Horn, *Robot Vision,* MIT Press, 1986.
[2] F. Wawak, N. Katevas and F. Matía, Co-operation between Omni-Directional Camera and Mobile Camera for the Localisation of a Mobile Platform, *SIRS'99,* Portugal (1999).
[3] H. F. Durrant-Whyte, Integration, *Coordination and Control of Multi-Sensor Robot Systems,* Kluwer Academic Publishers, 1988.
[4] H. R. Everett, *Sensors for Mobile Robots: Theory and Application,* A.K. Peters, Ltd., Wellesley, 1995.
[5] J. Borenstein, H. R. Everett and L. Feng, Where am I?, *Sensors and Methods for Autonomous Mobile Robot Positioning*. University of Michigan, 1996.

[6] P. Maybeck, The Kalman Filter: An Introduction to Concepts, *IEEE International Workshop on Intelligent Robots and Systems,* (1991), pp.194-204.
[7] R. C. Luo, M. G. Kay, Multisensor Integration and Fusion in Intelligent Systems, *IEEE Transactions on Systems, Man, and Cybernetics* Vol.19, (1989), pp.901-931.
[8] U. Larsson, J. Forsberg and A. Wernersson, Mobile Robot Localization: Integrating Measurements from a Time-of-Flight Laser, *IEEE Transactions on Industrial Electronics* 43 (1996) 422-431.

Chapter 15

Workspace Mapping for Mobile Robots

by Fernando MATÍA, Nikos KATEVAS, Cedric PEIGNOT

Mobile Robotics in Healthcare
N. Katevas (Ed.)
IOS Press, 2001

Chapter 15

Workspace Mapping for Mobile Robots

Fernando MATÍA, Nikos KATEVAS, Cedric PEIGNOT

1. Perception and Planning under Uncertainty

Figure 1 shows the perception framework already described in previous chapters. This framework is intended for sensor fusion, for localisation and mapping purposes. Regarding the latter, four boxes within the figure are related with: *environment models*, *local mapping*, *global mapping* and *geometric information updating*.

The *environment model* is a 2D map that contains information about the world in which the robot is operating. Three main mapping techniques exist: geometric maps, occupancy grids and certainty trees. In the first case, walls, doors and obstacles are represented by polygons. In the second, a grid with fixed sized cells models the same objects with a free or occupied value stored in each cell. In the last case, the grid cells have variable size in a tree structure.

Sensor values may be used to construct local maps, after a simplified data filtering, e.g. thresholding. The instantaneous maps are updated as soon as new sensor information is available. They are not correlated to their past instances therefore the new sensor data are applied directly to the local maps. This information is used mainly for obstacle avoidance. This is similar to the use of proximity raw sensor data, but the difference is that the noise and other sporadic errors are being filtered by the map update process.

After the matching process, erroneous sensor data is rejected by the Kalman filter. This means that, in the building process of a local map, erroneous data are eliminated. These maps must be updated in lower rates compared to the previous ones, since in these cases the aim is not to react to obstacles, but to elaborate a precise map of the environment. The local map may be easily integrated on-line with the environment model. This is what we call a global model and that could be used for global path planning (*see also* Chapter 8).

All these maps, local and global, may be elaborated with any of the above mentioned mapping techniques.

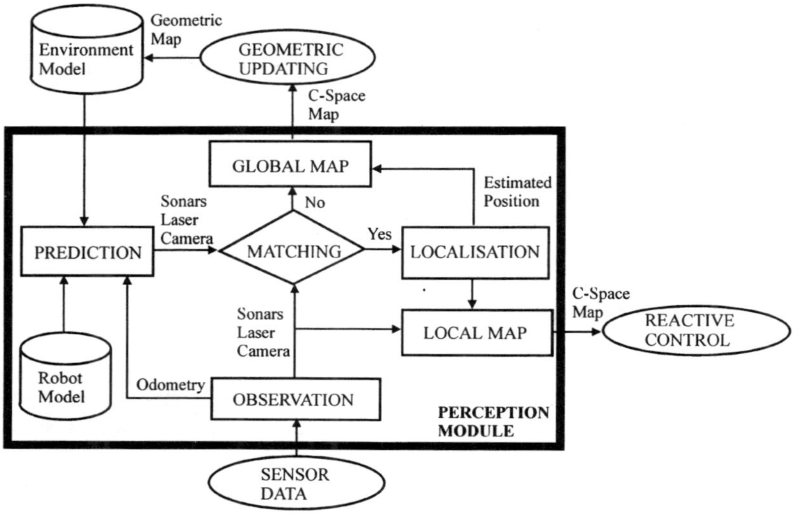

Figure 1. Perception framework

The mapping problem is strongly related with uncertainty. This topic will be presented throughout this chapter. But it must also be kept in mind that maps are built for path planning. Each mapping technique has advantages and disadvantages from the path planning point of view.

Along the chapter the three mapping techniques are discussed: *occupancy grids*, *quad-trees* and *geometric maps*. First we will see how geometric maps generated by an active vision sensor are used to add new objects to the environment. The main difficulties when identifying segments and objects are commented. Secondly, occupancy grids generated from both ultrasound sensors and an active vision sensor are introduced as an appropriate technique for workspace modelling in unstructured environments. Spatial and temporal map fusion techniques are commented, as well as the main problems when identifying static objects. Thirdly, advantages of quad-trees are described.

Also, some experimental results with a real mobile robot elaborating maps dynamically are commented. We finish with the conclusions comparing the mapping techniques, and explain how to make use of their advantages in path planning by unifying the mapping models.

2. Geometric Maps

2.1 Building Geometric Maps

An example of a geometric map is shown in Figure 2.

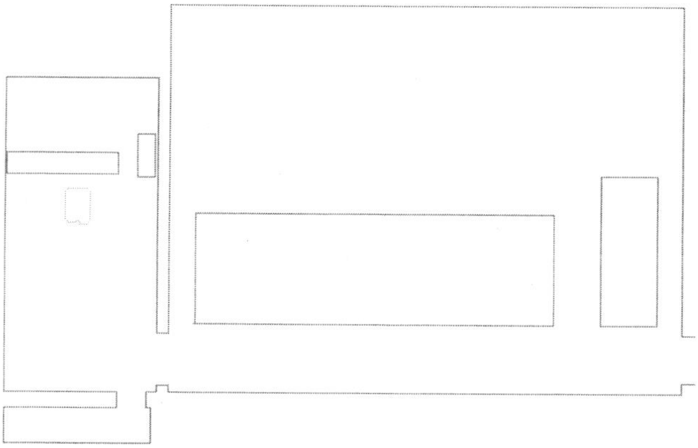

Figure 2. Geometric map

The most appropriate sensors for building geometric maps are the vision based sensors. Figure 3 shows a pair of an infrared laser and a black & white camera that is used for this purpose. The laser illuminates the environment with infrared light. The intersection of this light with the obstacles (in most of the cases, segment like) is observed by the b&w camera that uses an infrared filter in order to focus only on the segments of interest.

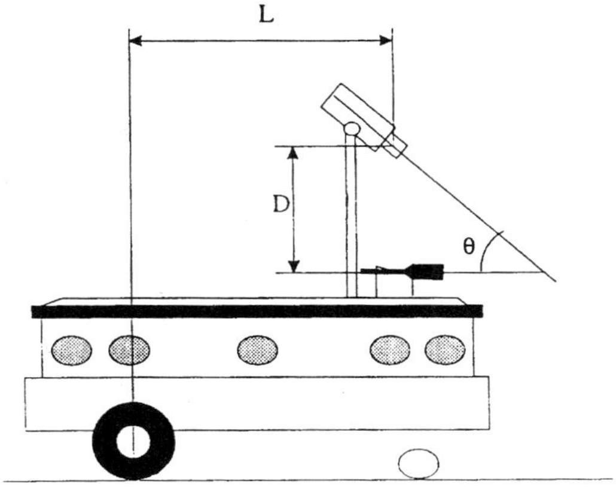

Figure 3. Infrared laser with camera

Using this sensor, the robot has a limited field of view (front view only) (*see* Figure 4).

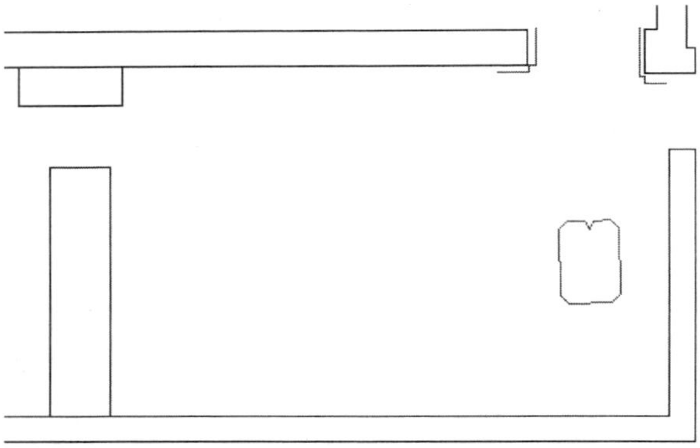

Figure 4. Robot's point of view

Nevertheless, the process of identifying segments is not so direct as it seems in the previous figure. In Figure 5, it is clearly shown that the b&w image is composed of a set of pixels which may be illuminated (corresponding to the intersection of light with objects) or not. From these points, which include noise, segments must be extracted.

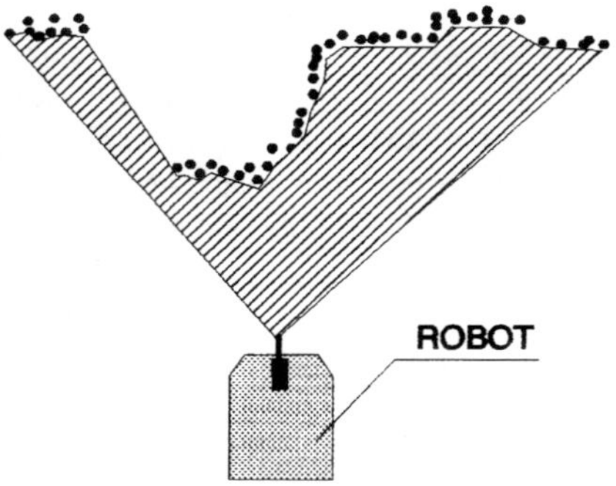

Figure 5. Perception framework

The process steps are as follows: i) elimination of noise, ii) identification of segments, and iii) fusion of segments into objects. The noise is usually due to the interaction of other sources of infrared light, as the sun light infrared component. In the first step, the noise filtering may be done just by deleting isolated sets of points from the image. As regards the identification of segments in the image, this is done by building a set of regression lines that minimise the error (*see* Figure 6). Special care must be taken with circular shape obstacles. In those cases the algorithm does not provide an efficient solution.

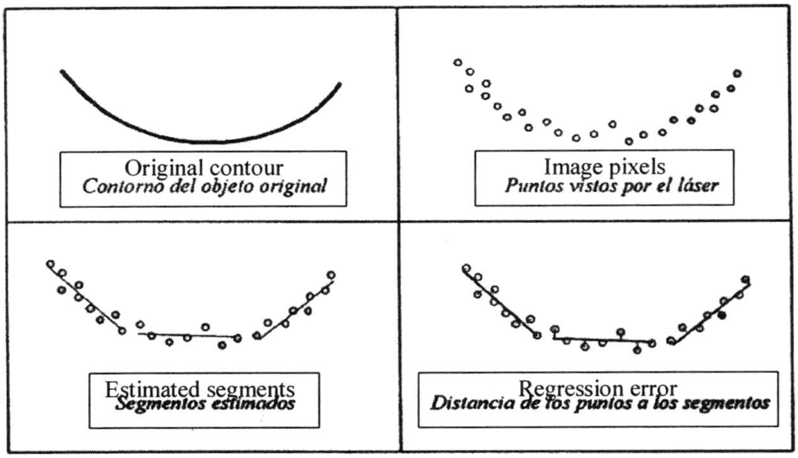

Figure 6. Segments identification

For the last step (the fusion of segments), Figure 7(a) shows a sequence of frames with the segments that are obtained at each moment. Objects that appear again increase their probability of existence, so segments may also disappear. The result is a set of segments without coherence. Figure 7(b) shows the same segments but using an algorithm to fuse them. The segment fusion consists of cutting the extra length of segments that intersect, and joining the end of segments that are too short, but have intersection lines. The result is an "open" polygon.

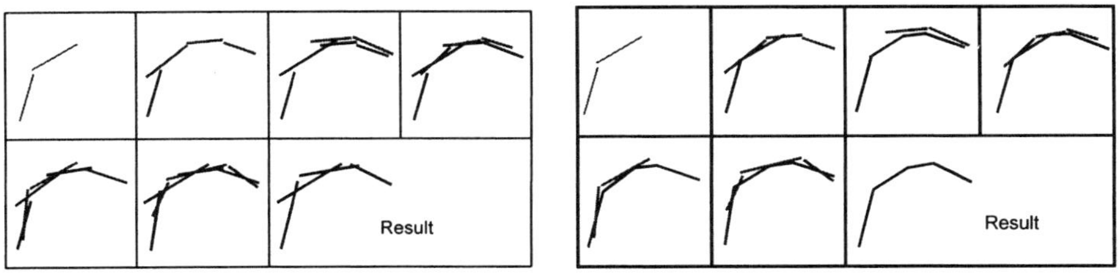

(a) *(b)*

Figure 7. (a) Original segments; (b) Segments with fusion

It must be also taken into account that a Kalman filter is running while the robot moves. This is important in order to match segments in the image with segments in the environment model. Only segments that clearly do not appear in the fixed map are considered in the segment fusion process, while the others are rejected, supposing that noise is present. Figure 8 shows an example of a new set of segments that have appeared after the robot has moved around the room, and after eliminating noise from segments that were in fact the wall or previous known obstacles.

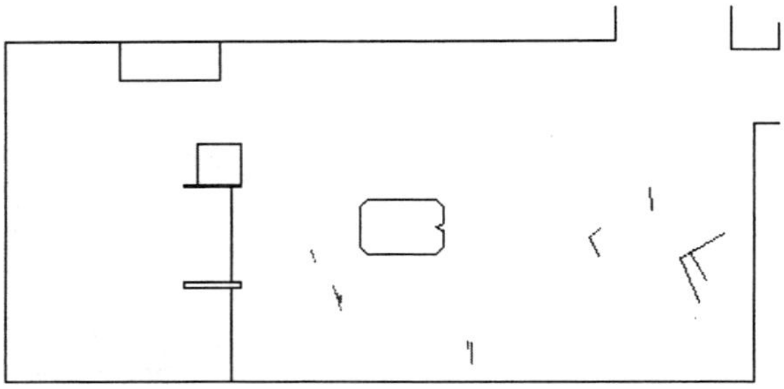

Figure 8. Set of new segments

2.2 Objects Recognition

The identification of objects from the previous sets of continuous segments is not easy. Suppose the obstacle shown in Figure 9 exists.

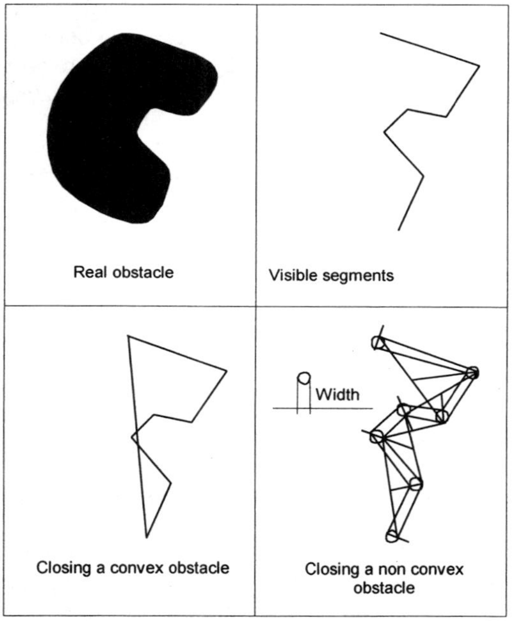

Figure 9. Closing objects

The first problem that arises is that the robot does not obtain a complete view of its contour during its movement around the room. The problem here is how to close the polygon. There are two different ways to do it. The first one is to join the two external vertices. This approach is not suitable for non convex objects, as those in the case of Figure 9. The alternative solution is to give a uniform width to the shape of the segments. Elevation maps may be obtained using this kind of sensor, by just pointing the laser to the floor with an inclination angle different from zero.

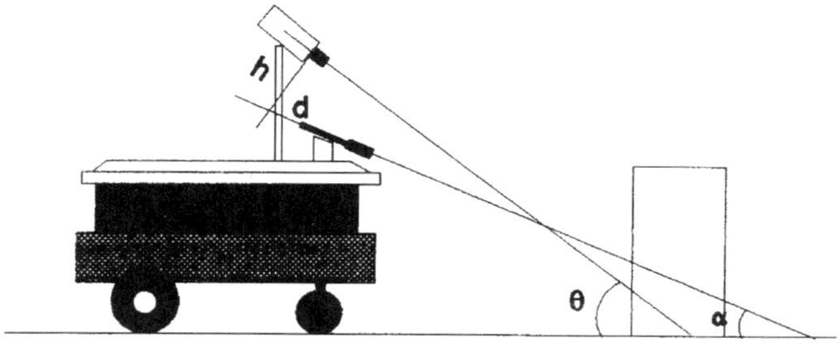

Figure 10. Building elevation maps

3. Occupancy Grids

3.1 Map Generation

An example of an occupancy grid map is shown in Figure 11.

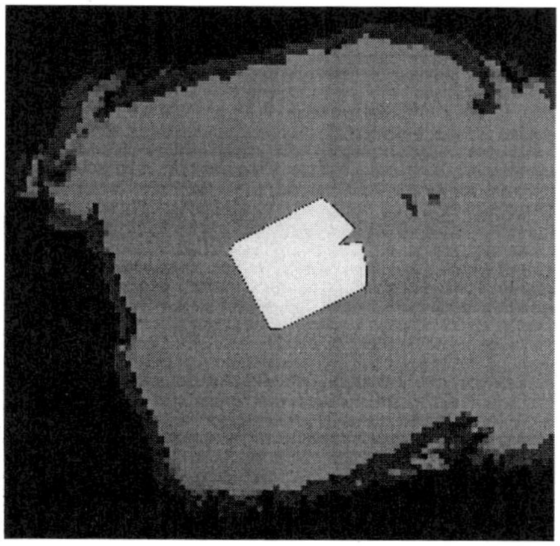

Figure 11. Occupancy grid map

Updating maps maintained by the perception module involves three steps. The first step of sensor interpretation consists of transforming the raw sensory data into grid representation, to form an instantaneous occupancy grid. In a second step, the previously constructed instantaneous map is used to update in real time both the local and global occupancy grids. In a third step, which might take place off-line, the geometric map is updated using the global occupancy grid. We will present a case of map elaboration according to these steps.

Occupancy grids may be generated using different sensors, like proximity sensors or the active vision system used in the previous section. We will focus on the use of sonars, which is the most common case. In such a case, a ring of ultrasound sensors is used (see Figure 12).

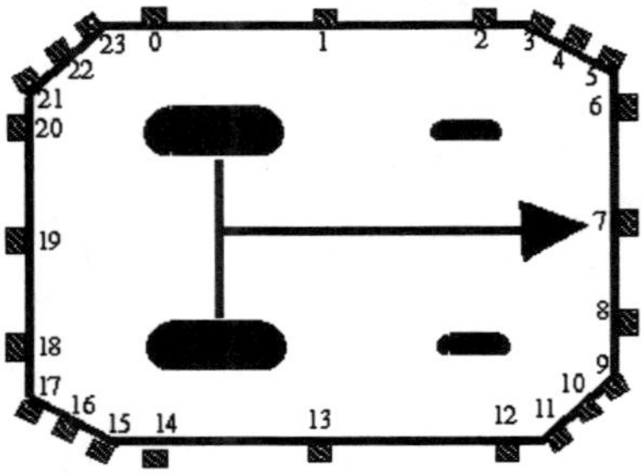

Figure 12. Ring of sonars

If we only consider the raw data obtained from the sensors, the information provided is forming a circumference arc. In order to take into account the high uncertainty inherent to ultrasonic ranging we model the sonar beams with a probabilistic model. In principle, an ultrasonic sensor returns a range measurement corresponding to the distance of the nearest object standing within the sensor's field of view (see Figure 13).

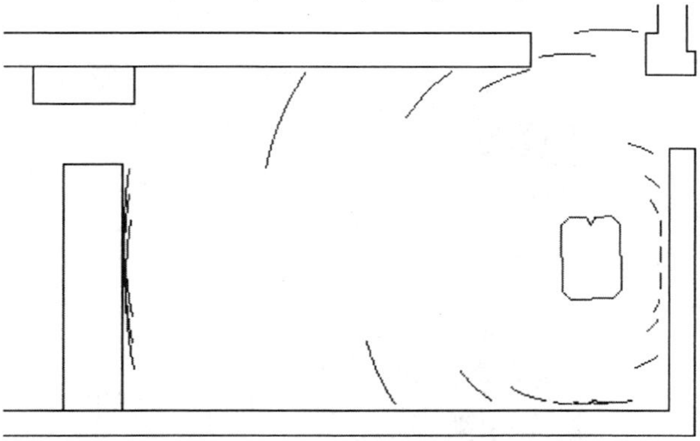

Figure 13. Perception framework

In practice however, the only assumption that can be made is that there is a probability that an object lies somewhere along the arc of given width at the distance returned by the sensor [8]. The transformation into grid representation consists of determining which are the cells that lie in the free space, i.e. which part of space lies in the ultrasonic beam at a distance inferior to the returned range, and which cells lie on the detection arc.

The map update consists of fusing the actual map with the instantaneous map just derived from sensor measures. There is a strong tradition in using *Bayes' theorem* to perform this step of data fusion when simple probabilities are involved. This is due to the fact that, given the prior probability of occupation of a cell, its conditional probability to be occupied, the sensor measure and its inverse model, Bayes's formula directly gives the probability of occupation of a cell located at a known distance. Bayes' theorem allows to calculate the new occupation probability optimally (i.e with the smallest probability of error).

Various attempts have been made also to apply the *Theory of Evidence* to this temporal fusion problem, because this paradigm allows to maintain a quantitative estimate of the uncertainty of the data associated to a given cell.

At any instant, the global map represents the most up-to-date knowledge of the environment, and the instant map the piece of data we need to integrate. When the integration of new data is performed through application the of Bayes' theorem, it is required that we get for each cell of the map a new estimate of its probability of occupation, in order to update it using also the prior probability.

Unknown cells are influenced by a probability of occupation of the order of 50%, which means that the posterior probability calculated will equal the prior one. The free and occupied values are two parameters of the updating procedure.

When the integration of new data is performed through the utilisation of the Theory of Evidence, each cell is affected by two values, one corresponding to the belief that it is empty, and one corresponding to the belief that it is occupied. These two values are determined within the updating procedure, provided the instant map tells whether each cell belongs to the free space, the detection arc or is outside the beam.

3.2 Experimental Results

In order to experiment various types of map generation techniques, and to be able to compare them, we performed an experiment with a robot following a short trajectory in a known environment (the mobile robotics room of our laboratory) (see also [16]). A few unknown obstacles were: a cardboard box in the middle of the room, a power supply box in the middle of the left wall and another robot in the top left-hand corner.

The initial knowledge of the environment is the transformation in grid representation of a geometric map. In the occupancy grid of the example, walls have the maximal probability of occupation. Additional objects not available in the original map are also present in the actual floor.

A map was obtained by processing the data through the temporal fusion operator derived from Bayes' theorem, where all of the expected features of the environment appear: the walls and various obstacles. However, the contour of the second robot is very imprecise and only a single segment can be seen from the two boxes.

Having the respective occupation probability of an empty and an occupied cell vary symmetrically in respect to the value 0.5, is equivalent to controlling the speed of the update algorithm. Having these non symmetric values, is equivalent to rely more on either the free space or the detection arc in the sonar model. It seems preferable to have the global map evolve as slowly as possible in order that high occupation areas correspond to features that have been detected a large number of times, and in order that temporary or moving obstacles not to appear at all. Concerning the local map however, the requirements are exactly the opposite, since we want it to integrate any existing obstacle as quickly as possible, even if it is moving, since this local map will be dedicated for use by the reactive control module.

Another map was obtained by processing the data through a fusion operator derived from the Theory of Evidence. This method should give more reliable results, for two major reasons. The first is that we have separate estimates for the state of occupancy and freedom of a given cell, but also an estimate of their reliability, given the map of uncertainty. While in the first method all cells that belonged to the detection arc were considered to have the same probability of occupation, in the second method the probability is uniformly distributed over the detection arc.

At a first sight, this method seems to lead to more satisfactory results. We can localise the same features as in the two previous maps, though they do not appear in the same way. The contour of the central cardboard box is better described, but the top left-hand corner robot and the power supply box barely appear. Walls appear much thinner. In our case however, the uncertainty map seems to indicate that the whole area within the hall has been explored, which means that the sensors happen to have seen 'through' the cardboard box.

Looking at intermediate steps of the global map construction, reveals that the central obstacle alternatively appears and disappears, as the information coming from the sensors is processed. This is due to the fact that the obstacle has not always been *seen* by the ranging system, and that the area it occupies has been updated as free area

At some steps, sonar measures are fairly reliable, but at others, part of the obstacles happen to belong to the free space area of one of the sonar beams. Others are indeed much more problematic, since the obstacle is not even detected, and clearly belongs to the free space reported by one or more beams. This is exactly what causes the obstacle to alternatively appear and disappear from the global map. Such false measure are due to a well-known phenomenon in ultrasonic ranging, called specular reflection. If a sonar faces a surface having a oblique angle in respect to the beam's direction, the sonar pulse might not return directly to the sensor but undergo various reflections on other features of the environment, thus causing the measured range to be much larger than expected.

Finally, the objective of the global map is to determine the new environmental features so that the geometric map may be updated. As we have seen above, the mapping procedure causes the walls to appear on the occupancy grids as thick segments which does not exactly coincide with the geometric map, due to the imprecision of sonar ranging and the sonar model we implemented. It is necessary to filter the incoming data, in such a way that ranging measures that correspond to already known features of the environment, are not used to update the global occupancy grid. Provided we could simulate the values returned by the sonars in an environment corresponding exactly to the geometric map, we could eliminate the actual sonar values that are equal to their simulated one, thus updating the map with the range measures that correspond to unknown obstacles.

Experimentation demonstrates that occupancy grids that were generated by elimination produce much better results. Walls are much finer and have even nearly disappeared in some sides. On the other hand, the central obstacle seems to be better described, but this might not be very reliable, since it suggests that some range measures have been considered by the matching filter to correspond to a wall, and thus discarded, while they were measures due to specular reflections.

4. Certainty Trees

4.1 Quad-trees Representation

The section presents a novel environment representation method and its use for mobile robotics motion planning applications. We introduce a new representation method called *Certainty Tree*. In addition, we give a complete path planning solution incorporating the Certainty Tree environment representation method and present the features of the certainty tree method in relation to all modules involved in the path planning procedure. The presentation includes a global path planner – based on the Approximate Cell Decomposition method and its extension called Approximate Cell Decomposition with Local Node Refinement -, a local path planner – based on Vector Force Field method -, and the newly introduced environment representation Certainty Tree method. Examples of the of the Certainty Tree application are depicted using a special purpose simulation environment.

A new method for probabilistic representation of obstacles has been developed. The method is based on the certainty grid world model concept for the accommodation of inaccurate sensor data such as range measurements from ultrasonic sensors [2][8]. The novel approach introduced, implements a multi-resolution representation of the sensors measurements in a quad tree data structure, called *Certainty Tree*. The concept relies on the employment of a quad tree rather than a fixed two dimensional array for the representation of the certainty acquired regarding the presence of obstacles in the workspace. Sensor measurements are refreshing the environment image contained in the Certainty Tree.

In more details, a new sensor reading results: I) to an increment of certainty values of an existing set of the certainty tree nodes or even to the creation of new node(s), if the corresponding node(s) belong to the obstacle detected by the sensor measurement, and II) to a decrement of the certainty value or deletion of an existing set of certainty tree nodes, if the corresponding node(s) belong to area reported as free of obstacles by the sensor reading.

Thus, a sensor reading is projected on the certainty tree and results in increment of the certainty values of those tree nodes that correspond to the sensor detection area. If some tree nodes are not available for the sensor detection area to be updated as described above (indicating no certainty regarding obstacle presence in the corresponding area), new nodes are created to hold the certainty values reported by the current sensor reading.

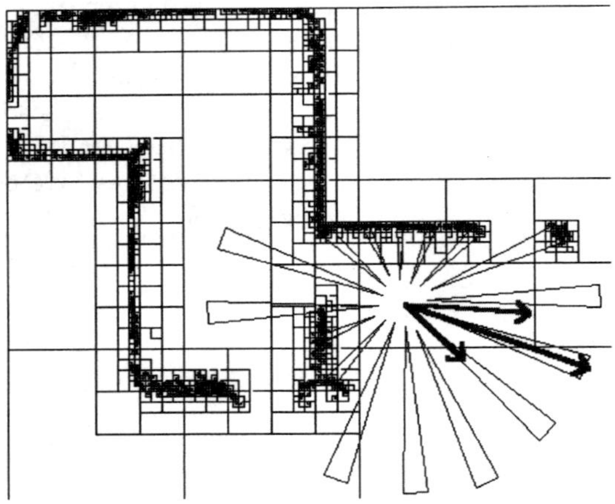

Figure 14. Certainty tree obstacle representation. Sensor projection and virtual force field vectors

On the other hand, a sensor measurement provides also information for the obstacle free area. This information is projected on the certainty tree resulting in a decrement of the certainty values of certainty tree existing nodes, even in a deletion of those nodes whose certainty has reached the lowest level. The Certainty Tree multi-resolution features conclude to reduction of the space required for a given maximum resolution and obstacle configuration in comparison to that required by the typical certainty grid representations. Also, the hierarchical nature of the quad tree enables hierarchical cost efficient updating, where the children nodes inherit their parent's certainty value and provide more detailed information regarding the area they are corresponding to. The Certainty Tree approach provides an efficient way for representing new sensor data, as the mobile robot moves. Updates (insertions and deletions) are performed with relatively low cost in comparison to former approaches.

In addition, the hierarchical nature of the tree is beneficial for the path planning algorithms complexity in terms of the representation cost involved. Also, the path planning cost is much lower compared to the fixed size certainty grid approach where the cost increases with grid size rather than with the number of obstacles present. The Certainty Tree adapts the environment representation to the volume of obstacles reported, rather than having a fixed predefined size. The environment representation image develops along with the actual environment. Finally, the searching procedure using the quad tree proves to be very efficient since it usually involves nodes corresponding to large areas of equal certainty.

The Certainty Tree has been used to represent the environment for global path planning purposes. The two dimensional workspace is modelled using a quad tree data structure on which the static polygonal obstacles are mapped. The decomposition of the workspace is performed by decomposing the quad tree and labelling its nodes. The approach takes full advantage of the workspace's modelling and applies computationally efficient algorithms widely used in computer graphics. A connectivity graph hosting the adjacency relations of the decomposed cells is produced and searched for a free path (Approximate Cell Decomposition) [13]. The node points of the produced paths are refined with respect to local workspace characteristics in order to produce potentially free paths of the highest degree at the current configuration. The refinement method considers the detailed information available only for those path nodes that are adjacent to obstacles. The method modifies the path nodes positions, in order to ensure production of paths according to a set of criteria defined within the algorithm (path length, preference on cell sizes etc.). Finally, the refined node points are smoothed by fitting a cubic spline curve. The spline curve is created using a knot vector selection method which produces curves that match the characteristics of the mobile robot motion. The physical analogue incorporates the centripetal motion behaviour (Approximate Cell Decomposition with Local Node Refinement) .

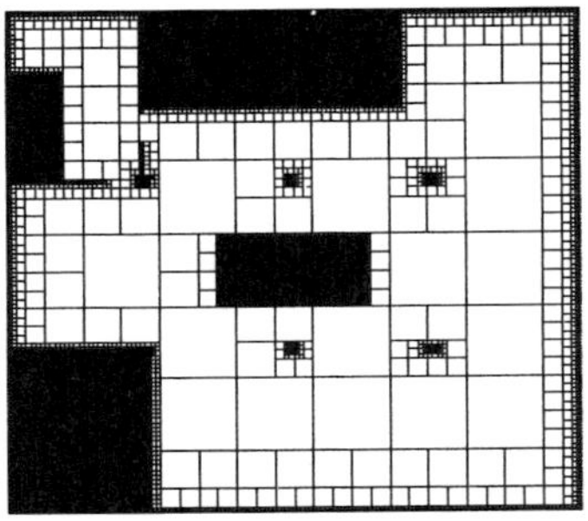

Figure 15. Global path planning with the approximate cell decomposition method

The global path planner is involved in two cases: (1) if the workspace is known the global path planner is invoked to produce intermediate goals for the local path planner, and (2) in order to resolve a local-minima situation. In this case, a temporary "global map" is obtained from the sensor based obstacle representations, and a global path planning procedure is initiated in order to resolve the local minima situation. The specific workspace modelling is used to obtain quick and accurate simulations of the sensors measurements. Using the sensors models and the workspace geometry, represented in the quad tree data structure, we are able to obtain the obstacles or the parts of obstacles that are *visible* to the sensory sub-system at any moment.

4.2 Management

The widely known *Virtual Force Field (VFF)* local path planning method was implemented and evaluated combined with the *Certainty Tree* representation in a special purpose simulation environment. Khatib [6] and Brooks [4] have suggested the principle of having obstacles conceptually exerting forces onto a mobile robot. Borenstein uses the Virtual Force Field planning approach using fixed size certainty grid [2,3].

In the simulation environment the VFF governs the robot motion while sensor readings derived are projected onto the Certainty Tree, which in sequence are fed into the VFF. The certainty tree nodes contributing in VFF calculation are those corresponding to a robot centred square area, well know as *active window*.

Each occupied node inside the active window applies a repulsive force to the robot, "pushing" the robot away from the corresponding area. The magnitude of this force is proportional to the node's certainty value and dimension, and is inversely proportional to the square of the distance between the node and the robot. At any time during the motion, a constant-magnitude attracting force pulls the robot toward the target. As shown in Figure 16, the vectorial sum of all forces, repulsive from occupied nodes and attractive from the target position, produces a resultant force vector ***R***. The direction of ***R***, is used to obtain the next configuration.

The simulation environment developed is a graphical Windows™ application. By the use of our simulation environment, one can perform simulation experiments to study and evaluate various sensor configurations, or new sensor designs, in relation with the certainty tree and the path planning approaches addressed.

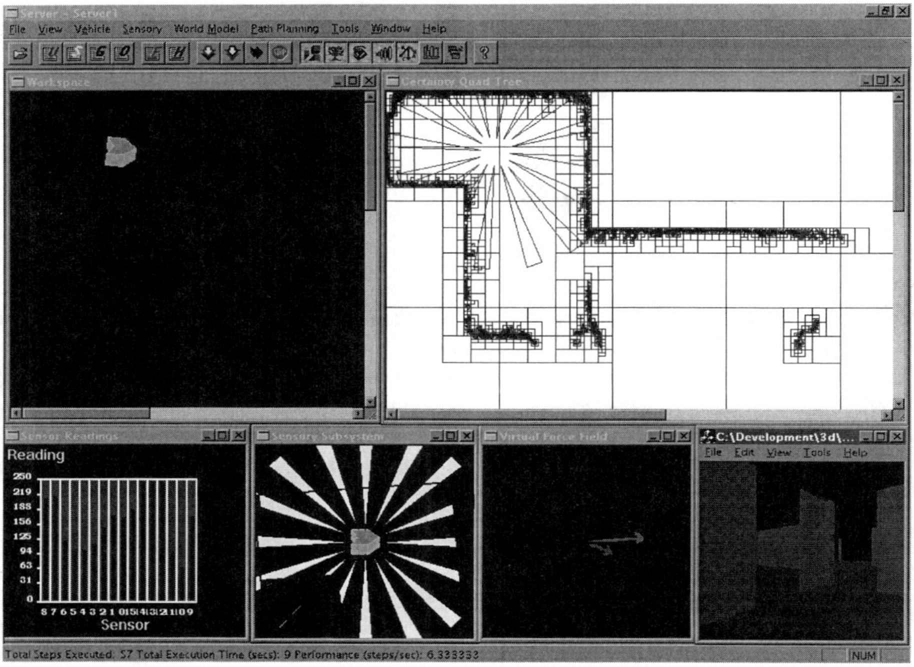

Figure 16. Simulation environment

The user may interactively define all the simulation parameters, such as robot configuration, sensor types, attributes and configuration, global map, global path planning, local path planning, motion execution, and obstacle representation parameters, starting and goal configurations. A set of windows can be enabled to monitor robot action and path execution, sensor measurements, virtual force field vectors, and sensor based map building.

The user can also view an actual 3D representation of the world as the robot navigates from the starting position to the target configuration. The next figure presents a snapshot of the simulation environment.

Various sensor configurations may be chosen or even created for the robot's navigation. These include ultrasonic sensors as well as laser scanners. The user can employ user-defined sensors or choose from a list of predefined sensor types. Sensor types, number and positioning may be interactively defined. Sensors configuration heavily affects the effectiveness (path characteristics, robot motion parameters etc.) of the path planning method incorporated. The sensors are modelled by a list of vertices that form the active area of the sensor (sensor field of view see Figure 17).

Figure 17. Two sensor congigurations and the corresponding simulated visible obstacles at a given time

The representation is supported by the certainty tree (quad tree) used to model the workspace & enables accurate and fast calculation of obstacles *visible* portions. Information obtained – measurements on simulated obstacles by sensors modelled – is projected on the certainty structure used for obstacle representation for map building. The same information is used for both for planning and visualisation purposes. The major components of the simulation environment developed for testing and evaluation purposes are integrated into a well defined iterative procedure presented in Figure 18.
The researcher – user of the simulation environment - initiates a simulation cycle after defining the simulation parameters. If the workspace is known, then the global path planning module searches for a collision-free global path and if one is found a sequence of intermediate goal configurations is calculated and fed to the local path planning module. Given a goal, the local path planning module starts an iterative procedure where new simulated measurements are produced with respect to the current configuration, the world model and the sensory sub-system. These measurements are then projected onto the certainty tree, thus continuously updating the world image as the robot moves. The robot is driven by the virtual force field produced by the certainty tree in the active window of the robot. The local path planning module is searching for a probable local-minima situation by keeping a list of the most-recent configurations. If the robot is trapped in a local-minima situation then the global path planning module is involved in order to obtain a new set of goal configurations based on the most recent sensor-based information mapped onto the certainty

tree. The local path planning module is then restarted. In the normal case, the next robot configuration is calculated and visualised.

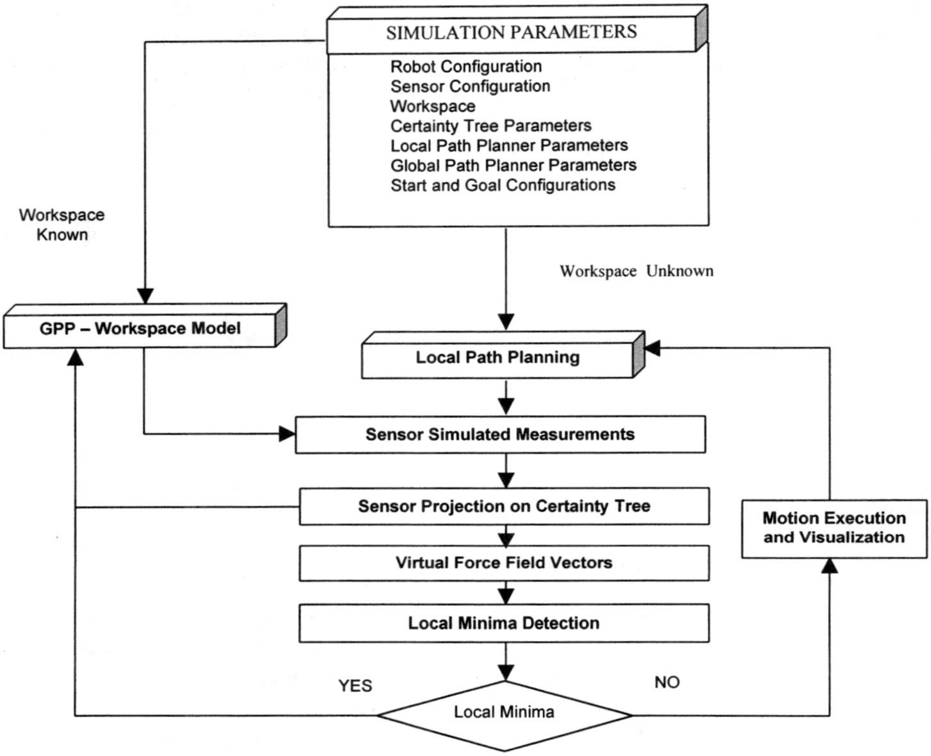

Figure 18. Simulator components integration

5. Conclusions

A discussion about the advantages and disadvantages of each method can be carried out from the results presented above. Geometric maps provide a very precise description of the environment, as well as an easy and a low memory consuming manner to codify the geometry of a given environmental feature. However they provide a very rigid and abstract description of the world with requires heavy computation of the sensory data.

On the other hand, occupancy grids are a much more intuitive representation of the environment, since they directly associate a given region of the space with the knowledge we have of its characteristics, in terms of information relevant to path-planning and reactive control. It also provides a very suitable frame for handling uncertainty, and representing the spatial information returned by the sensors, a consequence of which is that little computation required to transform sensor data into grid information. A quick comparison of the two updating methods we have presented seems to indicate that the one derived from Bayes' theorem is adequate for maintaining local occupancy grids, while for global grids, better results are obtained with the method involving the Theory of Evidence.

However the sonar model we implemented seems quite inadequate, since it assumes that the distance to the detected object is situated in an interval centered on the value actually returned. The solution to this problem will certainly involve multi-sensory data fusion. A first step in this direction will consists in considering groups of sonars both for the matching steps and the generation of the instantaneous maps. Another one is to incorporate data coming from other sensors such as an active vision system.

Furthermore, memory requirements in occupancy grids increase geometrically with the size and resolution of the map, rather than with the quantity of relevant information it contains. Certainty trees solve this memory consuming problem, but require more sophisticated algorithms for the dynamic computation and update of the tree nodes.

As we have seen, environment definition is highly related with the manoeuvrability capabilities of the robot. The best way to attack the *mapping for planing* problem is to establish the guidelines for model unification, taking into account the advantages of each method. Global mapping will close the highest loop of the robot control architecture, by supplying updated and accurate information to the global path planning system. But, to do this, several map transformations must be done.

First, the user prefers a geometric map to enter the environment definition, to visualise it, as well as to set targets for the robot, because he/she manages better this kind of representation. These maps may be directly used for building on-line maps, with the restrictions we have seen in one of the above sections. In parallel, an occupancy grid mapping system may build a fast local map for obstacle avoidance (simulating virtual measures from sensors), that may be matched with the a priori information to obtain a slower global map. This, can be fused with the geometric map to obtain a unique representation in occupancy grid format. This closes the loop in two ways. On one hand, the map may be transformed into a quad tree for path planning. On the other hand, it may be transformed into a geometric map to be stored as a new departure information to be used by both, the user and the environment model system.

6. References

[1] "The quad tree and related hierarchical data structures," Technical Report 23, Center for Automation Research, University of Maryland, College Park, November 1983.

[2] Borenstein J., and Koren Y., "Histogramic In-Motion Mapping For Mobile Robot Obstacle Avoidance." *IEEE Journal of Robotics and Automation*, Vol. 7.

[3] Borenstein J., and Koren Y., "Real-time Obstacle Avoidance for Fast Mobile Robots." *IEEE Transactions on Systems, Man, and Cybernetics*, Vol. 19, No. 5, Sept./Oct. 1989, pp. 1179-1187.

[4] Brooks R. A. and Lozano-Perez T., “A subdivision algorithm in configuration space for find path with rotation,” in *Proceedings of the Eight International Joint Conference on Artificial Intelligence*, 1983.
[5] Brooks R. A., "A Robust Layered Control System for a Mobile Robot." *IEEE Journal of Robotics and Automation*, Vol. RA-2, No. 1, 1986, pp. 14-23.
[6] Khatib O., "Real-Time Obstacle Avoidance for Manipulators and Mobile Robots." 1985 *IEEE International Conference on Robotics and Automation*, March 25-28, 1985, St. Louis, pp. 500-505.
[7] Durrant-Whyte, Dynamic Map Building for an Autonomous Mobile Robot, *Int. Journal of Robotics Research*, Vol. 11, 1992.
[8] Elfes A., "A Sonar-Based Mapping and Navigation System." Carnegie-Mellon University, The Robotics Institute, Technical Report, 1985, pp. 25-30.
[9] Elfes A., A 3D World Model Builder with a Mobile Robot, *Int. Journal of Robotics Research*, Vol. 11, 1992.
[10] Elfes A., Maintaining Representations of the Environment of a Mobile Robot, *IEEE Trans. on Robotics and Automation*, Vol. 3, 1989.
[11] Katevas N., Tzafestas S. G. and Pnevmatikatos C. G., “The Approximate Cell Decomposition with Local Node Refinement Global Path Planning Method: Path Nodes Refinement and Path Parametric Interpolation”, *Journal of Intelligent and Robotic Systems, Special Issue on Autonomous Mobile Robots in Health Care Services,* Kluwer Academic Publishers, 1998, Vol. 22, No. 3-4, pp. 289-314.
[12]Chen D., Szczerba R. and Uhran J., “A Framed-Quadtree Approach for Determining Euclidean Shortest Paths in a 2-D Environment.” *IEEE Transactions on Robotics and Automation*, Vol, 13, No. 5, October 1997.
[13] Latombe, J-P., “Robot Motion Planning”, Boston, MA: Kluwer Academic, 1990.
[14] Paul, *Robot Manipulators. Mathematics, Programming and Control*, MIT Press, 1982.
[15] Samet H., “An Algorithm for converting rasters to quadtrees,” *IEEE Transactions on Pattern Analysis and Machine Learning*, Vol.3, 1981, pp.93-95.
[16] Wawak F., Matia F., Katevas N., Peignot C., Pnevmatikatos C. “A Generic Perception Framework for Autonomous Mobile System”, *TMR Networks Conference*, Graz, Austria, 7-9 May, 1998.

The Authors

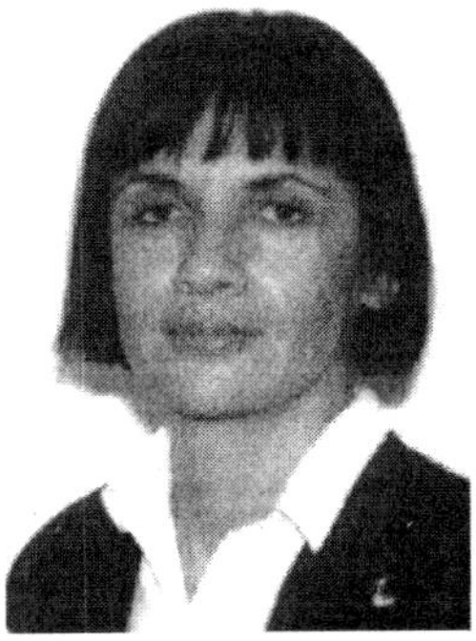

Dr. Marie-José ALDON graduated in 1982 as Doctor in Robotics and Automation from the University of Montpellier II. She joined the LAM-CNRS (Laboratory for Robotics and Microelectronics of the National Center for Scientific Research) in 1983, where she was primarly interested in modelling and control of manipulators. She is currently a Research Scientist at LIRMM-CNRS (Laboratory for Computer Science, Robotics and Microelectronics of Montpellier) in the Robotics Group and she is in charge of courses in Computer Vision at the University of Montpellier. Her research interests include Computer Vision, Range Image Processing, and Sensor Fusion for Robotics. Her main expertise is in sensor integration and data processing for navigation, localization and environment modelling of autonomous mobile robots (specially in underwater, agricultural, and service fields).

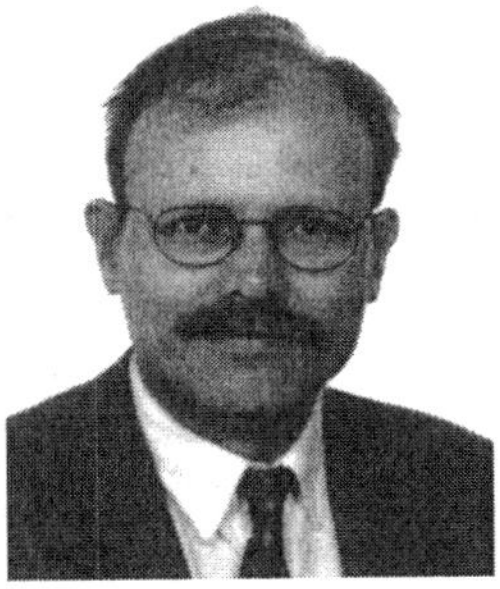

Prof. Gunnar BOLMSJÖ received the M.Sc. and PhD degree in Mechanical Engineering from Lund University, Lund, Sweden in 1981 and 1986 respectively. From 1986 he was a research associate at the Dept. of Mechanical Engineering, Lund University, and is since 1987 Professor in Robotics at the same department. His research interest include service robotics such as robotics in rehabilitation and industrial processes such as arc welding and grinding. Research include high level control structures including task level programming, multi-sensor feed-back, process models and robotic modeling and simulation.

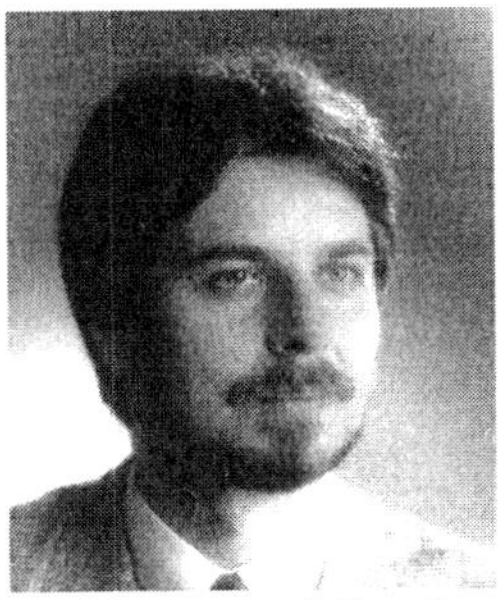

Dr. Ulrich BORGOLTE, holds a Master in Computer Science from Dortmund University (1984), Germany. In years 1984-1985 was appointed as Research Associate at Hagen University and in 1985-1989 as Research Associate at Dortmund University, Germany. From 1989 till the present time is a Lecturer/Research Associate at Hagen University, Germany. He finished his PhD in Electrical Engineering from Hagen University, Germany in 1990. From 1993-1999 was assigned as assistant head of automation department within AIP GmbH, Hagen, Germany. He is active in applied robotics including multi-robot systems, collision avoidance, mobile robots, rehabilitation robots. He is the project manager in national projects as well as the European projects OMNI and MOBIL.

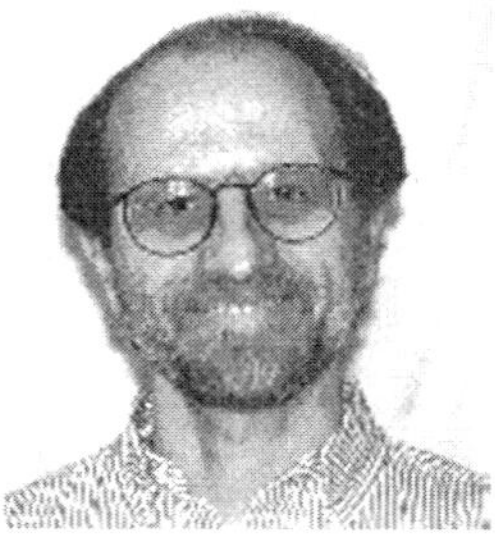

Prof. Paolo DARIO received the Dr. Eng. Degree in mechanical engineering from the University of Pisa, in 1977. He is Full Professor of Biomedical Robotics at the SSSA. He is the Director of the ARTS Lab and of the MiTech (Microengineering and Microfabrication Technologies) Lab of the SSSA, where he supervises a team of about 70 researchers and Ph.D. students. He has been a Visiting Professor at the Ecole Polytechnique Federale de Lausanne (EPFL), Switzerland, and at Waseda University, Tokyo, Japan. His main research interests are in the fields of medical robotics, mechatronics and microengineering. He is the co-ordinator of many national and European projects, the editor of two books on the subject of robotics, and the author of more than 200 scientific papers. He is President-Elect of the IEEE Robotics & Automation Society, in which he also serves as Associate Editor of the Transactions and co-chair of the Technical Committee on Medical Robotics.

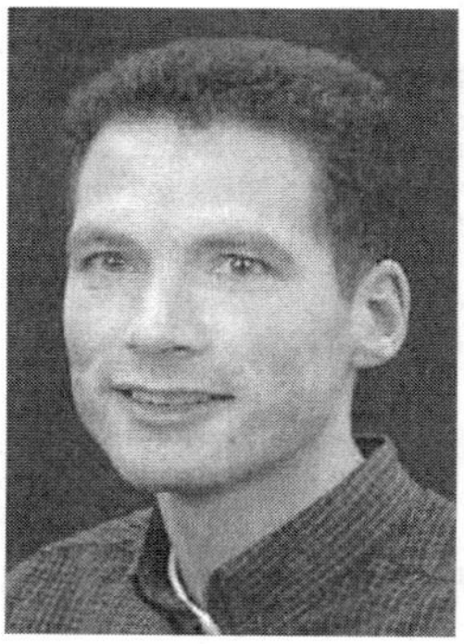

Ir. Bart J.F. DRIESSEN is with TNO-TPD in the Netherlands. He was born on 31st July 1966. He studied electrical engineering in Delft from 1984-1990. His graduation subject was the design of a control architecture for the MANUS wheelchair mounted manipulator. At TNO he is senior project manager in the mechatronics field. He worked on several projects such as: the development of semi-active shock absorbers for automobiles, the autonomous transport of container transport in the harbour of Rotterdam, the control of fast packaging machines in the food industry, and the design of harvesting robots for chrysanthemums. Currently he is active in physiotherapy robotics for people recovering from stroke, and in the redesign of the MANUS wheelchair mounted manipulator.

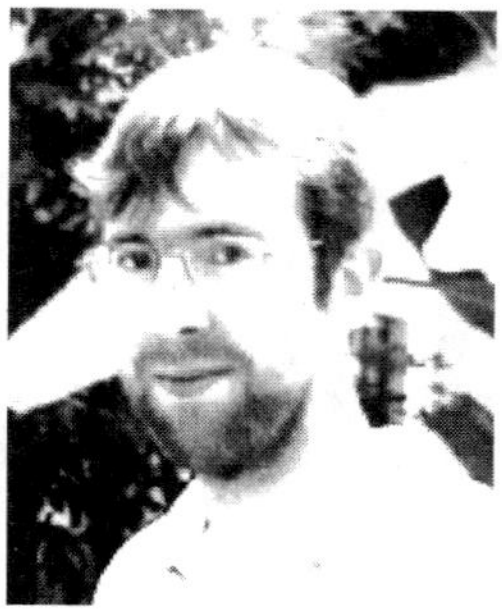

Mr. Fergal O'HART has received B.Sc. degrees in Computer Science from University College Dublin in 1994(Gen.) and 1996(Hons.). He is currently pursuing a Ph.D in Computer Science at Trinity College Dublin. During this time he has also worked as an EU TMR MOBINET researcher at the University of Reading. His research interests include mobile robotics, distributed computing and Petri Nets. His research advocates the incorporation of intelligent resources distributed throughout a building to facilitate the planning and scheduling activities of mobile robots.

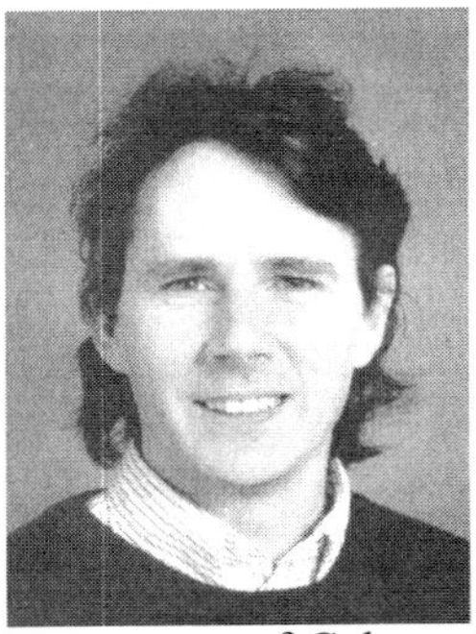

Dr. William HARWIN received a BA in engineering from Cambridge University in 1982, and MSc in Bioengineering from Strathclyde University in 1983 Following a period as a research assistant at the Engineering Department of Cambridge University be began a PhD on computer recognition of the head gestures made by people with cerebral palsy, work he completed in 1991. His research interest is in machines and the human system. In 1983 be worked at the Cambridge University Engineering Department on rehabilitation robotics research. Between 1990 and 1995 he directed rehabilitation robotics research at the Applied Science and Engineering Laboratories in Delaware, USA. He moved to the Department of Cybernetics at the University of Reading, England in 1996 where he directs work at the Human-Robot Interface Laboratory (thrill www.cyber.rdg.ac.uk/W.Harwin). Current research work includes robot assistance of human movements, information content of haptic interfaces and lumped parameter modelling of human interactions involving power exchange.

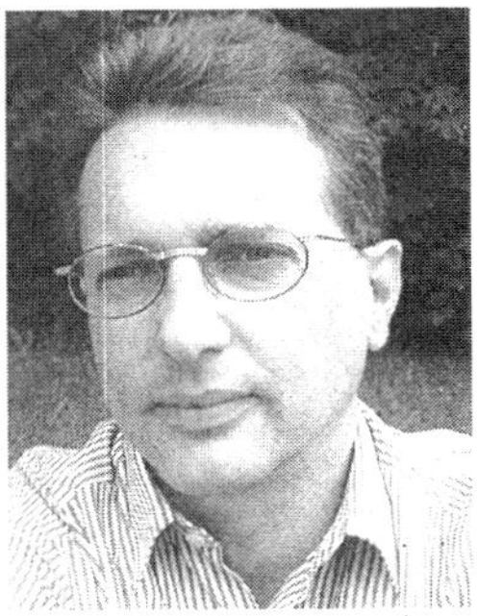

Dr.-Ing. Helmut HECK holds a diploma degree in Computer Science from the University of Dortmund, Germany, and a Dr.-Ing. degree in Electrical Engineering for his work in "Task-Oriented Robot Programming". He has been a research associate at the Institute of Robotics Research (IRF), University of Dortmund, where he was involved in research on programming and control of industrial robots (Volkswagen) and space robots (second German space mission, D2). Since 1991 Helmut Heck has been involved in the development of rehabilitation technology. He is head of the Development Centre at Forschungsinstitut Technologie-Behindertenhilfe (FTB) of Evangelische Stiftung Volmarstein (ESV), a rehabilitation centre in Germany. His current interests relate to the fields of computer/robotic applications and human-machine-interaction for people with motor and/or mental impairments, especially in the fields of augmentative and alternative communication and environmental control. He has been involved in various national and international projects.

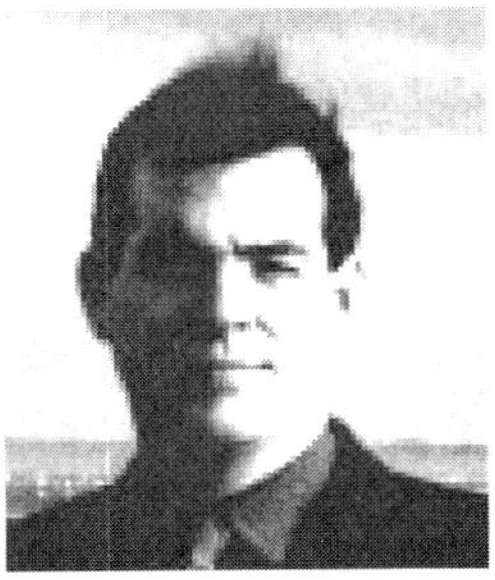

Mr. Richard GREENANE (23) was born in the South-East of England. He gained a degree in Cybernetics and Computer Science from the University of Reading in 1995. In the summer of that year, he helped build the hardware "installed" into Professor Kevin Warwick which featured heavily with news and media, gaining more status when it appeared on the front cover of “WIRED”, a popular magazine with technicians. In 1998 Mr. Greenane joined the Computer Robotics and Vision Group at Trinity College Dublin, to start a new programme of Smart Environment research. His chief involvement was the design and installation of "smart space" technology throughout the Department's main building, constructing a heterogeneous network infrastructure to support experiments in mobile context-sensitive computing. Mr. Greenane is now completing his Masters thesis and is a director of the Internet software company Conceptual Drift Ltd.

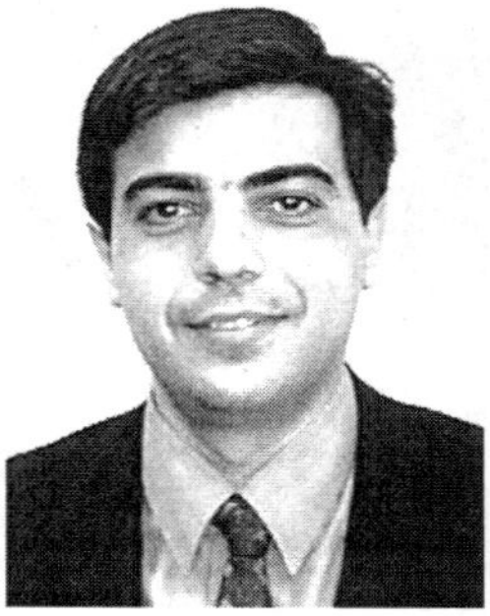

Dr. Nikos I. KATEVAS received the Diploma degree in Electrical and Computer Engineering in 1991, and the Ph.D. degree for research on Intelligent Autonomous Mobile Robots in 1997, from the National Technical University of Athens (NTUA). He joined Zenon SA Athens, Greece, in 1991 and he has been involved in over 25 projects under the ESPRIT, TELEMATICS, BRITE / EURAM, TMR, Innovation, IST, etc. programmes of the EC. Since January 1995, he is the head of R&D Dept. of Zenon SA. Currently he is the project leader and/or technical manager of 4 major EC projects, he participates in 5 other EC projects and he is associated scientist to National Technical University of Athens. Dr. Katevas, is the founder of Noemon Ltd., Halkida, Greece, dedicated to mobile robotics for services. He has published 46 papers in international journals and conferences in mobile robotics. He is a member of the IEEE Robotics and Automation Society.

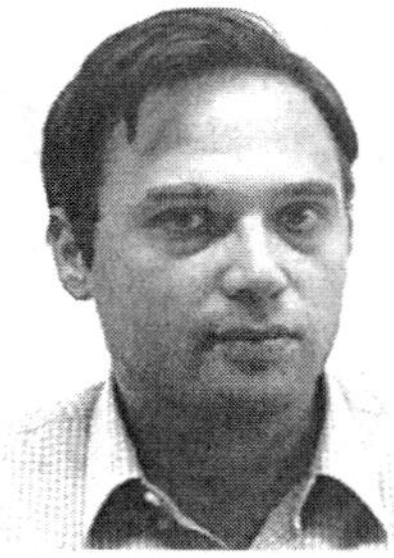

Mr. John KONTOULIS received his B.Eng(Hons) in Electrical & Electronic Engineering from the University of Sunderland in 1994, and MSc. in Control Systems from the University of Sheffield in 1995. He is a Graduate Member of the Institute of Measurement & Control, and a member of the Technical Chamber of Greece (TEE). He has been with Zenon S.A. since July 1999. He is being involved in numerous European Union research projects. Application areas of the work include telematics, robotics, and control technologies. Application of robotics in the health care sector consist one of his principal interests.

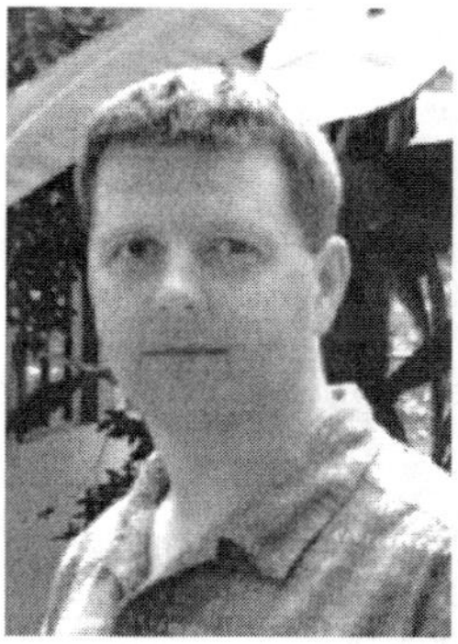

Dr. Gerard LACEY, received the B.A.I., MA. and Ph.D. degrees from Trinity College Dublin, Ireland. From 1991 to 1994 he was a Research Assistant in automated industrial inspection at Trinity College Dublin. In 1995 he was a visiting researcher at the University of Edinburgh, and subsequently returned to TCD to pursue a Ph.D. on Robot Guides for the Blind. This work was awarded a scholarship by the NRB in 1995 and became the EU project PAM-AID in 1997. At the RESNA'99 conference he and Shane Mac Namara he won the Paralyzed Veterans of America (PVA) Design Competition for their work on PAM-AID. From 1996-2000 he was a Lecturer in Computer Science in Trinity College Dublin and was head of the Computer Vision and Robotics

Group. He is now CEO of the Vartry Research Ltd which designs technology for elderly people. He has over 25 publications in computer vision, robotics and adaptive interfaces

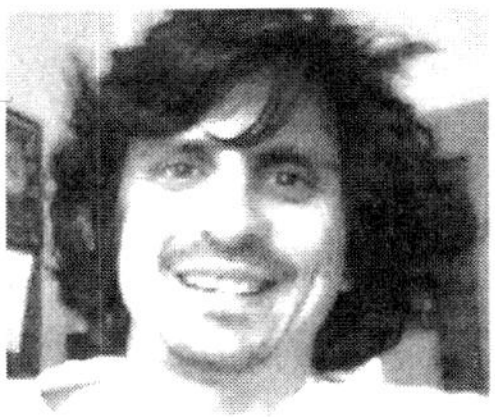

Dr. Stanislao LAURIA (PhD, Reading, UK) is a Research Fellow in the Centre for Neural and Adaptive Systems (CNAS) in the School of Computing at the University of Plymouth, UK. He is currently working on an EPSRC-funded project on 'Instruction-based Learning for Mobile Robots' in collaboration with the University of Edinburgh, Scotland. He has previously been involved in research projects on Neural Networks and Robotics at the University of Naples, Italy and the University of Reading, UK. His research interests are Neural Networks, Computer Vision and Robotics and he has published papers on these topics (Email address stasha@soc.plymouth.ac.uk).

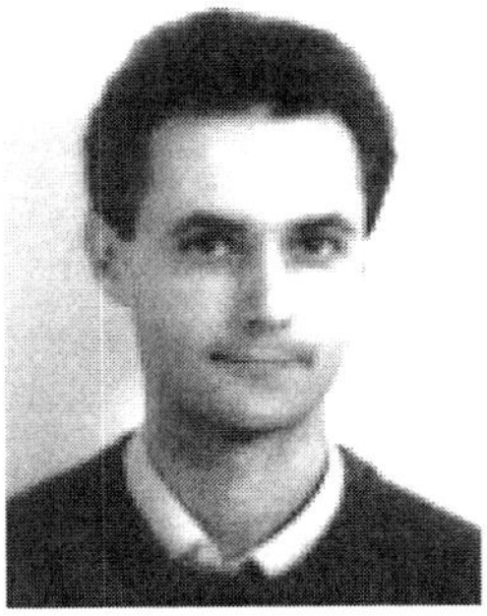

Dr. Fernando MATIA is Associate Professor at Universidad Politécnica de Madrid (UPM). He was born in Madrid, Spain, in 1966. He became Industrial Engineer at the UPM in 1990 and received his Ph.D. degree at the UPM in 1994, in the area of Control Engineering. He works in Process Control Engineering and Artificial Intelligence since 1988, and also leads the Autonomous Robots group since 1994. His main R&D activities are Intelligent Control, Fuzzy Control, Software Integration, Control Architectures, Robotics, Autonomous Systems and Uncertainty Management in Perception Systems. He has experience in ESPRIT-6447 HINT, ESPRIT-6450 ROCCO, ECLA-004-76102 CIMIS.net, ESPRIT 22130 DIXIT, TMR MOBINET, INCO-962074 PROQUS and IST-10258 DOTS among other projects. He has published one book, as well as many book chapters, articles in journals and papers in conferences. Presently, he is reviewer of five international journals.

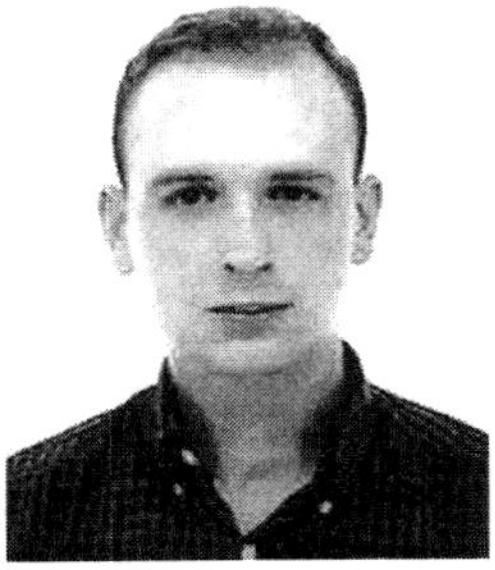

Mr. Cédric PEIGNOT obtained the Engineering Degree in Electricals and Automation in 1997, at Ecole Nationale Supérieure d'Electrotechnique, Electronique, Informatique et Hydraulique de Toulouse (ENSEEIHT). He has backgound in power electronics, automation, control, operations research and robotics. He has been a postgraduate researcher at Universidad Politecnica de Madrid, Spain, for two years, working in autonomous robots (OOP techniques, sensor data fusion and Autonomous navigation). Presently he is software engineer at CR2A-DI (TRANSICIEL), Toulouse, France, developing product data management systems for the aerospace industry.

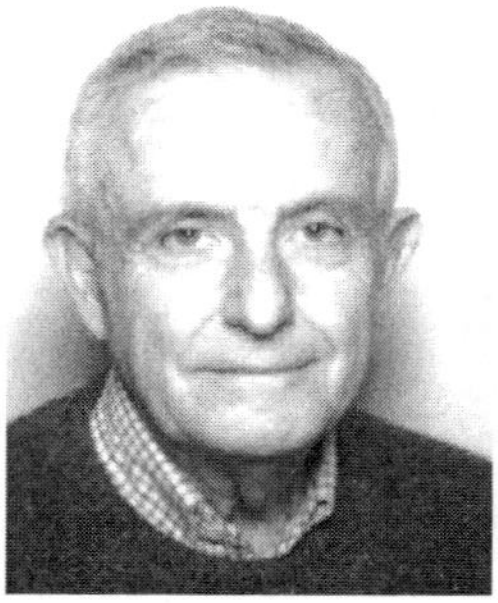

Mr. Edouard PERUCHON was born in France in 1939. He graduated from the Uninersity of Sciences of Montpellier, and received a Doctorate in Automatics and System Designing. Since 1971 he has been a researcher at the French Institut National de la Santé et de la Recherche Médicale (INSERM) in the fields of Biomechanics, Human Motor functions analysis and Rehabilitation Technologies. Since 1991, he was involved in various European research projects: AIM/CAMARC (1991-1995), AIM/BRITER 1993-1995), TIDE/SENARIO (1994-1997), TIDE/MOVAID (1994-1996), Human Capital and Mobility/CAMARN (1994-1997), TAP/ABCMALE (1997-1999), TAP Educational Multimedia/MODASPECTRA (1998-2000), TMR/MobiNet (1996-2000). He is member of the European Society of Biomechanics.

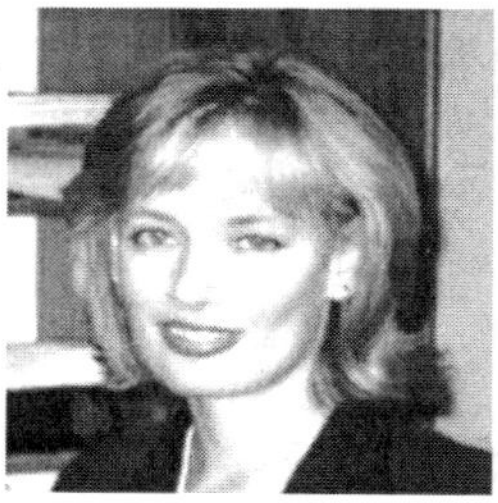

Dr. Andriana PRENTZA was born in Sydney, Australia in 1968. She received her Diploma degree in Computer Engineering and Information Sciences and her M.Sc. in Biomedical Engineering in 1991 and 1993 respectively from the University of Patras, Greece, and her Ph.D degree in Biomedical Engineering from the Eindhoven University of Technology, Eindhoven, the Netherlands, in 1997. During 1993-1997 she was a teaching and research assistant in the Department of Electrical Engineering at Eindhoven University of Technology. In 1997, she joined the Biomedical Engineering Laboratory, Department of Electrical and Computer Engineering, National Technical University of Athens, Athens, Greece, as a Research Scientist. She has published 13 scientific papers in international journals and conferences. Her current research interests include Biosignal Processing, Neural Networks, Internet Technology, and Applications of Computers and Telecommunications in Medicine. Dr. Prentza has been active in a number of European and National R&D programs in the field of Telematics Applications in Healthcare. She is a member of the Institute of Electrical and Electronics Engineers and a member of the Technical Chamber of Greece and the Greek Society of Biomedical Technology.

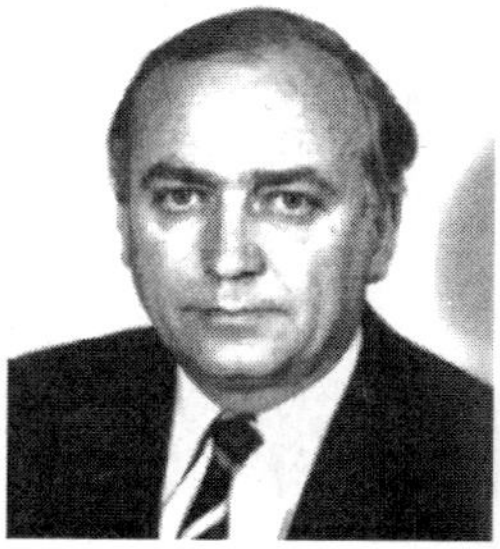

Prof. Pierre RABISCHONG was born on March 1st, 1932 in Nancy, France. He graduated in Medicine, from University of Nancy, School of Medicine in 1955, in Neuropsychiatry in 1958 and he appointed by the Faculty of Medicine in Montpellier (Anatomy) as Professeur Agrégé des Facultés de Médecine, in 1961. Prof. Rabischong the following positions: Chief assistant, University of Lausanne , Switzerland 1959-1961, Full Professor, Chairman of the Department of Anatomy, Faculty of Medicine of Montpellier 1964, Chief of the Functional Exploration of Motor Function Service in the Teaching Hospital (C.H.U.) of Montpellier 1965. Director of the Biomechanical research unit 103 of the National Institute for Health and Medical Research (INSERM) 1971-1995, Dean of the Faculty of Medicine of Montpellier

1978 - 1981. Member of the Consultative Committee of French (CCU) 1969 - 1981. Currently, he is Professor and Director of the Anatomy Lab, Faculty of Medicine of Montpellier since1964. Prof. Rabischong is the founding Member and Board Member of the Propara Center for treating spinal cord injuries since 1980, cCoordinator for the EUREKA-CALIES project (1989) and the SUAW project (Stand Up and Walk), demonstration project of the BIOMED II program of the European Community since 1996, president of ESEM (European Society for Engineering and Medicine) since 1995, president de ISCAS (International Society for Computer Aided Surgery) since 1995, vice President of the WABT (World Academy of Biomedical Technologies) at UNESCO since 1997. He is author of more than 150 scientific and medical articles in international magazines

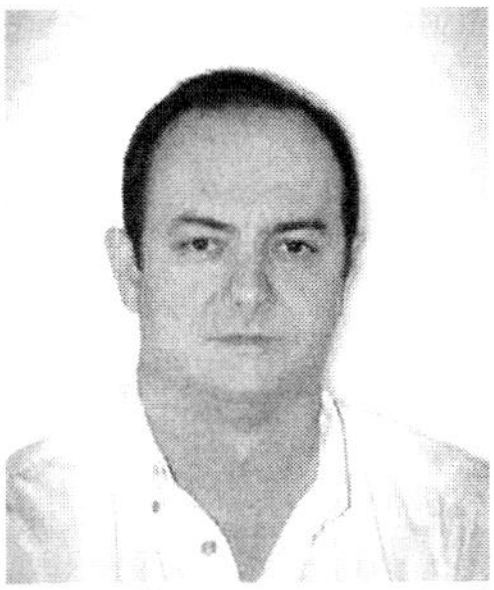

Dr. Ricardo SANZ is PhD in Engineering from the Universidad Politecnica de Madrid. During the last years, his work has concentrated in the design of large, complex controllers with heterogeneous information processing technologies: artificial intelligence, soft computing, blackboard systems, real time agent systems, etc. He is member of IFAC's TCs "Algorithms and Architectures for Real-time Control" and "Large Scale Systems" and OMG TC on "Real-time Distributed Object Systems". His current interests are the design of large modular controllers based on composable technologies, the structure of robotic minds, and the use of patterns, ontologies and frameworks as core technologies for control system construction.

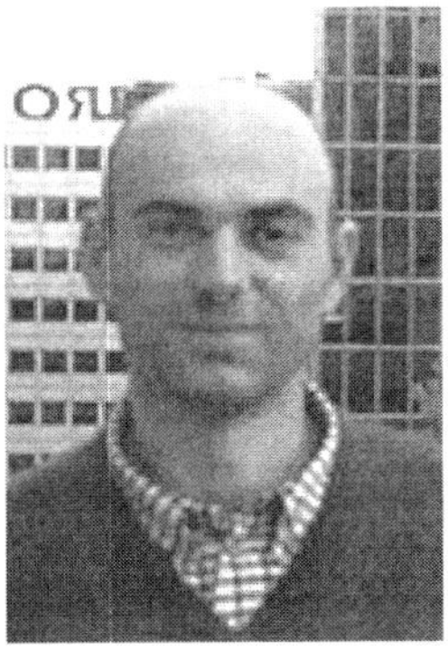

Mr. Miguel SEGARRA graduated in industrial engineering at Universidad Politecnica de Madrid (UPM) where he is also a candidate for doctorate. He is also a partner of SCILabs Ingenieros where he is in charge of the distributed object computing area. He is a frequent speaker about the OMG at conferences and writer of several books and articles in computing technology and development of complex systems. He has also imparted several courses at UPM in computer technology and automatics. His current work is focused towards software architecture of complex systems for process control. The objective of his work is the obtention of frameworks for industrial applications that guarantee the final properties and behavior of the system.

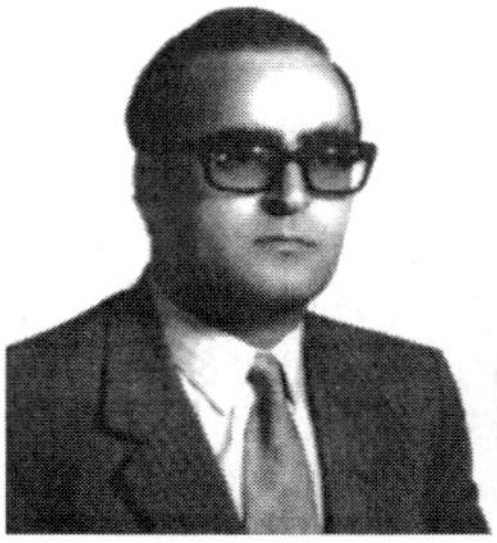

Prof. Spyros G. TZAFESTAS received the B.Sc. degree in Physics and Electronics from Athens University , the D.I.C. degree in Electrical Engineering from Imperial College, the M.Sc. degree in Automatic Control Systems form London University, and the Ph.D. and D.Sc. degrees in Systems, Control and Automation from Southampton University.

He is currently Professor of Control and Robotics, Director of the Intelligent Robotics and Automation Laboratory and Director of the Institute of Communication and Computer Systems at the National Technical University, Athens, Greece. From 1969 to 1973 , he was leader of the computer control group at the Computer Science Department of the Nuclear Research Center "Democritos" in Athens , and from 1973 to 1984 , he was Professor of Systems and Control Engineering at Patras University, Patras, Greece. His current interests include robust and adaptive control, robot modeling and control, knowledge-based systems, neural-fuzzy control systems and computer-aided manufacturing systems. He has published 30 books and over 600 journals and conference technical papers. He is an active reviewer of 20 journals, associate editor of 6 journals , the Editor-in-Chief of the Journal of Intelligent and Robotic Systems, and the Editor of the Kluwer book series entitled Microprocessor-Based and Intelligent Systems Engineering. He has served as guest editor for fifteen special issues on distributed systems, large-scale systems, orthogonal expansions, robotics , neural networks and soft-computing and has organized and/or chaired many international conferences on systems , computing , robotics and control.

Dr. Tzafestas is a member of the New York Academy of Sciences, a Fellow of the IEEE (CSS, CS, IES, RAS), a Fellow of IEE (London) , a member of ASME (N.Y.) and Chairman of the Control Systems and Robotics Committee of the International Association for Mathematics and Computers in Simulation (IMACS). He is recipient of a D.Sc. (Hon) from the International University Foundation and an Honorary Doctorate (Dr.-Ing. E.h) from the Technical University of Munich, Honorary President of SIRES (Society of Intelligent Robotics and Expert Systems, Brussels), and a member of the IFAC SECOM and MIM Technical Committees. He is coordinator for the part of NTUA in several European Community Projects (ESPRIT CIM, Stimulation Action, BRITE, TIDE, STRIDE, INTAS, Erasmus, Comett) on Information Systems Technology.

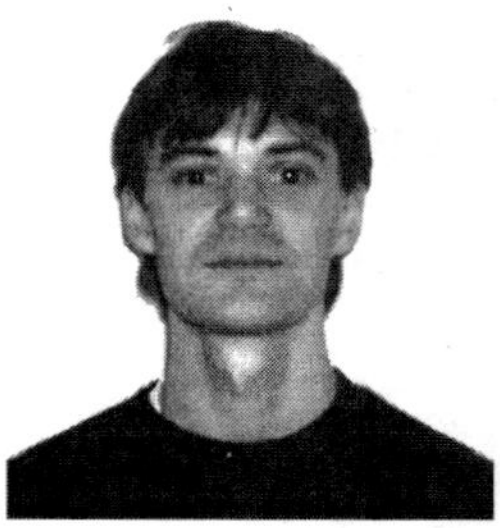

Dr. Fabrice WAWAK received his M.S in Electronics, Electrotechnics and Automation from the University of Science and Technology of Lille (France) in 1991. Then, he became Teaching Assistant at the University of Science and Technology of Lille and Researcher at the Automation Laboratory of Lille (CAL). He studied uncertainty problems in decision making for man-machine systems. He obtained his Ph.D in Information Processing, Soft Computing and Robotics in 1996. He joined the MobiNet project in 1997 at the Automation Laboratory (DISAM) of the

Polytechnic University of Madrid, where he studied sensors modelling, data fusion and autonomous control for mobile platforms.

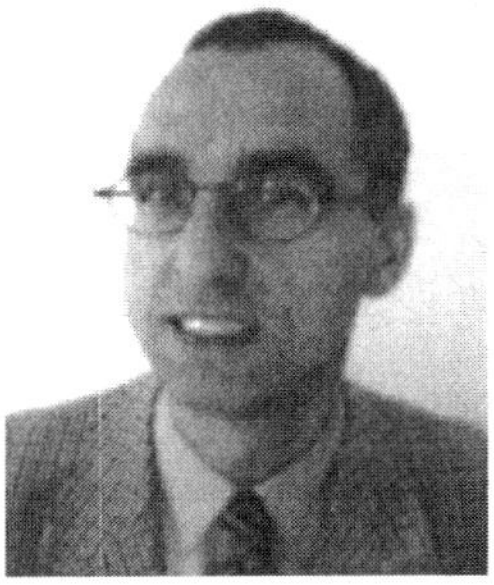

Mr. Frithjof WEBER studied production engineering at the University of Bremen. Before starting his studies, he gained several years of experience as electro mechanican on shopfloor level. After his studies, he joined BIBA in 1995 as a research scientist in the Department of Computer-Aided Design, Planning and Manufacturing. Since 1998 he is heading the Department. He has been involved in various European projects in the area of Concurrent Engineering. His current research is in the area of CE and information management. His special interests are process design, information logistics, bid preparation and problem solving in product development.

Author Index

Aldon, M.J. 73
Bolmsjö, G. 227,253,269
Borgolte, U. 73,161
Dario, P. 269
De Antonio, A. 137
Driessen, B. 227,253,269
Greenane, R.J. 211
Harwin, W. 73,227,253,315
Heck, H. 17,45,73
Katevas, N.I. v,1,17,73,101,161,187,295,315,349
Kontoulis, J. 73
Lacey, G. 17,45,73,211,295,315
Lauria, S. 227,315
Matía, F. 137,187,295,315,349
O'Hart, F.J. 211
Peignot, C. 349
Peruchon, E. 17,45,73
Prentza, A. 17,45,73
Rabischong, P. 45
Sanz, R. 137
Segarra, M. 137
Tzafestas, S.G. 101,187
Wawak, F. 295,315
Weber, F. 227,253
Wenn, D. 211